The Dentist's Drug and Prescription Guide

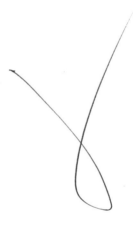

The Dentist's Drug and Prescription Guide

Mea A. Weinberg, DMD, MSD, RPh

Diplomate of the American Board of Periodontology
Clinical Associate Professor
Department of Periodontology and Implant Dentistry
New York University College of Dentistry
New York, New York

Stuart J. Froum, DDS

Diplomate of the American Board of Periodontology
Clinical Professor and Director of Clinical Research
Department of Periodontology and Implant Dentistry
New York University College of Dentistry
New York, New York

Consulting Editor:

Stuart L. Segelnick, DDS
Diplomate of the American Board of Periodontology
Clinical Associate Professor
Department of Periodontology and Implant Dentistry
New York University College of Dentistry
New York, New York

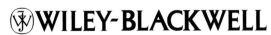
A John Wiley & Sons, Inc., Publication

This edition first published 2013 © 2013 by John Wiley & Sons, Inc.

Wiley-Blackwell is an imprint of John Wiley & Sons, formed by the merger of Wiley's global Scientific, Technical and Medical business with Blackwell Publishing.

Editorial Offices
2121 State Avenue, Ames, Iowa 50014-8300, USA
The Atrium, Southern Gate, Chichester, West Sussex, PO19 8SQ, UK
9600 Garsington Road, Oxford, OX4 2DQ, UK

For details of our global editorial offices, for customer services and for information about how to apply for permission to reuse the copyright material in this book please see our website at www.wiley.com/wiley-blackwell.

Library of Congress Cataloging-in-Publication Data

Weinberg, Mea A.
   The dentist's drug and prescription guide / Mea A. Weinberg, Stuart J. Froum.
      p.   cm.
   Includes bibliographical references and index.
   ISBN 978-0-470-96044-8 (pbk. : alk. paper)   1. Dental pharmacology–Handbooks, manuals, etc.   2. Drugs–Prescribing–Handbooks, manuals, etc.   3. Drugs–Dosage–Handbooks, manuals, etc.   I. Froum, Stuart J.   II. Title.
   RK701.W44 2012
   617.6′061–dc23

                                            2012012164

A catalogue record for this book is available from the British Library.

Wiley also publishes its books in a variety of electronic formats. Some content that appears in print may not be available in electronic books.

Cover design by Buffy Clatt

Set in 9/11.5 pt Times by SPi Publisher Services, Pondicherry, India
Printed and bound in Malaysia by Vivar Printing Sdn Bhd

1   2013

Disclaimer: The prescriber should use his/her own judgment in prescribing for particular patients. The prescriptions and suggested dosages in this guide are not absolute numbers, only suggestions.

Dedication

This book is dedicated to my family, especially to my parents Dr. Abraham and Gertrude Weinberg, because of their wonderful thought provoking ideas regarding medicine and pharmacy.

Contents

Preface

The *Dentist's Drug and Prescription Guide* is a reference book for those concerned with prescribing medications to dental patients. Pharmacology deals with many sciences and one outstanding purpose, which are to provide a scientific basis for the sensible and appropriate use of drugs in human therapeutics. Essentially, the book presents a basic rationale for understanding current drug therapy including how to write prescriptions and how to adjust dosages in the elderly, pediatric and certain medically compromised patients. How to manage potential drug interactions is reviewed with several tables explaining drug–drug, drug–food and drug–disease interactions that are most commonly encountered in dentistry.

The goal of writing this book is to explain the rationale for prescribing various medications for different dental conditions and to aid the dental practitioner in choosing the appropriate antibiotics, antifungal or antiviral drug. Understanding how drugs produce their effects allow the practitioner to better understand the different pharmacologic actions and adverse effects that drugs produce. The *Dentist's Drug and Prescription Guide* is intended to be a pocket book for rapid reference.

The book is presented in an easy-to-follow question and answer format. Many tables are included which summarizes the information in the text and makes it easier to refer back. Included in the book is evidenced based pharmacologic therapy with current and up-to-date references regarding adjunctive pharmacologic treatment of the dental patient. The book is divided into nine sections: Introduction to Pharmacology; The Prescription and Drug Names; Drug Dosing; Formulary Sections; How to Manage Potential Drug; Evidenced Based Theory for Drug Prescribing; Management of the Medically Compromised Dental Patient Herbal; Natural Remedies; and Appendices (Smoking Cessation Therapy, Oral Manifestations of Drugs, American Heart Association Antibiotic Prophylaxis Guidelines, List of Tables, Pharmacology Pearls in Dental Practice, Dental Drug Formulary). Drug therapy for each dental discipline including periodontics, implantology, oral surgery and endodontics is presented.

Features of the *Dentist's Drug and Prescription Guide* include:

- Readability: short, easy question and answer format linking pharmacy theory to clinical dental practice.
- Need-to-know information: The content of this book was written in regard to the many questions practitioners have about prescribing drugs to patients.
- Drug tables: There are many tables included in the book which not only summarizes the main pharmacologic features of the different disciplines but also allows the reader to review the key drugs and theories at a quick glance.

Contributors

The author would like to thank the following people for their assistance while writing this book:

James B. Fine, DMD
Assistant Dean for Postdoctoral Education
Associate Professor of Clinical Dentistry and Postdoctoral Director of Periodontics
College of Dental Medicine of Columbia University
New York, New York

Larry Gupta, RPh
Clinical Pharmacist
Englewood, New Jersey

David Hershkowitz, DDS
Clinical Assistant Professor
Associate Chair Clinical Education
Department of Cariology & Comprehensive Care
New York University College of Dentistry
New York, New York

Howard D. Silverman, DDS
Associate Professor
Department of Endodontics
New York University College of Dentistry
New York, New York

Surrendra M. Singh, BSc, BDS, MDS
Professor
Department of Periodontology
New Jersey Dental School
Univeristy of Medicine and Dentistry of New Jersey
Newark, New Jersey

Chapter 1

Introduction to pharmacology

I. Definition of terms

Absorption   the movement of a drug from its site of administration (oral, topical, or injection) into the systemic circulation (bloodstream).

Adverse drug event (ADE)   injury resulting from the use of a drug. It is an unfavorable and unintentional response resulting from an administered medication. Includes medication errors such as miscalculation of dosage or misreading a prescription.

Adverse drug reaction (ADR)   harm to the body due to a medication that was properly prescribed (e.g., drug taken at normal doses and the correct route of administration). Examples of an ADR are allergy to penicillin or adverse (side) effect of a drug.

Affinity   the ability of a drug to bind to the receptor to cause a therapeutic response.

Antibiotic prophylaxis   antibiotic given to prevent an infection.

Bioavailability   the amount of a drug (expressed as a percentage) that reaches the systemic circulation. For example, any drug administered intravenously has a 100% bioavailability

Biologics   agents that are naturally produced in an animal or human body.

Clearance   quantitative measure of the rate of drug elimination from the body divided by the concentration.

Creatinine   a waste product in skeletal muscle by the breakdown of creatinine phosphate.

Creatinine clearance (CrCl)   a test that compares the level of creatinine in the urine with that of creatinine in the blood and it determines normal functioning of the kidneys.

Cytochrome P450 (CYP) enzymes   found primarily in the liver that are responsible for the metabolism of many drugs. Many drug interactions occur because some drugs are inhibitors or inducers of the substrate (drug being metabolized) resulting in high or low blood levels of one or the other drug.

Distribution   movement of a drug through the body to the various target tissues/organs (site of action) after it enters the bloodstream.

Dose   the amount of drug taken at any one time.

Drug   any substance which changes a physiological function or modifies a disease process.

Drug action   the response of living matter to administered chemicals. Levels of drug action include cellular or molecular. Cellular site of drug action is defined as all foreign parts that enter the body, will react with at least one portion of the cell. The initial reaction occurs here. At the molecular level the molecules of the drug will react with the molecules of the body.

Efficacy   the ability of a drug to stimulate the receptor and produce the maximum response achievable by the drug. Two drugs can have the same efficacy but different potencies where one drug is more potent (stronger strength) than the first drug but both will have the same effect.

The Dentist's Drug and Prescription Guide, First Edition. Mea A. Weinberg and Stuart J. Froum.
© 2013 John Wiley & Sons, Inc. Published 2013 by John Wiley & Sons, Inc.

Elimination half-life ($t_{1/2}$):   The time required to reduce the amount of drug in the body or concentration of drug in blood by 50%. However, once the first 50% is gone, it will take the body more time to clear 50% of the remaining medication. Usually it takes about 5 half-lives to clear 99% of the medication. To determine the time it takes for a drug to be 99% eliminated from the body multiply the half-life of the drug by 5.

First-pass effect (or first-pass metabolism)   before an orally administered drug enters the systemic circulation it goes to the liver to be metabolized or biotransformed. Some oral drugs can undergo extensive first-pass effect that they are ineffective by the time of entering the bloodstream while other drugs undergo little first-pass effect and maintain the original efficacy. Drugs that undergo extensive first-pass effect cannot be given orally because it becomes pharmacologically ineffective by the time it enters the general circulation. Lidocaine is an example of a drug that cannot be given orally because it undergoes extensive first-pass effect.

First-order kinetics   the rate of drug elimination decreases with time. That is, the rate if drug elimination falls as the concentration falls. Most drugs are removed from the body by first-order kinetics.

Loading dose (LD)   an initial higher dose of a drug that may be given at the beginning of a course of treatment (to get initial quick plasma levels) before dropping down to a lower maintenance dose afterward. A loading dose is given on the first day of drug treatment.

Maintenance dose (MD)   a lower drug dose allowing the dose that keeps the plasma drug concentration continuously within the therapeutic range. The maintenance dose is given starting after the loading dose on day 1 of drug therapy.

Metabolism (biotransformation)   the primary mechanism of drug elimination from the body. Biotransformation will usually end the pharmacologic action of the drug.

Pharmacodynamics   describes how the drug actually works; mechanism of action. How drug interact with receptors and what happens once the drug binds to the receptor.

Pharmacokinetics   study of the action of drug once it is in the patient. It describes the absorption, distribution, metabolism and elimination of the drug from the body

Pharmacology   is a Greek word defined as the science dealing with drugs and their interaction with the body's components

Pharmacogenetics   the convergence of pharmacology and genetics that deals with genetic factors that influence an organism's response to a drug.

Pharmacognosy   study of drugs derived from herbal and other natural sources.

Pharmacotherapeutics   the medical use of drugs in the prevention, diagnosis, treatment of diseases.

Polypharmacy   many different medications including over-the-counter (OTC) and prescription drugs are taken by the patient.

Potency   strength of the drug.

Prodrug   a drug that becomes active only after it is ingested and metabolized in the liver. Codeine is converted from an inactive form to the pharmacologically active form, morphine, by first pass metabolism.

Protein binding   attachment of a drug to proteins in the plasma. Drugs that are protein bound are inactive and become active in the free unbound form.

Steady state   The point at which the rate of input of drug into the body is equal to the rate of elimination. As such, the amount or concentration in the body reaches a plateau.

Therapeutics   branch of medicine that deals with the treatment of disease.

Therapeutic index (TI) (therapeutic ratio)   a measure of the relative safety of a drug. Therapeutic index is expressed as the ratio of the lethal or toxic dose (LD) to the therapeutic dose (TD). For example, lithium has a narrow therapeutic index so if the dose is just slightly more than the therapeutic range toxicity can occur. Patients must be on chronic lithium maintenance treatment to avoid toxicity. On the other hand, penicillin has a wide therapeutic index so that slightly more than the usually dose will not cause toxicity.

Therapeutic range   the dosage range of a drug that achieves the desired pharmacologic response.

Toxicology   study of poisons and poisonings.

Zero-order kinetics   the drug is removed at a constant rate regardless of the drug concentration; it is linear with time. The elimination from the body of a large concentration of alcohol is an example of a drug that follows zero-order kinetics. (Weinberg, 2002; Gossel, 1998a, b).

II. Pharmacokinetics

Q. What is the definition of pharmacokinetics and why is it important to know?

A. Pharmacokinetics describes the actions of the drug as it moves through the body and how the body influences drug concentrations. It is easiest to remember pharmacokinetics by the acronym: ADME (A = absorption into the systemic circulation; D = distribution to the target tissues and organs; M = metabolism or biotransformation; E = elimination from the body). It is important to know the basics of pharmacokinetics in order to understand the basic principles of prescribing medications. Pharmacokinetics (e.g., absorption of the drug into the blood) may be altered when certain antibiotics prescribed in dentistry are taken with food. Instructions must be verbally expressed to the patient and documented in the patient's chart on how to take medications that are prescribed by dentists (e.g., antibiotics, antimicrobial agents, analgesics, antifungal agents, antiviral agents, fluorides).

Q. What factors affect the rate of drug absorption?

A. In the gastrointestinal tract, many factors can influence the rate of drug absorption into the systemic circulation including acidity of the stomach and food in the stomach.

Some medications used in dentistry should be taken with food to reduce gastrointestinal irritation, some medications should be taken on an empty stomach because the food could delay the absorption of the drug and some medications can be taken with or without food because food would not interfere with absorption. Usually the absorption of the total amount of drug is not reduced but rather it will just take longer to get absorbed. Usually antibiotics have the most restrictions regarding taking with meals. Nonsteroidal anti-inflammatory drugs such as ibuprofen must be taken with food to avoid gastric irritation. Specific drugs will be discussed within the chapters.

Q. What does "take on an empty stomach" mean?

A. Take on an empty stomach means to take the drug within 1 hour before eating or 2 hours after eating. Take on an empty stomach is not interpreted as not eating.

Q. What is the pharmacokinetics of an orally administered drug?

A. The pharmacokinetics of a drug administered orally such as penicillin VK is as follows (Weinberg, 2002; Gossel 1998a, b):

1. An orally administered drug is swallowed and goes through the esophagus. It is important to take a tablet/capsule with a full glass of water to facilitate its passage through the esophagus into the stomach.
2. In the stomach the tablet/capsule must be released or liberated from its formulation. Once a tablet is "broken up" and a capsule is "opened" and the active ingredients are released there is dissolution of the drug from the liberated drug particles. Some acidic drugs are enteric-coated to protect the stomach lining. Dosage forms such as syrups or solutions are already a liquid which are immediately available for absorption and transport. A liquid gel capsule (Aleve, Advil) is formulated to dissolve quickly which allows the liquid inside the capsule to be absorbed fast.
3. Drug goes into the upper part of the small intestine (duodenum) where most absorption into the systemic circulation occurs because the small intestine has a large surface area due to microvilli on the surface which drugs may diffuse.
4. From the small intestine the drug molecules are *absorbed* into the bloodstream. Many factors can affect the rate and extent of absorption of the drug including foods and minerals. For example, tetracycline should not be given at the same time as dairy products or minerals (e.g., iron, calcium, magnesium) because insoluble complexes form in the intestinal tract, which slows down absorption. This can be avoided by taking the tetracycline one to two hours before or after the dairy/mineral product. Some antibiotics (e.g., tetracycline) must be taken on an empty stomach (one hour before or two hours after meals) which increases the rate of absorption. Most antibiotics can be taken without regard to meals (with or without food) but if stomach upset occurs food should be taken (Huang *et al.*, 2009).
5. Absorption occurs when a drug is nonionized or charged form and if it is more lipid-soluble. Most drugs are combined with a salt to enhance its absorption (e.g., lidocaine HCl, tetracycline HCl, doxycycline hyclate, amoxicillin trihydrate).

6. Before an orally administered drug reaches the systemic circulation it goes to the liver via portal vein whereby it is immediately exposed to metabolism by liver enzymes (Huang *et al.*, 2009). This first exposure is referred to as **first-pass effect**. Some drugs such as lidocaine and morphine that undergo extensive first-pass embolism will become inactive so they cannot be given orally. Diazepam (Valium) has close to 100% bioavailability (low first-pass metabolism) so it has similar oral and intravenous doses. Alternate routes of drug administration that bypass the first-pass effect include sublingual, rectal or parenteral (intravenous, intramuscular, and subcutaneous) (Pond & Tozer 1984; Fagerholm 2007).

7. Once reaching the systemic circulation, the drug is distributed in the blood to the various organs. Many drugs are bound to circulating proteins such as albumin (acidic drugs) and glycoproteins (basic drugs). Highly protein bound drugs are not active and only the free drug that is not bound to proteins is active.

8. Once the drug has exerted its actions it must be eliminated from the body. The first part of drug elimination involves **metabolism** or **biotransformation**, which occurs mostly in the liver. It may take a drug several passes through the liver before it is entirely metabolized. Biotransformation converts lipid-soluble drug molecules to metabolites or end products that are more water-soluble and easier to be eliminated from the body. Most of process of conversion of drugs occurs in the liver by metabolizing enzymes called microsomal enzymes. These enzymes, which are also called **cytochrome P450 (CYP)** enzymes are the primary enzymes responsible for the oxidation of many drugs. There are many different isoenzymes for different drugs (e.g., CYP3A4 is involved with many dental drugs). Many drug–drug and drug–food interactions occur via the microsomal enzymes. Some drugs called **prodrugs** (e.g., codeine is metabolized by the liver enzyme CYP2D6 to the active morphine), have no pharmacologic activity unless they are first metabolized to the active form in the body (Weinberg, 2002).

9. **Drug elimination**: now the more water-soluble metabolite must be eliminated from the body. The main route of drug elimination is excretion via the kidneys. Diseases of the kidney can significantly prolong the duration of drug action and dosage adjustment may be needed from the patient's physician. Some elimination occurs through the lungs, breast milk, sweat, tears, feces and bile. Some drugs (e.g., tetracycline) undergo biliary excretion whereby the drug is eliminated in the bile and enters the small intestine and eventually leaves the body in the feces. Most bile is then circulated back to the liver by **enterohepatic recirculation** and eventually metabolized by the liver and excreted via the kidneys. This route of reabsorption is helpful in prolonging the activity (increasing the half-life) of some antibiotics (Weinberg, 2002).

Q. What is the definition of drug absorption?

A. Drug **absorption** is the movement of a drug from the site of administration to the systemic circulation.

Q. What does it mean when a drug has 100% bioavailability?

A. **Bioavailability** describes the portion of an administered drug that reaches the systemic circulation. It is the rate and extent of absorption and how fast and how much of the drug is absorbed. It indicates that the drug is 100% absorbed into the blood. Only intravenously administered drugs have 100% bioavailability because 100% of the drug enters directly into the blood. A drug administered orally that undergo extensive first-pass metabolism (or first-pass effect) by traveling first to the liver, where it is metabolized and can become almost inactive by the time it reaches the systemic circulation. This drug would have low bioavailability.

Q. What is the first step involved in drug absorption?

A. Disintegration of the dosage formulation into a formulation that can easily be absorbed is the first step before a drug can be absorbed in the small intestine. The stomach should be the first site of absorption, but in reality, very little absorption occurs in the stomach because the surface area is very small. A tablet must break up to expose the active ingredient which takes some time. A capsule must open up which takes less time than a tablet. A solution is already in a liquid, easily absorbed form and takes the least time for disintegration and absorption of all dosage forms. The order of bioavailability is oral solution > oral suspension > capsule > tablet (Lloyd *et al.*, 1978).

Q. Is there any systemic absorption of a topical anesthetic applied on the surface of the gingiva?

A. Yes. The purpose of topical agents is to maximize the concentration of the drug at the target site while minimizing potential systemic adverse effects. Although drug absorption is not desired there could be some systemic absorption especially if the agent is applied on abraded gingiva or skin.

Because of its lipophilic nature, the stratum corneum of the skin may act as a reservoir for many drugs. Consequently, the local effects of the drug may be sufficiently long to allow once-daily application. For example, once-daily application of corticosteroid preparations is as effective as are multiple applications in most circumstances. Direct access to the skin may predispose the patient to frequent topical applications, increasing the risk of systemic adverse effects.

Q. How does a drug get absorbed into the systemic circulation?

A. A drug must pass through many cell membranes to get into the blood. A drug must have some water solubility to go through aqueous fluids and some lipid solubility to get through the cell membrane, which has 2 layers of phospholipids.

Q. What is the purpose of epinephrine added to local anesthetics?

A. Epinephrine is a vasoconstrictor that acts to constrict blood vessels to decrease blood flow in the area that the local anesthetic solution was injected. This allows the anesthetic solution to stay the site of action longer, which slows absorption of the anesthetic solution. Also acting as a vasoconstrictor reduces bleeding at the surgical site.

Q. What is drug distribution and what factors affect distribution?

A. Drug **distribution** is the movement of an agent through the blood or lymph to various sites of actions in the body. An important factor affecting drug distribution is **protein binding**. Many drugs in the blood are bound to circulating proteins such as albumin for acidic drugs (e.g., penicillin, barbiturates, aspirin, vitamin C) and acid glycoproteins and lipoproteins for basic drugs (e.g., narcotic analgesics, erythromycin). When drugs are bound to plasma proteins they are inactive circulating in the blood. This binding to proteins is temporary and reversible and can convert to free drug. Only drugs that are not bound to plasma proteins are "freely active" and bind to specific receptors on the target tissue/organ. Another factor that affects drug distribution is blood flow to the target organs.

Q. What is the definition of minimum effective concentration (MIC) of a drug?

A. The **minimum effective concentration (MIC)** is the amount of drug required to produce a therapeutic effect. This is important to know because a drug should not be given that is above the MIC that will produce toxic concentrations. The ideal concentration of a drug should be between the MIC and the toxic concentration. This is referred to as the **therapeutic range**. For example, after periodontal surgery the patient is recommended to take ibuprofen (Motrin, Nuprin). The patient decides to take only one 200 mg tablet during the day. The patient still experiences pain because the therapeutic range was not reached. The patient should take two or three tablets which will increase the plasma level of ibuprofen into the therapeutic range. If the patient takes 5 or more tablets at one time then adverse effects may occur because the plasma level of ibuprofen is outside the therapeutic range and the maximum dose has been reached beyond which the analgesic effect does not increase.

Q. What does the term "dose" mean?

A. The **dose** of a drug is the amount of drug taken at any one time. Dose is expressed as the weight of drug (e.g., 500 mg), the number of dosage forms (e.g., one capsule), or the volume of liquid (e.g., two drops).

Q. What is the definition of elimination half-life of a drug?

A. The **elimination half-life ($t_{1/2}$)** of a drug is essentially the duration of action of a drug. Also, it is used to determine the dosing of a drug. The elimination half-life of a drug is defined as the amount of time required for a drug to decrease its original concentration by 50% after it is administered. The second half-life is when it removes another 50%, leaving 25% in the blood. The third half-life is when it removes another 50%, leaving 12.5% in the blood. Drugs have different predetermined half-lives. The $t_{1/2}$ of a drug is used to determine the dosing of a drug and duration of drug action. As repeated doses of a drug are administered the plasma concentration builds up and reaches "**steady-state**". Steady-state occurs when the amount of drug in the plasma builds up to a level that is considered to be therapeutically effective. In order to achieve steady state the amount of drug that is administered must balance the amount being cleared from the body. It usually takes about between four and five half-lives to reach clinical steady-state and about six half-lives before 98% of the drug is eliminated from the body. For example, if a drug has a $t_{1/2}$ of 2 hours it will take about 8 to 10 hours to reach the clinical steady state.

Drugs with a short $t_{1/2}$ are eliminated faster than drugs with a long $t_{1/2}$. For example, tetracycline HCl has a $t_{1/2}$ of 6–12 hours and doxycycline hyclate has a $t_{1/2}$ of 14–24 hours. Thus, tetracycline dosing is one capsule every 4 hours while doxycycline is dosed 100 mg every 12 hours on day 1, then 100 mg every day. On the average, doxycycline's half-life is around 19 hours. By multiplying 19 hours by 6 hours (average $t_{1/2}$ to be 98% eliminated from the body) ($19 \times 6 = 114$ hours) it takes 114 hours, or about 5 days, before 98% of the doxycycline has been removed from the body. Penicillin VK has a $t_{1/2}$ of 30 minutes and amoxicillin $t_{1/2}$ 1-1.3 hours. Thus, penicillin is doses every 6 hours and amoxicillin is dosed every 8 hours (Thomson, 2004a, b).

Ibuprofen has a short $t_{1/2}$ and is cleared from the body more rapidly than a drug with a longer $t_{1/2}$. Ibuprofen requires a more frequent, regular dosing regimen of 200 to 400 mg every 4 to 6 hours in order to build up and maintain a high enough concentration in the plasma to be therapeutically effective.

Q. What is the definition of volume of distribution (V_D)?

A. **Volume of distribution** (V_D) refers to the distribution of the drug in the various body tissues. Volume of distribution is a calculated value referring to the volume of fluid [e.g., plasma, interstitial fluid (fluid between the cells), and lymph] in which a drug is able to distribute to the organs. The volume of distribution can be used to calculate the clearance of a drug (Aki *et al.*, 2010; Thomson, 2004a, b).

Q. What is drug biotransformation?

A. Drug biotransformation (or metabolism as it is sometimes referred to) is a method to terminate the action of a drug. Usually drug biotransformation occurs in the liver by enzymes, but can also occur in the plasma and kidney.

Q. What is the importance of drug clearance?

A. **Clearance** refers to the volume of fluid (e.g., plasma) that would be completely cleared of drug if the entire drug being excreted were removed from that volume of fluid. Essentially, clearance is the removal of a drug from the plasma. It is a calculated value and measured in liters/hour. Clearance indicates the ability of the liver and kidney to eliminate a drug. Clearance may be reduced in the elderly. Both clearance and V_D are important values in determining the half-life of a drug (Gossel, 1998a, b).

Q. What must happen in the body to a drug in order to have a drug effect to occur?

A. The rate of absorption must be greater than the rate of elimination in order for the drug to have an effect on the body. Usually the rate of elimination is slower than the rate of absorption so that it is the rate of elimination that is the controlling factor in the presence of the drug in the body (Fujimoto, 1979).

III.   Pharmacodynamics

Q. What is the definition of pharmacodynamics and its significance in dentistry?

A. **Pharmacodynamics** deals with the mechanism of action of drugs or how the drug works in the body to produce a pharmacologic response and the relationship between drug concentration and response. It is important to know the mechanism of action of drugs because it will help with understanding the reason for prescribing the drug.

Q. What is the definition of drug affinity?

A. **Affinity** is the ability of a drug to bind to the receptor to elicit a therapeutic response. If one drug has a greater affinity than another drug it means that that drug binds more readily to the receptor. A drug with a "high affinity" means that even a small dose can produce a response.

Q. Do drugs bind strongly to a receptor?

A. Most drugs bind weakly to their receptors via hydrogen, hydrophobic and ionic bonds. Because it is a weak bond, the drug can come on and off the receptor. Some drugs do bind strongly to the receptor via covalent bonds.

Q. Can drugs bind to other receptors besides their specific receptors?

A. Yes. For example, atypical antipsychotic drugs bind to dopamine receptors for its antipsychotic response but also bind to alpha receptors which cause adverse effects such as weight loss and binding to muscarinic receptors causes xerostomia.

Q. How do most drugs cause a therapeutic response?

A. Most drugs have an affinity for a specific receptor. Most receptors are proteins. Once the drug binds to the receptor a therapeutic response occurs. Receptors have a steric or three-dimensional structure so that as the substrate or drug binds to that receptor the receptor undergoes steric realignment or changes which allows for the drug to bind more precisely to the receptor and have better efficacy.

Q. Do all drugs interact with receptors to cause a therapeutic response?

A. No. Epinephrine does bind to alpha and beta receptors on the organs but also it produces some of its effects by activating an enzyme called adenyl cyclase. Also, anesthetic gases do not bind to receptors in the central nervous system and antacids do not work by interacting with receptors.

Q. What are a drug agonist and antagonist?

A. Drugs produce their effects by altering the function of cells and tissues in the body or organisms such as bacteria. Most drugs have an affinity for a target receptor, which is usually a protein on the cell surface. Once a drug binds to a receptor it can act as either as an **agonist** (produces a stimulatory response) or an **antagonist** (sits on the receptor site and prevents an agonist from binding to the receptor; an antagonist does not produce a therapeutic response).

For example, epinephrine in low doses as used in dentistry is an agonist that when bound to $beta_2$-receptors results in vasodilation of skeletal muscle. This vasodilation tends to reduce peripheral resistance and therefore diastolic blood pressure. At the same time, the $beta_1$ (and $beta_2$)-receptors in the heart are activated to increase cardiac output and systolic blood pressure. These two influences cancel each other out regarding mean blood pressure.

An example of an antagonist is flumazenil (Romazicon), which is a benzodiazepine receptor antagonist that is used in benzodiazepine overdose. It will sit on the receptor and prevent the benzodiazepine from attaching. Naloxone (Narcan) is a narcotic receptor antagonist.

Q. What is the difference between drug potency and efficacy?

A. **Potency** is the relationship between the dose of a drug and the therapeutic effect; it refers to the drug's strength. **Efficacy** refers to the ability of a drug to exert an effect. For example, 500 mg of acetaminophen and 200 mg of ibuprofen both produce the same analgesia and have the same efficacy but ibuprofen is more potent because it requires a lower dosage.

Q. What is the therapeutic index of a drug?

A. The **therapeutic index** (TI) is the median effective dose (ED_{50}) is the dose required to produce a specific therapeutic response in 50% of patients. The median lethal dose (LD_{50}) refers to the dose of drug that will be lethal in 50% of a group of animals, not humans. To determine drug safety the drug's TI is calculated as the ratio of a drug's LD_{50} to its ED_{50}. Some drugs (e.g., lithium, digoxin) have a narrow TI whereby routine blood tests are necessary to assure the plasma drug level is within the therapeutic range.

Q. What is an adverse drug reaction and why is it important to know?

A. An **adverse drug reaction** (ADR) is defined by the World Health Organization (WHO) as any response to a drug that is noxious, unintended, and *occurs when a drug is properly prescribed at doses normally* used in humans for the prophylaxis, diagnosis, or therapy of disease. Medical errors are not included in this definition. Bisphosphonate-induced osteonecrosis of the jaws is an ADR. Other examples of adverse drug reactions include drug interactions, allergic reactions and irritating adverse effects of a drug such as gastrointestinal problems (nausea, diarrhea). A drug interaction occurs when the effects of one drug are altered by the effects of another drug resulting in an increase or decrease of the drug. An allergic reaction due to a drug is an abnormal and unwanted response that range from a mild rash to life-threatening anaphylaxis. An allergic reaction does not often happen the first time you take a medication. A reaction is much more likely to occur the next time you take that medication.

Q. How does an ADR differ from an adverse effect or allergy?

A. An adverse effect is a type of adverse drug reaction mediated by an immune response and is not the intended therapeutic outcome. It has been suggested to avoid using the term "side effect" and use the term "adverse effect or adverse drug reaction" instead (VA Center for Medication Safety and VHA Pharmacy Benefits Management Strategic Healthcare Group and the Medical Advisory Panel. 2006; Riedl & Casillas, 2003).

Q. What is an adverse drug event?

A. An **adverse drug event** (ADE) is an unfavorable and unintended response to a drug that includes medical errors (e.g., miscalculations, confusion with handwritten prescriptions). The dentist has the responsibility to report any ADE that occurs through the FDA's Adverse Event Reporting System (MedWatch). (Mayer *et al.*, 2010). (http://www.fda.gov/Safety/MedWatch/default.htm)

Q. What is the definition of tolerance?

A. **Tolerance** to a drug is the development of resistance to the effects of a drug whereby in order to have the desired response more of the drug must be taken. Overdose is very common. Narcotics and alcohol are common examples of drugs that produce tolerance.

References

Aki, T., Heikkinen, A.T., Korjamo, T., *et al.* (2010) Modelling of drug disposition kinetics in in vitro intestinal absorption cell models. *Basic Clinical Pharmacology and Toxicology*, 106(3):180–188.

Fagerholm, U. (2007) Prediction of human pharmacokinetics–gastrointestinal absorption. *Journal of Pharmacy and Pharmacology*, 59:905–916.

Fujimoto, J.M. (1979) Pharmacokinetics and drug metabolism. In: *Practical Drug Therapy* (ed. Wang, R.I.H.), 1st edn, pp. 11–16. J.B. Lippincott Company, Philadelphia.

Gossel, T.A. (1998a) Pharmacology back to basics. *US Pharmacist*, 23:70–78.

Gossel, T.A. (1998b) *Exploring pharmacology US Pharmacist*, 23:96–104.

Huang, W., Lee, S.L.,Yu, L.X., (2009) Mechanistic approaches to predicting oral drug absorption. *Journal of the American Association of Pharmaceutical Sciences*, 11:217–224.

Lloyd, B.L., Greenblatt, D.J., Allen, M.D., *et al.* (1978) Pharmacokinetics and bioavailability of digoxin capsules, solutions and tablets after single and multiple dose. *The American Journal of Cardiology*, 2:129–136.

Mayer, M.H., Dowsett, S.A., Brahmavar, K., *et al.* (2010) Reporting adverse drug events. *US Pharmacist*, 35:HS-15-HS-19.

Pond, S.M., Tozer, T.N. (1984) First-pass elimination. Basic concepts and clinical consequences. *Clinical Pharmacokinetics*, 9:1–25.

Riedl, M.A., Casillas, A.M. (2003) Adverse drug reactions: types and treatment options. *American Family Physician*, 68:1781–1790.

Thomson, A. (2004a) Back to basics: pharmacokinetics. *The Pharmaceutical Journal*, 272:796–771.

Thomson, A. (2004b) Variability in drug dosage requirements. *The Pharmaceutical Journal*, 272:806–808.

VA Center for Medication Safety and VHA Pharmacy Benefits Management Strategic Healthcare Group and the Medical Advisory Panel. Adverse drug events, adverse drug reactions and medication errors. Frequently asked questions. November 2006. (www.pbm.va.gov/vamedsafe/Adverse%20Drug%20Reaction.pdf) Accessed online December 15, 2011.

Weinberg, M.A. (2013) Fundamentals of drug action. In: *Oral Pharmacology* (eds. Weinberg M.A., Westphal, C., Fine, J.B.), 2nd edn, pp. 18–40. Pearson Education Inc., New Jersey.

Chapter 2

The prescription and drug names

I. Parts of a prescription

Q. What are the different parts of a written prescription?

- Heading:
  - Prescriber's name, address, phone number, license number, DEA number and NPI (national provider identifier) number (the DEA number can also be located at the bottom of the prescription by the prescriber's signature)
  - Patient's information (name, address, age, weight)
  - Date of the order (must be written or it is not legal).
- Body:
  - Rx symbol
  - Medication prescribed (drug name, strength and formulation) and quantity to be dispensed
  - Instructions to the pharmacist. For example: Dispense 10 capsules.
- Closing:
  - Signature (Sig): directions to the patient
  - Signature of prescriber
  - Substitution permissible
  - Number of refills
  - Label (informs the pharmacist how to label the medication).

Q. What does "Rx" mean?

A. Rx is a symbol referring to "prescription". Rx is the Latin meaning "recipe" or "take thou" or "take thus" or "to take". Essentially, it is a command to take a specific compound.

Q. What does "Sig" mean?

A. Sig is an abbreviation for the Latin *signatura*, meaning "write", "make" or "label". These should always be written in English; however, prescribers sometimes use Latin abbreviations, e.g. "1 cap tid pc," which the pharmacist translates into English, "take one capsule three times daily after meals."

Q. Does the age of the patient need to be written on the prescription?

A. Yes. Generally, it is helpful to write in the age (in years) of the patient. For pediatric prescriptions it is recommended to write in the age of the child if the patient is less than twelve and the age in years and months if less than five. Including the weight of the child is also helpful. For Schedule II drugs it is mandatory to include the age of the patient on the prescription. The reason for writing the age of the patient is that in some cases the dose may need to be adjusted.

The Dentist's Drug and Prescription Guide, First Edition. Mea A. Weinberg and Stuart J. Froum.
© 2013 John Wiley & Sons, Inc. Published 2013 by John Wiley & Sons, Inc.

Q. Is my DEA number required on all prescriptions?

A. The DEA number must have a space on the prescriber's prescription blank. It is required to write the DEA number on the prescription blank when prescribing controlled substances. A separate DEA number is required in each state the dentist is licensed and the DEA license is renewed every 2 years.

Q. What is the NPI?

A. NPI stands for national provider identifer. It is an identification number given to health care providers by the CMS (Centers for Medicare and Medicaid Services). Health care providers must apply for an NPI number through an application process on the CMS website. Health practitioners need to have this number in order to receive reimbursement from insurance companies and to prescribe medicines.

Q. What is the label box at the bottom of the prescription mean?

A. Any information about the medication to be dispensed is provided on the label that is affixed to the drug container.

II.   Generic substitution

Q. When does a brand name drug become generic?

A. A brand name drug can become generic when the patent for that drug expires. Once the brand name drug goes off-patent, several drug companies can begin to manufacture a generic equivalent drug. In the United States, one company is given 180 days of exclusivity to manufacture a generic version of a drug. After 180 days, other manufacturers of generic medications can then start to make their own generic form of the drug. For example, the patent on Celebrex® expires in 2013. Until then, Celebrex is not available in a generic form (www.fda.gov/Drugs/DevelopmentApprovalProcess/ucm079031.htm).

Q. At the bottom of the prescription there is a section that says "dispense as written" or "substitution permissible". What is the difference between a generic drug and a brand name drug?

A. A generic drug is manufactured and distributed usually without a patent. However, the generic drug may still have a patent on the entire formulation but not on the active ingredient. A drug that has a trade (brand) name is protected by a patent whereby it can only be manufactured and sold by the company holding the patent. Once the patent expires (between 7 and 12 years) on a brand name drug the generic form will be available (Welage *et al.*, 2001).

Q. What is generic equivalency mean?

A. Generic equivalency was developed to save consumers and insurance companies high costs. Generic drugs are much cheaper because of competition between drug manufacturers once the patent has expired. Also, it costs less to manufacturer generic drugs. Many brand name drugs have less expensive generic drug substitutes that according to the FDA are therapeutically and biochemically equivalent to the brand name drug. The FDA requires the bioequivalence of the generic drug (active ingredient) to be between 80% and 125% of that of the brand name drug. Generics are considered by the FDA to be identical in dose, strength, safety, efficacy, and intended use (Balthasar, 1999; Greene *et al.*, 2001).

Q. Is a generic drug always equivalent to a brand name drug?

A. According to the law, drug companies are required to prove bioavailability. Many drugs that are available generically are equally efficacious with the equivalent brand name (Birkett, 2003).

Q. What is generic substitution and how do I know if a generic drug substitute is available?

A. Generic substitution is the process by which a generic equivalent is dispensed by the pharmacist rather than the brand name. There is a book called the "Orange Book: Approved Drug Products with Therapeutic Equivalence

Evaluations" that all pharmacies have, and since February 2005, there is a daily Electronic Orange Book (EOB) product information for new generic drug approvals. The downloaded Annual Edition and Cumulative Supplements are also available in a paper version (Approved Drug Products with Therapeutic Equivalence Evaluations, ADP 2008) from the US Government Printing Office: http://bookstore.gpo.gov/; toll free telephone number 866-512-1800.

Q. How do I write for a generic substitute on a prescription?

A. Prescriptions have instructions on whether the prescriber will allow the pharmacist to substitute a generic version of the drug. This instruction is communicated in a number of ways which differs among States. Usually, the prescription contains two signature lines. One line has "substitution permitted" or "substitution permissible" printed at the bottom of the prescription and the other line has "dispense as written" or "do not substitute". The prescriber signs either line. Some States have a "daw" (dispense as written) box printed at the bottom of the prescription. This means that the prescription will be filled generically unless the prescriber writes "daw" in the box in which case the prescription will be filled the way it is written by the prescriber. For example, if you write a prescription for the trade name of a drug such as Vibramycin (the patient only wants to take a brand name drug) and signs the line "do not substitute" or write "daw" in the box, the prescription will be dispensed with the brand name drug (Vibramycin) rather than the generic substitute (doxycycline) (Meridith, 2003).

Q. When should a generic drug rather than a brand name drug be prescribed?

A. Anytime. It is the decision of the patient. Generic substitution is intended for the pharmacist to use a form of the drug which may be less expensive to the patient. It is usually the cheaper drug yet still has same FDA guidelines in manufacturing and should be equal in efficacy to the brand name drug. However, if the prescriber writes a prescription for the brand name drug and signs "do not substitute", the patient cannot request the generic (Food and Drug Administration – Center for Drug Evaluation and Research (CDER). Statistical approaches to Establishing Bioequivalence, 2001).

Q. Who decides to choose a generic substitute?

A. The patient makes the decision as long as the prescription is signed by the prescriber to allow for substitution. If the prescriber does not sign the appropriate place to allow for generic substitution, the pharmacist has to dispense the generic.

III. Controlled drugs

*Note: Always confirm any drug laws with your state regulations because *the most restrictive clause will prevail, whether state or federal.*

Q. What are controlled substances?

A. Controlled substances come under the jurisdiction of the Controlled Substances Act of 1970. The Federal agency is the Drug Enforcement Administration (DEA. and the State agency is the Division of Narcotics and Dangerous Drugs of DHHR. The Controlled Substances Act of 1970 was developed to educate and monitor the prescribing and dispensing of potentially addictive substances into five Schedules according to their potential for abuse or physical or psychological dependence.

Q. What is the definition of physical dependence?

A. Physical dependence is a physiological state characterized by the development of an abstinence syndrome on abrupt withdrawal of the medication. Physical dependence does not imply abuse or addiction.

Table 2.1 Controlled drugs.

Schedule	Abuse potential	Examples
C-I	Highest	Not accepted for medical purposes: heroin, lysergic acid diethylamide (LSD), methaqualone, peyote, 3,4, methylenedioxymethamphetamine ("ecstasy")
C-II	High	oxycodone/acetaminophen (Percocet®, Tylox®), meperidine (Demerol®), codeine, cocaine, morphine, oxycodone (OxyContin®), methadone (Dolophine®)
C-III	Less potential than C-II	Hydrocodone/acetaminophen (Vicodin®, Lorcet®), acetaminophen w/ codeine, phenobarbital
C-IV	Less potential than C-III	Zolpidem (Ambien®), diazepam (Valium®), alprazolam (Xanax®)*
C-V	Limited abuse	Cough syrups with codeine, antidiarrheals such as diphenoxylate/atropine (Lomotil®)

*Note: in certain states like New York, Schedule IV benzodiazepines (e.g., Valium, Xanax) are treated as Schedule II.

Q. What is the definition of tolerance?

A. Tolerance is a physiological state characterized by the need to increase doses of a drug to produce the initial effects of the drug or a markedly diminished effect with continued use of the same amount of the substance. Tolerance does not imply physical dependence or addition (Vilensky, 2002).

Q. Sometimes controlled substances are seen as written as Schedule III or "C-III". Is there a difference?

A. No. The *C* refers to controlled substance. Drugs which are subject to control under the Controlled Substances Act are assigned to one of five schedules: Schedule I, Schedule II, Schedule III, Schedule IV and Schedule V depending on the abuse potential. These schedules are commonly shown as C-I, C-II, C-III, C-IV, and C-V.

Q. What are the different controlled (Scheduled) drugs?

A. Refer to Table 2.1.

Q. Is a DEA number required to prescribe a narcotic?

A. Yes. A dentist is required by law to register with the Drug Enforcement Administration (DEA) in Washington, to dispense, store or prescribe controlled drugs. A DEA number will be issued to the prescriber in the State where he/she is practicing dentistry. If the State where the dentist is practicing requires that the dentist have a State Controlled Substance Number, in addition to the DEA number, then the DEA will require that this number be issued before the DEA number can be issued. Twenty-six States that require a Controlled Substance Number and a DEA number including New Jersey, Alabama, South Carolina, Nevada, Iowa, District of Columbia, Utah, Oklahoma, Massachusetts, Michigan, Illinois, Connecticut, South Dakota, Louisiana, Guam, Wyoming, Puerto Rico, Rhode Island, Missouri, Indiana, Delaware, Texas, New Mexico, Maryland, Hawaii, and Idaho. There must be a space on the prescription to write in the DEA number.

Q. Are prescription writing rules for controlled substances state or federal regulated?

A. Both. Regulations can be under state or federal. Prescriber must review individual laws in the state he/she is a prescriber. For example, under federal law, a prescription for Schedule II substances most be filled within 30 days of the written prescription. *A state could establish rules tighter than the federal rules and the most restrictive clause will prevail, whether state or federal.*

Q. According to state and federal law, are there limits to the amount of controlled drugs that can be prescribed?

A. While states may have more restrictive rules, the federal law does not limit the amount prescribed. *The most restrictive clause will prevail, whether state or federal.*

Q. Can Schedule I substances be prescribed by a private practitioner?

A. No. Schedule I substances have the highest abuse potential and there are no indications to prescribe them and are not legally available to the public. This is a federal law and does not vary from State to State.

Q. Can Schedule II substances be prescribed by a private practitioner?

A. Yes. Schedule II drugs have a high abuse potential and include narcotics, and amphetamines. There cannot be any refills and the prescription becomes invalid after **a** certain number of days which is state regulated. For example, in New Jersey any controlled substance prescription can be filled in a pharmacy within 30 days of writing the prescription. After the limit a new prescription is required. A Schedule II drug can be phoned into the pharmacy only in emergency situations and must be followed up by a written prescription immediately within 72 hours. Only a 3 day supply is allowed to be dispensed.

Q. What are the regulations for schedule III drugs?

A. Schedule III drugs have a lesser abuse potential than Schedule II drugs. Prescriptions for Schedule III substances expire 6 months after the date written. Refills are allowed but only five refills within 6 months. Refill authorization can be transferred from one pharmacy to another once within the 6-month period. A practitioner may issue a new prescription for the Schedule III substance within a 6-month period if necessary.

Q. What is the refill regulation for Schedule IV and V drugs?

A. Five refills in 6 months.

Q. Can the prescriber presign prescriptions for controlled substances?

A. No. Federal law prohibits prescribers from presigning prescriptions. All prescriptions for controlled substances have to be dated and manually signed on the day the prescription was written.

Q. What are Prescription Drug Monitoring Programs?

A. Diversion of controlled substances that have a high potential for abuse or profit when sold illegally is a serious problem. Different ways for diversion include: illegal selling of controlled substance by physicians, dentists and pharmacists; prescription theft; and inappropriate prescribing by physicians and dentists to themselves, family members or others. Drug monitoring programs were developed to control diversion. Some States that have a drug monitoring system include: California, Hawaii, Idaho, Illinois, Indiana, Massachusetts, Michigan, New York, Oklahoma, Rhode Island, Texas, and New Jersey (will be in effect as of September 1, 2015). Information of controlled drug, primarily Schedule II substances, prescribing, dispensing and purchasing is sent via electronic means to the State and analyzed. New York State also has extended their program to include benzodiazepines that are schedule IV controlled substances. So, in New York State, all benzodiazepines including alprazolam (Xanax) or diazepam (Valium) require a new prescription every month and no refills.

Q. Are there controlled substances in Schedule VI?

A. Yes. Massachusetts and North Carolina have controlled substances in Schedule VI where all other drugs which are not federally classified (C-II to C-V) but require a prescription to be classified as a Schedule VI (C-VI) drug. Five refills in 6 months. Penicillin, cimetidine (Tagamet) and ibuprofen (Motrin) are classified in Massachusetts as Schedule VI drugs. In North Carolina Schedule VI drugs include marijuana, hashish, hash oil, and tetrahydrocannabinol. Possession of these substances carries a prison term of 2 to 5 years.

IV.   Principles of prescription writing

Q. What is a legend drug?

A. A legend drug is a drug that can only be dispensed by a pharmacist with a prescription. Labels on these medications carry the legend: "Caution! Federal law prohibits dispensing without a prescription."

Q. What is the chemical name of a drug?

A. The chemical name describes the chemical makeup of a drug. For example, the chemical name for acetaminophen is *N*-acetyl-*p*-aminophenol.

Q. What is the proprietary name of a drug?

A. Other terms for proprietary name are brand or trade name and refer to the assigned drug name by the specific manufacturer and is protected by copyright. For example, one of the brand names for ibuprofen is Motrin (McNeil).

Q. How long is a prescription valid until it is filled?

A. Every state has different rules which apply to prescriptions. A non-narcotic prescription is valid for 60 days (1 year) from the date on the prescription. Check with the local state boards of the specific state.

Q. How is the quantity of the drug being dispensed written?

A. The symbol # is acceptable to indicate *number* and informs the pharmacist to dispense tablets, capsules or liquid ounces. Sometimes the prescriber will write *Disp*: before the # meaning dispense. For example: Disp: # 12.

Q. What does "*Sig*" refer to?

A. *Sig*. refers to the Latin word *signature*, which means *write on the label*. This is the directions to the patient on how to take the medication.

Q. Should the dosage form of the drug be indicated on the prescription?

A. Yes. Tablets, capsules, or suspension/solution must be indicated on the prescription. For example, amoxicillin 500 mg Disp: # 28 capsules.

Q. Should the drug strength be written on the prescription?

A. Yes. The correct strength of the drug prescribed must be clearly written on the prescription. For example, amoxicillin 500 mg/

Q. Should the route of administration be specified on the prescription?

A. Yes. The dentist must indicate the correct route of administration of the drug prescribed even if it is orally.

Q. Should the duration of the drug prescribed be specified on the prescription?

A. Yes. The number of days or weeks must be written on the prescription. For example, penicillin VK, 500 mg tid for 7 days.

Q. Does the number of refills need to be written on the prescription?

A. Yes. If no refills are required then "NR" or "zero" should be checked or written on the prescription. The number of refills should be spelled out. Do not just write "0". Some prescriptions have a checkoff box for "None".

Q. How many refills are allowed for non-scheduled and schedule drugs?

A. The prescriber can write for no refills which are indicated by NR (no refills). Prescription drugs may be refilled for only 1 year after the date of the prescription. A prescription for a controlled substance listed in schedule III to V can only be refilled for 6 months or 5 refills, whichever comes first, after the date on such prescription. After five refills or 6 months, whichever occurs first, a new prescription is required. For Schedule II drugs there are no refills allowed. Insurance companies and Medicaid will limit the number of refills allowed.

Q. What is the law for dispensing a controlled substance for office use?

A. A blanket prescription cannot be written to provide a medical/dental office with medications for administration. If the office requires C-II medications a DEA 222 form must be used to transfer the C-II stock. For all other medications an invoice must be utilized.

Q. What does "label" on the prescription mean?

A. When the prescriber wants the patient to know the name of the drug, the box on the prescription form marked "label" should be checked.

Q. Can I phone in a prescription for a medication?

A. Yes. A non-narcotic medication (e.g., antibiotics, nonsteroidal anti-inflammatory drugs such as Anaprox, Dolobid) can be phoned into the pharmacist and does not require a follow-up written prescription to be sent to the pharmacist.

When phoning in a controlled substance (e.g., Vicodin C-III, Tylenol with Codeine C-III, Percocet C-II) the rules are different. Schedule II drugs cannot be phone into the pharmacy except for an emergency and must be followed up with a written prescription usually within 72 hours (States may require that the prescription be sent to the pharmacist in a shorter time frame and the more restrictive clause prevails) and only a 3 day supply. Schedule III drugs can be dispensed by an oral (verbal) or written prescription and does not need a follow-up written prescription (the pharmacist writes all information which is equivalent to a written prescription). Renewal of Schedule III-V can be called-in to the pharmacy.

Q. Is there a limit on quantity prescribed for a Schedule II, III, or V narcotic?

A. Although, some states and many insurance companies limit the quantity of controlled substances dispensed to a 30-day supply or 120 doses, whichever is less, there a no specific federal limits to quantities of drugs dispensed by a prescription. Review the law in individual states. Remember the most restrictive clause will prevail, whether state or federal.

Q. Can a Schedule II narcotic (e.g., Percocet) be phoned into the pharmacy?

A. Yes, only for emergency situations only. Federal law requires the prescriber to follow up with a written prescription sent to the pharmacy within 72 hours but different states have different time limits. No refills are allowed.

Q. Can a prescription be sent via the computer (e-prescribe) to the pharmacist?

A. Yes. All non-narcotic prescriptions can be e-prescribed. There will be a digital electronic signature of the health-care provider. Either the prescription can be printed out and the patient brings it to the pharmacy or the prescription can be electronically transmitted directly to the pharmacy.

According to the DEA (federal law), as of 1 June 2010 it is permissible to have electronic prescriptions (e-prescribing) for controlled substances. *However, some states do not allow e-prescribing and that state rule will prevail*. The rule revises DEA (Drug Enforcement Administration) regulations to provide practitioners with the option of writing prescriptions for controlled substances electronically. The original Schedule II prescription must be presented to the pharmacist for review prior to the actual dispensing of the controlled substance. E-prescribing software must meet the new DEA requirements and have the required certifications before e-prescribing is allowed. In addition, some state laws and regulations will require changes before controlled substance e-prescribing will be fully legal. In dentistry few companies if any at this time have software that is capable of e-prescribing. One company "DoseSpot" has dental e-prescribing application directly from the web. E-prescribing helps to reduce medication error prescribing. For Schedule III-V a facsimile (fax) is considered to be equivalent to an original prescription.

Q. Can a Schedule II prescription be faxed to the pharmacy?

A. According to the DEA, in order to expedite the filling of a prescription, a prescriber may transmit a Schedule II prescription to the pharmacy by fax, but the original prescription must be presented to the pharmacist before the drug can be dispensed. The faxed copy is just an alert to the pharmacist that the patient is en route with an original prescription. Otherwise, a fax for a Schedule II drug is not accepted.

Q. In which situations can a faxed CII prescription serve as an original prescription?

A. A faxed CII prescription can serve as an original for patients in a long-term care facility (LTCF), community based care, enrolled in hospice, or receiving home infusion/IV pain management therapy. The fax MUST be signed by the prescriber.

Q. Can a Schedule III-V prescription be faxed to the pharmacist?

A. It depends. According to federal law Schedule III-V substances can be faxed but certain states do not allow faxing prescriptions for any controlled substance. The most restrictive clause will prevail. So, if federal law allows faxing but state law does not, the state law will succeed. According to the DEA, Schedule III-V can be communicated orally, in writing, or by fax to the pharmacist and may be refilled (not more than 5 times within 6 months) as written on the prescription or by call-in.

Q. Are preprinted prescriptions for controlled substances allowed?

A. No.

Q. What are the more common Latin abbreviations used in prescription writing

A. See Table 2.2.

Q. What are the different measurement systems used in pharmacy and for writing prescriptions?

A. Metric system which bases calculations on the base of 10. There is a metric unit of weight [e.g., gram (gm)] and a metric unit of volume [e.g., liter (L)]. The apothecary system, which is becoming obsolete, uses old measures of weights and volumes such as grains (gr). This system is also confusing because the abbreviation "gr" can be mistaken for gram, which is abbreviated "g". The avoirdupois system or household system of weights is used for ordinary commodities such as ounce, teaspoonful and tablespoonful.

Table 2.2 Commonly used Latin abbreviations used in dental prescription writing.

q	every hour
qhs	every night
qd	every day
q8h	every 8 hours
bid	twice a day
cap	capsule
tid	three times a day
qid	four times a day
stat	immediately
ac	at meal time
h	hour
hs	at bedtime
NR	no refills
pc	after meals
po	orally (by mouth)
prn	as needed
tab	tablet

Q. What is a milligram (mg)?

A. A milligram (mg) is a unit (metric system) of mass equal to one thousandth of a gram. Thus, 1 gram (gm) equals 1000 milligrams (mgs). It is advised to write "g" instead of "gm" as an abbreviation for gram because "gm" can easily be misinterpreted as "mg".

Q. What is a grain?

A. A grain (gr) is a unit of (apothecary) measurement of mass and 1 gr = 64.79 mg = 0.06479 g. It is often confused with grams, which is abbreviated g.

Q. What does the term "parts per million" mean when expressing permissible exposure to fluorides?

A. Part per million when referring to permissible exposure to fluorides means the number of grams (gm) per million ml of solution. For example, one part per million (ppm) is interpreted as one gram per million ml of solution.

Q. What does a 1:100 solution mean?

A. In calculating the amount of a drug that must be administered, especially if it is in solution, there is specific information that is required to do the calculations. The concentration of the drug in solution is expressed as gm/ml, or as a per cent or as a ratio such as 1:100, 1:1000 and so on. A percent solution means what percentage of 100 grams of a drug is in 100 milliliters of solution (www.ferretrealm.com; http://nursesearegreat.com/article/drugcal.htm):

- For example: 1:100 means that there is 1 g of drug in 100 mL of solution (1 g/100 mL) = 0.01 g/mL = 10 mg/mL = 1%
- 1:100 000 = 1 mg/100 mL = 0.01 mg/mL = 0.001%
- 5% solution means that there is 5000 mg/100 mL or 50 mg/mL. A simple way to figure this out is just to move the decimal one place to the right of the percent.
- 3% hydrogen peroxide means: 3 g of hydrogen peroxide in 100 mL of solution or 3000 mg/100 mL or 30 mg/mL.

Q. What is a **Black Box Warning** regarding certain drugs?

A. A **black box warning** (sometimes called a boxed warning) is a word of warning that is found on the package insert of a drug. It is given this name because a black border is found around the text of the warning. According to the FDA, a boxed warning is given to drugs that have a significant risk of serious or life-threatening adverse effects. Note that every **black box warning** has the date that the warning was announced by the FDA. Not all drugs have a boxed warning. Examples of some drugs related to dentistry with boxed warnings include:

- *March 2011*: fluoroquinolone antibiotics including levofloxacin (Levaquin) can exacerbate muscle weakness in persons with myasthenia gravis.
- *January 2011*: The Food and Drug Administration (FDA) asked drug manufacturers to voluntarily limit the strength of acetaminophen in prescription drug products, which are predominantly combinations of acetaminophen and opioids. This action will limit the amount of acetaminophen in these products to 325 mg per tablet, capsule, or other dosage unit, making these products safer for patients.

In addition, a *Boxed Warning* highlighting the potential for severe liver injury and a *Warning* highlighting the potential for allergic reactions (e.g., swelling of the face, mouth, and throat, difficulty breathing, itching, or rash) are being added to the label of all prescription drug products that contain acetaminophen. These actions will help to reduce the risk of severe liver injury and allergic reactions associated with acetaminophen.

Note: OTC products containing acetaminophen (e.g., Tylenol) are not affected by this action. Information about the potential for liver injury is already required on the label for OTC products containing acetaminophen. FDA is continuing to evaluate ways to reduce the risk of acetaminophen related liver injury from OTC products.

- *April 2009*: OnabotulinumtoxinA (marketed as Botox®/Botox Cosmetic) and RimabotulinumtoxinB (marketed as Myobloc®) the possibility of experiencing potentially life-threatening distant spread of toxin effect from the injection site after local injection to produce symptoms consistent with botulism. Symptoms such as unexpected loss of strength or muscle weakness, hoarseness or trouble talking (dysphonia), trouble saying words clearly (dysarthria), loss of bladder control, trouble breathing, trouble swallowing, double vision, blurred vision and drooping eyelids may occur. The other botulinum toxin product in this class, AbobotulinumtoxinA (marketed as Dysport®), was approved on April 29, 2009 and included the Boxed Warning.

- *July 2008*: fluoroquinolone antibiotics [ciprofloxacin (Cipro), levofloxacin (Levaquin)] have an increased risk of tendonitis and tendon rupture that could cause permanent injury. This risk is further increased in patients over 60 years of age, in patients taking corticosteroid drugs, and in patients with kidney, heart or lung transplants.

- *November 2005*: Clindamycin; *Clostridium difficile* associated diarrhea (CDAD) has been reported with use of nearly all antibacterial agents, including clindamycin HCL and may range in severity from mild diarrhea to fatal colitis. Treatment with antibacterial agents alters the normal flora of the colon leading to overgrowth of *C. difficile*. *C. difficile* produces toxins A and B, which contribute to the development of CDAD. Hypertoxin-producing strains of *C. difficile* cause increased morbidity and mortality, as these infections can be refractory to antimicrobial therapy and may require colectomy. CDAD must be considered in all patients who present with diarrhea following antibiotic use. Careful medical history is necessary since CDAD has been reported to occur over two months after the administration of antibacterial agents. If CDAD is suspected or confirmed, ongoing antibiotic use not directed against *C. difficile* may need to be discontinued. Appropriate fluid and electrolyte management, protein supplementation, antibiotics or surgical intervention may be required.

- *April 2005*: Celebrex; FDA has concluded that the benefits of Celebrex outweigh the potential risks in properly selected and informed patients. Accordingly, FDA will allow Celebrex to remain on the market and has asked Pfizer to take the actions listed below.Revise the Celebrex label to:

  ○ Include a boxed warning containing the class NSAID warnings and contraindication (see below) about cardiovascular (CV) and GI risk, plus specific information on the controlled clinical trial data that demonstrate an increased risk of adverse CV events for celecoxib (Messerli & Sichrovsky, 2005).
  ○ Encourage prescribers to discuss with patients the potential benefits and risks of Celebrex and other treatment options before a decision is made to use Celebrex.
  ○ Encourage practitioners to use the *lowest effective dose* for the shortest duration consistent with individual patient treatment goals.

- *April 2005*: FDA asked manufacturers of all OTC products containing ibuprofen (Motrin, Advil, Ibu-Tab 200, Medipren, Cap-Profen, Tab-Profen, Profen, Ibuprohm), naproxen (Aleve), and ketoprofen (Orudis, Actron) to revise their labeling to include more specific information about the potential CV and GI risks and instructions about which patients should seek the advice of a physician before using these drugs.

- *July 2001*: warning about the abuse potential of OxyContin, a Schedule II controlled substance.

Q. How do I write for a prescription for doxycycline?

A. See Figure 2.1.

Interpretation of prescription: the salt form of doxycycline is hyclate or monohydrate. Doxycycline monohydrate (Adoxa®, Monodox®) is used the treatment of acne. Doxycycline hyclate is used for other bacterial infections. So it is necessary it identify the correct salt form. Also, in order to write a prescription you must know whether to write for capsules or tablets. Doxycycline is supplied as 50 mg, 75 mg and 100 mg capsule or tablets. In this prescription the prescriber prescribed capsules. Latin abbreviations were used but they were written legibly. It is probably safest not to use Latin abbreviations but rather write the prescription in English. The number of days the patient should take the medication for was indicated (× 10 days; the × refers to "for"). Also, it is important for the safety of the patient to write on the prescription "for dental infections" because the patient may be taking many different medications and may have a lot of pill containers in the medicine cabinet. Identifying this prescription bottle for use for a dental infection will make easier for the patient to pick up that container. Directions for use (Sig:): Take one capsule orally every 12 hours on day 1, then one capsule every day for 10 days for dental infections.

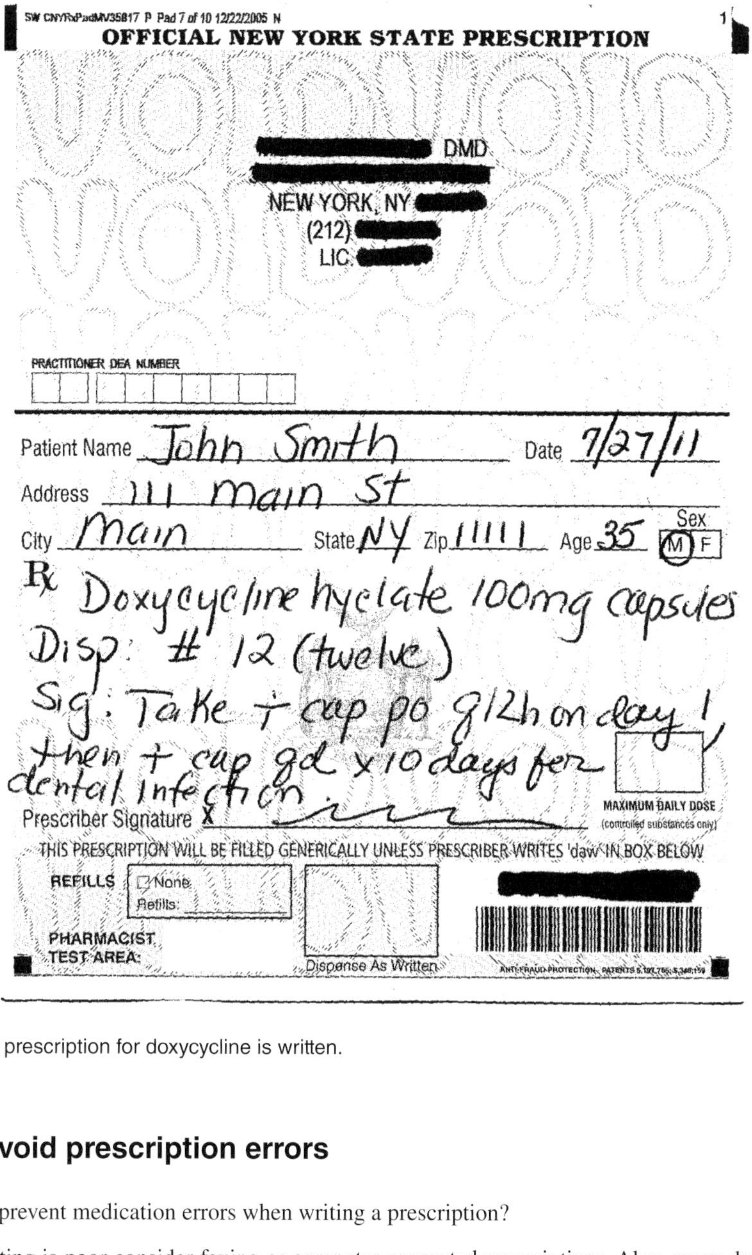

Figure 2.1　How a prescription for doxycycline is written.

V.　How to avoid prescription errors

Q. How can I help prevent medication errors when writing a prescription?

A. If your handwriting is poor consider faxing or computer generated prescriptions. Also, many drug names are very similar. To avoid misinterpretation names should be written clearly and the use of abbreviations avoided. Also, review the prescription and make sure the drug, strength and directions are correct.

Q. Should I review the prescription with the patient?

A. Absolutely. The dentist should go over the medication and how to take it including the number, frequency, and with meals or on an empty stomach. Also, make sure the patient is not allergic to the medication. Don't just review the medical history in the chart. You must ask the patient if he/she is allergic. If the patient confirms allergy, ask what happened when that drug was taken: was there a rash or hard to breath or just gastrointestinal upset (diarrhea). Document in the chart that you reviewed how to take the medication with the patient, allergies were denied and that the patient had no questions and understood everything.

A. Are the Latin abbreviations on how to take the medicine alright to use?

Q. Yes, but it is not advised because misinterpretation of abbreviations is a common source of error. Overdoses have occurred when "qd" used for every day was interpreted as "qid", four times a day. It is recommended not to abbreviate and to write out all instructions in English and avoid Latin abbreviations.

Q. Is it acceptable to write abbreviations of drugs?

A. No. The full name should be written legibly. For instance do not write PCN for penicillin VK.

Q. Is it acceptable to write "take as directed"?

A. No. The instruction, "take as directed," or "take as needed" is not satisfactory and should be avoided. Patients may fail to understand or forget the instructions given in the prescriber's office. Similarly, most insurance companies will only reimburse the patient or pharmacist for a specific number of doses or duration of treatment. Same thing holds true with writing "as needed". The directions to the patient should include a reminder of the intended purpose of the medication by including such phrases as "for relief of dental pain" or "for dental infection" (Warner & Mitchell, 2008).

Q. What else can I do to help avoid prescribing errors?

A. Always interview your patient thoroughly about allergies. For example, a patient with asthma who is allergic to aspirin may experience an acute bronchospasm after taking an NSAID (nonsteroidal anti-inflammatory drug) such as ibuprofen (Advil®, Nuprin®) or naproxen sodium (Aleve®). In adults, this reaction is called Samter's triad and it is a condition consisting of asthma, non-allergic aspirin sensitivity and nasal polyps. Recently a fourth symptom has been added, hyperplastic sinusitis and instead of Samter's triad it can also be called aspirin exacerbated respiratory disease. This occurs because NSAIDs block the production of prostaglandins, allowing arachidonic acid cascade to shut entirely to the production of leukotrienes, chemical substances involved in the inflammatory response resulting in severe allergy-like symptoms. Best to avoid aspirin and NSAIDs in asthmatics.

   Another example: clindamycin is prescribed to a patient that is allergic to penicillin. A review of the patient's history confirms she has a past history of ulcerative colitis. Clindamycin is contraindicated in an individual with a history of ulcerative colitis. An alternative choice would be azithromycin (Zithromax). Refer to Chapter 4.

Q. What about recommending over-the-counter drugs?

A. Even though over-the-counter (OTC) drugs are not prescription or legend drugs if the dentist recommends an OTC in the dental office the same responsibilities for proper prescribing are upheld. For example, after a surgical procedure the patient asks which OTC analgesic is good to take. Do not recommend any OTC drug without reviewing the medical history. If the patient has controlled hypertension and is taking a beta-blocker, NSAIDs (e.g., ibuprofen, naproxen sodium) in doses adequate to reduce inflammation and pain can increase blood pressure in both normotensive and hypertensive individuals. In addition, NSAID use may reduce the effect of all antihypertensive drugs except calcium channel blockers [nifedipine (Procardia), amlodipine (Norvac)]. The manufacturer recommends that NSAIDs be used for a maximum of 5 days in patients taking any antihypertensive drugs except for calcium channel blockers (White, 2007).

Q. Is there any special labeling of OTC drugs?

A. Yes. In the Federal Register of March 1999, the Food and Drug Administration published the OTC Drug Facts Label regulation. This regulation required most OTC drug products to comply with the new format and content requirements by May 2002. This "new" drug labeling of OTC was intended to inform the consumer about the medication in an easy to read label. OTC medicines also differ from prescription drugs in their labeling. The OTC Drug Facts label contains all the information a consumer needs in order to select an appropriate OTC medicine, to use the medicine safely and effectively, and to decide when to consult a physician, if needed. Some changes to the labeling include: the word "uses" replaces "indications," and terms such as "precautions" and "contraindications" have been replaced with more easily understood words. The label is written in large font and formatted with bullets so it is easier to read a type size large enough to be easily read.

Q. Can there be errors when writing decimal points and zeros on a prescription?

A. Yes. To avoid prescription misinterpretations avoid unnecessary decimal points. For example, when writing for 5 mL of a suspension or solution, it should be written as 5 mL not 5.0 mL because the 5.0 could be understood as 50. Also, always place a zero before quantities. For example, write 0.25 mg and not .25 mg because this could be misinterpreted as 25 mg.

References

Balthasar, J. (1999) Bioequivalence and bioequivalency testing. *American Journal of Pharmaceutical Education*, 63:194–198.

Birkett, D. (2003) Generics-equal or not? *Australian Prescriber*, 26:85–87.

Food and Drug Administration – Center for Drug Evaluation and Research (CDER). Statistical approaches to Establishing Bioequivalence. January 2001. Available from: http://www.fda.gov/downloads/Drugs/GuidanceComplianceRegulatoryInformation/Guidances/ucm070244.pdf. September 26, 2011.] (accessed 10 December 2011).

Food and Drug Administration. (2008) Approved drug products with therapeutic equivalence evaluations. 31th 31st edition. Available from http://www.fda.gov/cder/orange/obannual.pdf (2008) (accessed 26 September 2011).

Greene, W.L., Concato, J. & Feinstein, A.R. (2001) Claims of equivalence in medical research: Are they supported by the evidence. *Annual Annals of Internal Medicine*, 132:715–722.

Meridith, P. (2003) Bioequivalence and other unresolved issues in generic drug substitution. *Clinical Therapeutics*, 25:2875–2890.

Messerli, F.H. & Sichrovsky, T. (2005) Does the pro-hypertensive effect of cyclooxygenase-2 inhibitors account for the increased risk in cardiovascular disease? *American Journal of Cardiology*, 96:872.

Vilensky, W. (2002) Opioid "mythstakes": Opioid analgesics – current clinical and regulatory perspectives. *Journal of the American Medical Association*, 102:S11–S14.

Warner, T.D. & Mitchell, J.A. (2008) COX-2 selectively alone does not define the cardiovascular risks associated with non-steroidal anti-inflammatory drugs. *Lancet*, 371:270–273.

Welage, L.S., Kirking, D.M., Ascione, F.J., *et al.* (2001) Understanding the scientific issues embedded in the generic drug approval process. *Journal of the American Pharmaceutical Association*, 41:856–867.

White, W.B. (2007) Cardiovascular effects of the cyclooxygenase inhibitors. *Hypertension*, 49:408–418.

Additional references and websites

- http://www.massmed.org/AM/Template.cfm?Section=Home6&TEMPLATE=/CM/HTMLDisplay.cfm&CONTENTID=5751
- http://www.deadiversion.usdoj.gov/pubs/manuals/pract/section5.htm
- http://www.fda.gov/Drugs/DrugSafety/ucm239821.htm
- http://www.fda.gov/Safety/MedWatch/SafetyInformation/ucm194129.htm
- www.blackboxrx.com
- http://www.fda.gov/Drugs/DrugSafety/PostmarketDrugSafetyInformationforPatientsandProviders/ucm150314.htm
- FDA Guidance for Industry. Dissolution Testing for Immediate Release Solid Oral Dosage Form. US Department of Health and Human Services. Food and Drug Administration Center for Drug Evaluation and Research (CDER) August 1997.BP1.

Chapter 3

Drug dosing

I. Basic principles of drug dosing

Q. What is the difference between dose and dosage form?

A. The dose of a drug is a specified quantity of a drug; the size or frequency at which the drug doses are administered. The dosage form of a drug is the drug formulation such as a tablet, a capsule, syrup, a liquid suspension/solution or an ointment/cream that generally contains a mixture of the active drug substance, in association with one or more nonactive ingredients. The FDA has stated that a dosage form is the way of identifying the drug by its physical form, which is linked both to physical appearance of the drug product and to the way it is administered (http://www.fdalawblog.net/fda_law_blog_hyman_phelps/2009/05/fda-petition-response-reaffirms-fda-orange-book-dosage-form-nomenclature-policy.html).

   If the patient is instructed to take one 500 mg capsule po (orally) qid (four times a day) the total dose is calculated from the dose administered multiplied by the number of times a day the dose is administered; one tablet (500 mg) qid is 2000 mg or 2 g.

Q. Why are some tablets "candy coated"?

A. These "candy coated" tablets are referred to as enteric-coated. Some drugs are either irritating to the stomach lining or are inactivated, by different degrees, by acid in the stomach. To prevent the drug from dissolving in the stomach and allow it to get absorbed in the intestine the drug is available in enteric-coated tablets or are buffered to protect the drugs from gastric juices. Examples include erythromycin base, ibuprofen, and aspirin.

Q. Is it important to know the patient's baseline hepatic and renal function when deciding on the proper dosage for a patient?

A. Yes. Most drugs require adequate hepatic function for metabolism and adequate renal function for elimination. It is important to review the medical history and specifically ask the patient if he/she has any liver or kidney problems.

Q. What is the principle of selection of a therapeutic regimen?

A. Since the outcome of drug therapy is the product of a multifaceted interaction between drug and patient, the selection of an appropriate drug and regimen is depend on a thorough evaluation of the patient's medical and dental status and the actions and effects of the drugs to be used in treatment.

Q. What are the variabilities in drug dosage requirements?

A. There are many variabilities relating to alterations in drug dosing. The age of the patient, renal and liver function of the patient and pregnancy can change the way the body reacts to medications.

The Dentist's Drug and Prescription Guide, First Edition. Mea A. Weinberg and Stuart J. Froum.
© 2013 John Wiley & Sons, Inc. Published 2013 by John Wiley & Sons, Inc.

Q. What are the loading and maintenance doses of drugs?

A. Most drugs are not administered as a single dose. Rather, repeated doses resulting in an accumulation of the drug in the blood are needed to reach a plateau whereby the level of drug in the plasma is maintained constantly within the therapeutic range and avoid fluctuations in the concentration-time profile. A **steady-state** is achieved when the same amount of drug that is absorbed into the body equals the same amount of the drug leaving the body. To keep a proper steady-state, the drug dosing must be consistent and the drug must be taken at the same time every day. Not achieving and maintaining steady-state may make the drug ineffective. It must be emphasized to the patient that the drug must be taken as prescribed. The drug should be taken at the same time every day and no doses missed. In order to reach this steady-state, a **loading dose** is first administered on day 1, which is a higher amount of drug needed to quickly reach a therapeutic response. Without a loading dose it takes longer to reach steady-state. After the loading dose is administered and before the plasma levels drop, a **maintenance dose** is given to maintain plasma drug levels within the therapeutic range. This maintenance dose is given in sporadic doses after the loading dose. For example, penicillin VK is usually given as "1000 mg initially, followed by 500 mg every 6 hours". Doxycycline is given as "100 mg every 12 hours on day 1, then 100 mg every day afterward".

Q. How much loading dose is administered?

A. The loading dose is usually twice the regular dose.

Q. What drugs are given as an initial loading dose followed by a maintenance dose?

A. Antibiotics that are administered every 6 to 8 hours (also including azithromycin, which is dosed once every 24 h) usually require a loading dose in order to rapidly achieve a high tissue concentration for acute dental infections.

Q. How is a loading dose, followed by a maintenance administered?

A. The loading dose is given on day 1, followed by the maintenance dose on day 1, day 2 etc.…

Q. What is the proper duration of antibiotic treatment for dental infections?

A. Generally, the duration of antibiotic therapy has been variable and not evidence based. The current theory focuses on shortening the course of antibiotics, which might limit antibiotic resistance. Generally, most private practice and hospital-based dentists empirically prescribe antibiotics for 7 to 10 days. However, high-dose, short-term therapy has also been advocated. Prescribing antibiotics for 3 days has supported the fact of reducing the incidence of antibiotic resistance with prolonged antibiotic exposure. It is also important to take the antibiotic for the full course prescribed even if the patient is clinically responding in order to minimize the chance of the resistant bacteria not being targeted preventing a relapse. There are no dental guidelines or recommendations regarding the duration of antibiotic therapy. There are a few published medical guidelines that were found concerning the duration of antibiotic therapy. The Infectious Diseases Society of America/American Thoracic Society (IDSA/ATS) regarding hospital patients with pneumonia recommends that antibiotic therapy should be for a minimum of 5 days (Mandel *et al.*, 2007). Important information for dental infections can be extrapolated from these guidelines.

Q. What is the importance of knowing the peak concentration of a drug?

A. Peak concentration is the maximum plasma concentration of a drug which is seen during dosing intervals. At the time (usually hours) of peak concentration, the drug has the highest concentration in the plasma. Knowing the peak concentration of a drug (e.g., antibiotic) is important because this is the time that is desired if antibiotic prophylaxis is warranted. Antibiotic prophylaxis is defined as prevention of the development of an infection at the surgical site (Munckoff, 2005). For example, recommending antibiotic prophylaxis according to the American Heart Association (AHA) for the prevention of bacteria or before a sinus graft is performed in anticipation of possible perforation of the Schneiderian membrane (creating signs and symptoms of a sinusitis). At these times having the antibiotic already in the systemic circulation before the surgical procedure is performed is idea for optimum therapeutic effects. Thus, before

Table 3.1 Peak blood levels of antibiotics.

Amoxicillin	1–2 hours
Azithromycin (Zithromax)	704.25 pt2.5 to 4 hours
Clindamycin	45 to 60 minutes
Doxycycline	1–2 hours
Penicillin VK	30 to 60 minutes
Tetracycline	2 to 4 hours

Table 3.2 Peak levels of common analgesics.

Acetaminophen	0.5–2 hours
Codeine	1–1.5 hours
Diflunisal (Dolobid)	2–3 hours
Ibuprofen	1–2 hours
Meperidine (Demerol)	1 hour
Naproxen sodium (Aleve, Anaprox)	1 hour
Oxycodone	30–60 minutes

performing these surgical procedures the antibiotic needs to only be administered during the peak hours before the surgery and not days before.

Q. What are the peak blood levels of antibiotics used in dentistry?

A. See Table 3.1.

Q. What are the peak levels of common analgesics used in dentistry?

A. See Table 3.2

Q. What is the difference in prescribing capsules or tablets (e.g., doxycycline 100 mg comes in tablets and capsules)?

A. If a patient has difficulty swallowing capsules, prescribe tablets. To be absorbed capsules need to undergo dissolution or to be opened (usually takes about 4 minutes) and tablets need to undergo disintegration or to break up (takes slightly longer than a capsule) to release the active ingredient that will be absorbed. Both processes take time and absorption will occur in the duodenum (small intestine). A liquid gel capsule (Aleve, Advil) is formulated to dissolve quickly which allows the liquid inside the capsule to be absorbed fast. A gel capsule is a capsule-shaped tablet coated with gelatin for easy swallowing. Basically, it is a tablet and not a capsule. That means it will be absorbed like a tablet but it may take longer to disintegrate because the gelatin has to disintegrate first and then the tablet. Liquid drug form (e.g., solution) is absorbed the quickest, followed by liquid gel capsule, capsule, tablet and then gel capsule.

Q. What happens if a patient misses a dose of an antibiotic?

A. It is important not to miss a dose because drugs that require daily administration are only effective when they achieve steady-state in the blood, which is required for a medication to reach therapeutic and effective levels in the blood. This means that steady-state occurs when the same amount of drug entering the blood equals the same amount of drug being eliminated from the body.

Ideally, doses should be equally spaced throughout the day and taken at the same times each day. This will help to maintain a constant level of antibiotic in the bloodstream. If the patient misses a dose of an antibiotic it is best not to double the next dose because this could increase the incidence of adverse effects. If you miss a dose, take it as soon as remembered; do not take if it is almost time for the next dose. Instead, skip the missed dose and resume your usual dosing schedule. Do not "double-up" the doses.

Q. What does first-pass effect have to do with drug dosing?

A. First-pass effect is defined as the biotransformation of a drug in the liver that occurs before the drug enters the systemic circulation. For example, sublingual nitroglycerin has a high first pass metabolism because 90% of it is inactivated by the liver before it enters the blood. Morphine and lidocaine are other drugs with high first-pass effect when administered orally. Because of a high first-pass metabolism these drugs cannot be given orally because it would be totally inactive before it reached the site of action.

Q. How does age affect drug metabolism?

A. Age often affects drug metabolism and drug dosages may need to be adjusted in children and the elderly. Years ago pediatric dosing was determined using pediatric formulas such as Clark's Rule, Young's Rule and Fried's Rule, which were based on the weight of the child in pounds or on the age of the child in months. Today, these formulations are not used but rather the dose is based on body surface area or weight of the infant/child. In order to calculate the proper dosage the manufacturer's appropriate dose (in mg/kg) of the prescribed drug which is safe must be known. This dose is a given and predetermined value from the manufacturer.

Children and the elderly require lower drug doses than other individuals due to difference in their response to drugs.

II. Pediatric patient

*Note: The prescriber should use his/her own judgement in prescribing for a particular pediatric patient. The prescriptions in this section are not absolute numbers, only suggestions. These are just a few examples how you can calculate doses.

Q. Are there standardized dosage recommendations for children?

A. Yes. The dosage is dependent on the age and weight of the child. It should be noted that there is a wide range of correct dosages for a drug. Usually, drug information for pediatric dosage (mg/kg) is supplied by the drug manufacturers. For example, the dose recommendations for children on amoxicillin range from 20 to 45 mg/kg body weight per day depending on weight and height of the patient and the severity (mild or severe infection) of the medical condition. (http://www.emiphysicians.com/calculator1.html).

Q. Should a solid dose form such as tablets or capsules or liquid suspension or solution be given to a pediatric patient?

A. It depends on the age and the weight of the child but always ask the parent if the child can swallow a pill. Sometimes when doing dosage calculations it may be more accurate to give a liquid dosage form.

Q. What is the difference between mL and cc?

A. mL (milliliters) is sometimes referred to as cc or cubic centimeters. Sometimes, a medical dropper will have markers in cc, cc is the same as mL.

Q. How does the parent accurately measure out teaspoonfuls or mL?

A. A medicine dropper and spoon are available in the pharmacy. The dropper and spoon have measurements in medically or marked teaspoonful (tsp) and mL. The patient should be cautioned about a household teaspoon because it can vary in size.

Q. What should be prescribed if the calculation for a pediatric dose is, for example, 275 mg for penillicin VK?

A. Since there is no dosage strength available for 275 mg, it is recommended to always use the lower dose and then increase the number of days of therapy (prescribe the antibiotic for 10 days rather than 7 days) *or* to use the suspension instead.

Table 3.3 Calculation for correct dose to give to a pediatric patient.

Step 1. Convert pounds to kg:	70 lb×1 kg/2.2 lb=31.8 kg
Step 2. Calculate the dose in mg:	31.8 kg×15 mg/kg/day=477 mg/day
Step 3. Divide the dose by the frequency:	477 mg/day ÷ 3 (tid)=159 mg/dose q8h
Step 4. Convert the mg dose to mL:	¶159 mg/dose ÷ 125 mg/5 mL=6.36 mL qid
Step 5. Convert mL into teaspoonfuls*	6.36 mL ÷ 5 mL=1.27 teaspoonful (round to 1¼ teaspoonful)

*Each teaspoonful is 5 mL.
¶Calculation for 159 mg/dose ÷ 125 mg/5 mL is the following: 159 x 5 ÷ 125=6.36.

Table 3.4 How the prescription is written.

Rx Penicillin VK oral suspension 250 mg/5 mL
Disp: 1 bottle (100 mL)
Sig: Take 1¼ teaspoonful orally three times a day for 7 days for dental infection.

*Advise the parent to get a medicine dropper/spoon rather than using an ordinary teaspoon because of variations in measurements of a teaspoonful. After penicillin V solution is mixed, it is best to store it in a refrigerator between 2 and 7°C (36–46°F); do not freeze. Throw away any unused medicine after 14 days.

Q. What directions should be given to the parent about oral suspensions?

A. Oral suspensions should be shaken very well and stored in the refrigerator. Any unused medicine should be discarded after 14 days.

Q. Given the following case, what dosage of penicillin VK should be prescribed to this child?

A. *10-year-old male patient that weighs 32 kg (70 lbs) has an endodontic abscess that is not draining. An antibiotic should be prescribed. Penicillin VK is the drug of choice. The antibiotic can be prescribed as an oral suspension or as a tablet.*

a. Penicillin VK oral suspension

Steps to follow when prescribing for a pediatric patient: http://www.drugguide.com/ddo/ub/view/Davis-Drug-Guide/109514/0/Pediatric_Dosage_Calculations

- What is the dose required for the age of the child? This information can be obtained from a drug reference source. This is a set dosage for the child of that age and weight.
  - Dose required: <12 yr 15–30 mg/kg/d q6–8 h; max: 3 g/day×7–10 days (This is already established and a given dosage obtained from a drug reference source.)
- In this case if it is decided to give an oral suspension the amount of active ingredient in the oral suspension must be known. This information is also obtained from a drug reference book.
  - How supplied: oral suspension 125 mg/5 mL; 250 mg/5 mL (100 mL bottle)
- Now, the correct dose to give to the pediatric patient must be calculated (Table 3.3):
- How is the prescription written (Table 3.4)?

b. How is the dose calculated if the child could swallow tablets (Table 3.5)?

Penicillin VK tablets

- Dose required: <12 yr 15–30 mg/kg/d q6–8 h; max: 3 g/day×7–10 days (This is already established and a given dosage. There is a dose range so it depends on the weight of the patient and severity of the infection.)
- How supplied: 250, 500 mg tabs.

Table 3.5   How to calculate dose if the child could swallow tablets.

Step 1. Convert pounds to kg:	70 lb × 1 kg/2.2 lb = 31.8 kg
Step 2. Calculate the dose in mg:	31.8 kg × 15 mg/kg/day = 477 mg/day
Step 3. Divide the dose by the frequency:	477 mg/day ÷ 3 (tid) = 159 mg/dose q8h

*The total dose is 159 mg every 8 hours. Since the tablets only come in 250 and 500 mg then it is probably best to prescribe the oral suspension to be more precise.

Table 3.6   Calculating the dose of amoxicillin suspension in mL for a 10-year-old child weighing 70 lbs (amoxicillin oral suspension).

Step 1. Convert pounds to kg:	70 lb × 1 kg/2.2 lb = 31.8 kg
Step 2. Calculate the dose in mg:	31.8 kg × 40 mg/kg/day = 1272 mg/day
Step 3. Divide the dose by the frequency:	1272 mg/day ÷ 3 (tid) = 424 mg/dose bid
Step 4. Convert the mg dose to mL:	424 mg/dose ÷ 125 mg/5 mL = 3.39 mL bid
Step 5. Convert mL into teaspoonful*	3.39 mL ÷ 5 mL = 0.68 teaspoonful

*Each teaspoonful is 5 mL

Rx: amoxicillin oral suspension 125 mg/5 mL
Disp: 100 mL bottle
Sig: Take 3.4 cc orally three times a day for 7 days for dental infection.
Note: mL (milliliters) is sometimes referred to as cc or cubic centimeters. Usually, a medical dropper will have markers in cc's. CC is the same as mL. There is probably less misinterpretation when mL is used rather than cc.

Table 3.7   Calculating the dose of amoxicillin chewable tablets in mg for a 10-year-old child weighing 70 lbs.

Step 1. Convert pounds to kg:	70 lb × 1 kg/2.2 lb = 31.8 kg
Step 2. Calculate the dose in mg:	31.8 kg × 30 mg/kg/day = 954 mg/day
Step 3. Divide the dose by the frequency:	954 mg/day ÷ 3 (tid) = 378 mg/dose bid

Since chewable tablets only come in strengths of 125 and 400 mg it is recommended to always use the lower dose and then increase the number of days of therapy *or* to use the suspension instead, which may be more precise.

c.   *If amoxicillin were to be prescribed*

Amoxicillin oral suspension

Calculate the dose of amoxicillin suspension in mL for a 10-year-old child weighing 32 kg (70 lbs) (Table 3.6).

- Dose required: 25–45 mg/kg/day divided BID or 20–40 mg/kg/d q8h (this is given by the manufacturer).
- How supplied: suspension comes in a concentration of 125 mg/5 mL; 250 mg/5 mL; 250 mg/mL, 400 mg/mL (100 mL bottle).

*Advise the parent to get a medicine dropper/spoon rather than using an ordinary teaspoon because of variations in measurements of a teaspoonful. After penicillin V solution is mixed, it is best to store it in a refrigerator between 2 and 8°C (36–46°F); do not freeze. Throw away any unused medicine after 14 days.

Amoxicillin chewable tablets (Table 3.7)

- Dose required: 25–45 mg/kg/day divided bid or 20–40 mg/kg/d q8h (this is given by the manufacturer).
- How supplied: chewable tabs: 125, 400 mg.

Table 3.8 Calculating the dose of amoxicillin capsules in mg for a 10-year-old child weighing 70 lbs.

Step 1. Convert pounds to kg	70 lb × 1 kg/2.2 lb = 31.8 kg
Step 2. Calculate the dose in mg	31.8 kg × mg/kg/day = 1272 mg/day
Step 3. Divide the dose by the frequency	1272 mg/day ÷ 2 (bid) = 636 mg/dose bid

The dose is 636 mg bid; either 500 mg capsules can be prescribed and increase the number of days of therapy or it may be best to use the oral suspension.

Table 3.9 Calculating the dose of clarithromycin (Biaxin) in mL for a 10-year-old child weighing 70 lbs.

Step 1. Convert pounds to kg:	70 lb × 1 kg/2.2 lb = 31.8 kg
Step 2. Calculate the dose in mg:	31.8 kg × 15 mg/kg/day = 477 mg/day
Step 3. Divide the dose by the frequency:	477 mg/day ÷ 2 (bid) = 238.5 mg/dose bid
Step 4. Convert the mg dose to mL:	238.5 mg/dose ÷ 250 mg/5 mL = 4.77 mL q12h
Step 5. Convert mL into teaspoonful	4.77 mL ÷ 5 mL = 0.954 teaspoonful bid

Table 3.10 Pediatric dosage schedule.

Weight (kg)	Weight (lbs)	Dosage (q12h) (Tablets)	125 mg/5 mL* (Suspension)	250 mg/5 mL (Suspension)
9	20	67.5 mg q12h	2.7 mL q12h	1.35 mL q12h
18	40	136 mg q12h	5.4 mL q12h	2.7 mL q12h
25	55	187.5 mg q12h	7.5 mL q12h	3.75 mL q12h
34	75	255 mg q12h	10 mL q12h	5 mL q12h

Adapted from: http://www.rxlist.com/biaxin-drug.htm
*A teaspoonful is 5 mL.
This is an easy to follow table for prescribing clarithromycin to pediatric patients; the usual recommended daily dosage is 15 mg/kg/day divided q12h for 10 days

Table 3.11 How the clarithromycin (Biaxin) prescription should be written.

Rx: clarithromycin oral suspension 250 mg/5 mL
Disp: 1 bottle (100 mL)
Sig: Take 1 teaspoonful orally twice a day for 7 days for dental infection.

Amoxicillin capsules (Table 3.8)

- Dose required: 25–45 mg/kg/day divided bid (this is given by the manufacturer).
- How supplied: Capsules: 250, 500 mg.

Q. If the child in Case 1 (above) were allergic to penicillin, what other antibiotics could be prescribed?

A. Clarithromycin (Biaxin) (Table 3.9)

- Dose required (given): 15 mg/kg/day divided q12h (Table 3.10).
- Supplied: oral suspension comes in a concentration of 125 mg/5 mL; 250 mg/5 mL (100 mL bottle) (Table 3.11).

Table 3.12   Calculating the dose of azithromycin oral suspension in mL for a 10-year-old child weighing 70 lbs and how the prescription should be written.

Step 1. Convert pounds to kg:	70 lb × 1 kg/2.2 lb = 31.8 kg
Step 2. Calculate the dose in mg:	31.8 kg × 10 mg/kg/day = 318 mg/day
Step 3. Divide the dose by the frequency:	318 mg/day once a day = 318 mg/dose
Step 4. Convert the mg dose to mL:	318 mg/dose ÷ 200 mg/5 mL = 7.9 mL q24h

Rx: azithromycin oral suspension 200 mg/5 mL
Disp: 1 bottle (100 mL)
Sig: Take 7.9 mL orally once a day for 3 days for dental infection.

Table 3.13   Calculating the dose of azithromycin tablets in mg for a 10-year-old child weighing 70 lbs.

Step 1. Convert pounds to kg:	70 lb × 1 kg/2.2 lb = 31.8 kg
Step 2. Calculate the dose in mg:	31.8 kg × 10 mg/kg/day = 318 mg/day
Step 3. Divide the dose by the frequency:	318 mg/day once a day = 318 mg/dose once a day

*The strengths of tablets are 250, 500 or 600 mg. Since the dose is 318 mg once a day it is probably best and more precise to prescribe the oral suspension.

d.   *Azithromycin*

Oral suspension (Table 3.12)

- Dose required (given): 10 mg/kg/day q24h × 3 days.
- Supplied: oral suspension comes in a concentration of 100 mg/5 mL, 200 mg/5 mL; 1 g powder packet.

Q. When should the 100 mg/5 mL suspension be prescribed?

A. The 100 mg/5 mL strength is prescribed for younger children weighing less than 44 lbs (20 kg).

Azithromycin tablets (Table 3.13)

- Dose required (given): 10 mg/kg/day q24h × 3 days.
- Supplied: 250 mg, 500 mg, 600 mg tablets.

e.   *Clindamycin*

Clindamycin oral solution (Table 3.14)

- Dosage required (given): 10–30 mg/kg/day q6–8 h.
- How supplied: oral solution 75 mg/5 mL (100 mL bottle).

Clindamycin capsules (Table 3.15)

- Dosage required (given): 10–30 mg/kg/day q6–8 h.
- How supplied: 75, 150, 300 mg capsules.

Table 3.14 Calculating the dose of clindamycin oral solution in mL for a 10-year-old child weighing 70 lbs and how the prescription should be written.

Step 1. Convert pounds to kg:	70 lb × 1 kg/2.2 lb = 31.8 kg
Step 2. Calculate the dose in mg:	31.8 kg × 10 mg/kg/day = 318 mg/day
Step 3. Divide the dose by the frequency:	318 mg/day ÷ 3 (tid) = 106 mg/dose q8h
Step 4. Convert the mg dose to mL:	106 mg/dose ÷ 75 mg/5 mL = 7 mL tid
Step 5. Convert mL into teaspoonful	7 mL ÷ 5 mL = 1.4 teaspoonful*

*Each teaspoonful is 5 mL.

Rx: Clindamycin oral solution 75 mg/5 mL
Disp: 1 bottle
Sig: Take 1.4 teaspoonful orally three times a day for 7 days for dental infection.

Table 3.15 Calculating the dose of clindamycin capsules in mg for a 10-year-old child weighing 70 lbs.

Step 1. Convert pounds to kg:	70 lb × 1 kg/2.2 lb = 31.8 kg
Step 2. Calculate the dose in mg:	31.8 kg × 10 mg/kg/day = 318 mg/day
Step 3. Divide the dose by the frequency:	318 mg/day ÷ 4 (QID) = 80 mg/dose q6h

*The dose is 80 mg; either 75 mg capsules can be prescribed and increase the number of days of therapy, or it may be best to use the oral suspension.

III. Pregnant and nursing patients

Q. Why may dosage adjustment be required in the pregnant patient?

A. Pregnancy and the first weeks of life represent two physiologic situations in which there is a continual and significant change in the levels of plasma proteins, and it may therefore be necessary to adjust the doses of medication during these times (Moore, 1998).

Q. What is the importance of taking certain drugs in the nursing mother?

A. Nearly all drugs pass into human milk by passive diffusion. Almost all medication appears in very small amounts, usually less than 1% of the maternal dose. The higher the dosage, the more the drug transfers into milk. Different features of the drug including molecular weight, fat solubility, and the half-life will affect how much of the drug is transferred into the milk. The pH of milk is 7, which is slightly lower than plasma (pH 7.4) so that drugs that are weak bases (e.g., erythromycins, tetracyclines) will achieve high concentrations in breast milk and should be avoided.

Q. What are the FDA pregnancy categories?

A. The Food and Drug Administration requires that all prescription drugs absorbed systemically or that are known to be potentially harmful to the fetus be given a pregnancy category of A, B, C, D or X. Table 3.16 lists all categories (Lynch *et al.*, 1991).

Q. What drugs used in dentistry are safe during pregnancy and breast feeding?

A. See Table 3.17 (Turner *et al.*, 2006).

Table 3.16   FDA pregnancy categories.

During category	Description
A	Controlled studies in women fail to show a risk to the fetus
B	Animal or human studies have not shown a significant risk to the fetus. No controlled studies in pregnant women. Drugs that have been found to have adverse effects in animals but no well controlled studies of humans.
C	Drugs for which there are no adequate studies, either animal or humans, or drugs shown to have adverse fetal effects in animals but for which no human data are available.
D	Fetal risk in humans is evident.
X	Studies in animals or humans have shown definitive fetal risk. These drugs are contra-indicated in women who are or may become pregnant.

Table 3.17   List of common dental drugs during pregnancy and nursing.

Drug	FDA category	Can use during pregnancy?	Can use during nursing
Antibiotics			
Amoxicillin	B	Yes	Yes
Penicillin VK	B	Yes	Yes
Erythromycin base or ethylsuccinate	B	Yes (except for estolate form)	Yes
Clarithromycin	C	No	No data is available. Manufacturer cautions its use in nursing mothers.
Azithromycin	B	Yes; no human studies; give when benefits outweigh risk.	Not enough information. Manufacturer advises caution.
Ciprofloxacin	C	No	Discontinue breast feeding or do not use ciprofloxacin.
Clindamycin	B	Yes; when benefit outweighs risk	Excreted in mother's milk. Decision to either discontinue nursing or choose another antibiotic.
Metronidazole	B	Yes; but not in first trimester	Discontinue breast-feeding for 12–24 hours. Best to prescribe another antibiotic.
Tetracyclines	D	No	No
Analgesics			
Acetaminophen	B	Yes	Yes
Aspirin	C/D (risk for use during third trimester)	No. Aspirin use in pregnancy has been associated with alterations in both maternal and fetal hemostasis.	No
Ibuprofen (and all NSAIDs including Naprosyn and naproxen)	B/D (D in third trimester; do not recommend during the 3rd trimester)	After 1st trimester for 24 to 72 hours only. Best to avoid in third trimester due to effects on the fetal cardiovascular system (closure of the ductus arteriosus).	No data is available. Effects on nursing baby are not known.

(continued)

Table 3.17 *(cont'd)*

Drug	FDA category	Can use during pregnancy?	Can use during nursing
Codeine (e.g., acetaminophen with codeine)	C/D (in third trimester)	Only give if benefit outweighs the risks. Codeine is the only narcotic analgesic which has shown a statistically significant association with teratogenicity (involving respiratory tract malformations; depression)	Codeine is metabolized to morphine, which can result in morphine overdose in the baby especially if mothers are ultra-rapid metabolizers of codeine. Signs of morphine overdose in a nursing baby include limpness, increased sleepiness, or difficulty in breathing.
Hydrocodone (e.g., Vicodin)	C/D (in third trimester)	Neonatal respiratory depression	No. Codeine is metabolized to morphine which can result in morphine overdose in the baby especially if mothers are ultra-rapid metabolizers of codeine. Signs of morphine overdose in a nursing baby include limpness, increased sleepiness, or difficulty in breathing.
Antifungal agents			
Nystatin	B	Yes	Yes
Clotrimazole (topical)	B	Yes	Yes
Local anesthetics			
Lidocaine	B	Yes	Yes
Mepivacaine	C	No	Caution
Bupivacaine	C	No	Yes
Etidocaine	B	Yes	Yes
Prilocaine	B	Yes	Yes
Articaine	C	No	Caution
Marcaine	C	No	Caution
Anesthesia			
Nitrous oxide	Not classified	Not in first trimester; with caution in third trimester	Controversial; consult with patient's prenatal care provider
Antianxiety drugs			
Benzodiazepines (e.g., diazepam, alprazolam)	D	No	No
Triazolam and Temazepam	X	No	No

Adapted from: New York State Department of Health. Oral Health Care during Pregnancy and Early Childhood. Practice Guidelines. August 2006; Moore (1998) Selecting drugs for the pregnant dental patient. *Journal of the American Dental Association*, 129:1281–1286. (www.drugs.com/pregnancy)

Q. Why are there concerns about the use of antibiotics during pregnancy?

A. Some antibiotics have adverse effects on the developing fetus. Choosing the appropriate antibiotic requires consideration of the effects on both the mother and the fetus. The first trimester starts at conception and continues throughout the 11th week. During this period there is an increase in blood volume and hepatic and renal blood flow, which can alter the serum antibiotic concentrations. Thus, the safety of many antibiotics varies with the period of gestation and the maturity of the fetus. The time when the embryo is most vulnerable to a teratogenic agent occurs between days 18 and 60 (Lynch *et al.*, 1991; Moore, 1998; Lomaestro, 2009).

Q. What antibiotics are the safest for pregnant patients?

A. Penicillin VK and amoxicillin are thought to be safe to prescribe during pregnancy. If the patient is allergic to penicillin, erythromycin (except estolate form), metronidazole or clindamycin can be prescribed and these have been reported to have minimal risk. Tetracyclines including tetracycline HCl, doxycycline hyclate and minocycline HCl are category D and are contraindicated and should be avoided (Moore, 1998). Also, clarithromycin is a category C, but azithromycin is a category B drug.

Q. Are dosage adjustments required when prescribing a "safe" antibiotic or analgesic for the pregnant patient?

A. No. It is not needed to reduce the dose of an antibiotic prescribed to a pregnant patient.

Q. Is aspirin safe in pregnant patients?

A. Aspirin should be avoided especially late in pregnancy due to delivery complications and postpartum bleeding in the mother.

Q. Is ibuprofen safe in pregnant patients?

A. Almost for the same reason with aspirin, NSAIDs may prolong pregnancy and should be avoided especially in late pregnancy or after the 1st trimester and they can be used for 24 to 72 hours only.

Q. Which is the safest analgesic recommended for pregnant patients?

A. Acetaminophen alone, but not in combination with codeine, is safe for the pregnant patient and nursing mother.

Q. Is epinephrine safe to administer in pregnant patients?

A. Yes. Epinephrine (also known as adrenaline) is a natural hormone and neurotransmitter produced by the adrenal medulla (part of the adrenal gland). It is generally considered to have no teratogenic effects when administered in dental anesthetics. It must be emphasized that since epinephrine stimulates cardiac function, when administering careful technique (e.g., aspirate to avoid intravascular injection) and proper dosing is demanded (Fayans *et al.*, 2010).

Q. Can acetaminophen and codeine be prescribed safely to a nursing patient?

A. On 17 August 2007, the FDA warned breastfeeding mothers who take codeine, either in combination with another analgesic, or in any form of cough syrup, that babies are at increased risk for morphine overdose. Newborn babies are especially sensitive to the effects of the smallest dosages of narcotics. Codeine is metabolized to morphine and in women who are "ultra-rapid" metabolizers of codeine adverse effects of morphine can be seen very quickly versus women who normally slowly metabolize codeine into morphine. The FDA warns nursing mothers to observe for morphine overdose in their babies. Being an ultra-rapid metabolizer of codeine is due to a mutation in the gene coding for cytochrome P450 enzyme (*CYP2D6*) in the liver. It is relatively uncommon but could occur. (www.fda.gov/Drugs/DrugSafety/PostmarketDrugSafetyInformationforPatientsandProviders/ic,118108/htm)

Q. Can hydrocodone (Vicodin) be prescribed to a nursing mother?

A. It is best to limit the amount of narcotics to a nursing mother because the newborn is extremely sensitive to oral narcotics and a narcotic overdose with signs of breathing difficulties or limpness can occur. Hydrocodone is metabolized to active metobolites such as hydromorphone. It is recommended to use a nonnarcotic when possible. (www.drugs.com/breastfeeding/hydrocodone.html)

IV.　Elderly patient

Q. Are dosage adjustments necessary in the elderly patient?

A. Yes. Volume of drug distribution, drug clearance (renal function), protein binding, and metabolism are altered in the elderly necessitating the reduction in drug dosage. If necessary, contact the patient's physician. Additionally, there is a difference in body composition (decrease muscle mass) and function. The elderly may also have an increased sensitivity drugs because the liver metabolized and kidneys excrete the drug less efficiently.

Q. Is kidney function reduced in the elderly?

A. Yes. Renal function progressively declines as one ages even though there could be normal serum creatinine values. Since there are many drugs excreted through the kidneys a reduction in drug dosage is necessary.

Q. Is liver function reduced in the elderly?

A. Yes. There may be a significant reduction in hepatic function and it is important to reduce the dose of drugs that are metabolized by the liver.

V.　Renal-impaired patient

Q. Does renal disease alter the response to drugs?

A. Yes. The use of drugs in patients with reduced kidney function (e.g., patients on dialysis) may produce toxicity because of impaired elimination from the body. Whether the dose must be reduced depends on if the drug is eliminated entirely by renal excretion or is partly metabolized. Because the kidney is the major regulator of the internal fluid environment, the physiologic changes associated with renal disease have pronounced effects on the pharmacology of many drugs.

　Either the dose does not have to be altered but the dosing interval is increased or the dose is reduced while maintaining the same dosing interval (this is called the dose reduction method and is the preferred method because it keeps more constant plasma concentrations).

Q. What happens to the half-life of the drug in kidney disease?

A. As the plasma half-life of drugs excreted by the kidney is prolonged in renal failure it may take many days for the reduced dosage to achieve a therapeutic plasma concentration. Therefore, the loading dose should usually be the same size as the initial dose for a patient with normal renal function but the maintenance dose should be reduced. Consult with the patient's physician.

Q. What blood value must be known before prescribing for a patient with renal impairment?

A. Dose recommendations are based on the severity of renal impairment is expressed in terms of glomerular filtration rate (GFR), which is measured by the creatinine clearance. The serum creatinine concentration can be used as a measure of renal function (renal drug excretion), but is only a rough guide. The creatinine clearance test compares the level of creatinine in the urine with the creatinine in the blood. GFR is a measurement of how well the kidneys are processing wastes (Brockmann, 2010).

Table 3.18 Severity scale for renal disease.

Grade (severity)	GFR	Creatinine clearance (CrCl)
Mild	20–50 mL/min/1.73 m²	1.7–3.4 mg/dL
Moderate	10–20 mL/min/1.73 m²	3.4–7.9 mg/dL
Severe	<10 mL/min/1.73 m²	>7.9 mg/dL

Stage	Severity	GFR
Stage 1	Normal or increase GFR	≥90 mL/min/1.73 m²
Stage 2	Mild	60–89 mL/min/1.73 m²
Stage 3	Moderate	30–59 mL/min/1.73 m²
Stage 4	Severe	15–29 mL/min/1.73 m²
Stage 5	Kidney Failure	<15 mL/min/1.73 m²

Adapted from National Kidney Foundation (http://www.kidney.org/professionals/kdoqi/ guidelines_ckd/p1_exec.htm).

Q. When should antibiotics be given to a patient undergoing dialysis?

A. Antibiotics should be administered after dialysis to allow for therapeutic concentrations to be maintained.

Q. What is the severity scale for renal disease?

A. Currently, according to the National Kidney Foundation, there is no uniform classification of the stages of chronic kidney disease (Table 3.18). A review of textbooks and journal articles clearly demonstrates ambiguity and overlap in the meaning of current terms.

Q. Can tetracycline be prescribed to a patient with renal disease?

A. No. Tetracycline HCl is contraindicated in patients with kidney disease because it is 50–60% eliminated through the kidneys, whereas doxycycline hyclate is only 20–30% eliminated through the kidneys, so no dosage adjustment is needed.

The renal clearance of tetracycline is significantly affected in individuals with impaired renal function but not in individuals with normal renal function. Also, tetracycline may cause an increase in BUN (blood urea nitrogen; a measure of urea level in blood). However, excessive accumulation of doxycycline does not occur so that the dose of doxycycline does not to be altered in patients with kidney impairment but tetracycline does. So, doxycycline is the drug of choice when a tetracycline is indicated in patients with renal insufficiency (Brockmann, 2010).

Q. Can penicillin VK be prescribed to patients with renal impairment?

A. Penicillin VK is rapidly excreted through the kidneys in the urine. There is a delay in excretion in patients with impaired renal function. When GFR is <10 mL/min/1.73 m² then the dose of penicillin VK should be reduced to 250 mg every 6 hours.

Q. Which antibiotics require an increase in dosing interval in chronic kidney disease?

A. Amoxicillin, amoxicillin/clavulanic acid, cephalexin (Keflex).

Q. Which antibiotics *do not* require a change in dosing adjustment in chronic kidney disease?

A. Azithromycin, clindamycin, doxycycline, erythromycin, penicillin VK.

Q. Which antibiotic is contraindicated in chronic kidney disease?

A. Tetracycline.

VI.   Hepatic-impaired patient

Q. Does liver disease alter the response to drugs?

A. Yes. Liver disease, including hepatitis and cirrhosis, may alter the response to drugs. Drugs that are primarily cleared by the liver *may* require dosage adjustment in patients with hepatic impairment. However, liver disease has to be severe before changes in drug metabolism occur. Consultation with the patient's physician is necessary before drug prescribing.

Q. How can the dentist determine if dosage adjustment is necessary?

A. Unlike in renal disease whereby creatinine clearance and GFR can be used as a reliable indicator for adjustments in drug dosage, it is more difficult to determine indicators of liver function. The liver enzymes such as AST, ALT GGT and AP only indicate if there is liver cell damage but does not relate to the ability of the liver to metabolize drugs. Either the dosage has to be decreased or the dosing interval is increased. Consult with the patients' physician for any dosage adjustments (Golla *et al.*, 2004).

Q. Why do certain drugs require dosage adjustments in patients with liver insufficiency?

A. See Table 3.19. All drugs have to be eliminated from the body. Elimination happens either after the drug is metabolized into a water-soluble metabolite in the liver or eliminated unchanged (not metabolized). Most drugs are metabolized and excreted primarily by the kidneys in the urine. Other drugs that are not metabolized go through the liver intact or unchanged and are excreted in the bile (fluid secreted by the liver and stored in the gallbladder). From there, the bile with the drug enters the gastrointestinal tract and then is either eliminated in feces or reabsorbed back to the liver by **enterohepatic recirculation** (or enterohepatic cycling) and eventually metabolized by the liver and excreted via the kidneys in the urine. Some drugs can also change into metabolites in the liver and then excreted in the bile; these are eliminated in the feces and reabsorbed back into the blood. For example, tetracycline is not metabolized (unchanged) and undergoes enterohepatic recirculation being excreted in both the urine and bile and recovered in the feces. Doxycycline is also not metabolized in the liver but is partially deactivated in the intestines and primarily recovered in the feces.

   If the liver is not functioning normally, the dosage of a drug that is eliminated primarily in the liver may need to be adjusted. But as mentioned early, there is no way to determine liver function.

Q. What drugs used in dentistry have to have their dosage altered in patients with renal and liver impairment?

A. See Table 3.19.

Q. Can penicillins be prescribed to patients with liver disease?

A. Yes.

Q. Are local anesthetics metabolized in the liver?

A. Yes. Lidocaine, mepivacaine, bupivacaine and prilocaine are metabolized in the liver. These agents are still well tolerated by patients with mild to moderate liver disease; however, in severe disease changes may be necessary. According to Little *et al.* (2008) three cartridges of 2% lidocaine is considered to be adequate for these patients. Consultation with the patient's physician is recommended (Pamplona *et al.*, 2011).

Table 3.19 Drug dosages in renal and liver impairment.

Drug	GFR > 50 mL/ min/1.73 m²	GFR 10–50 mL/ min/1.73 m²	GFR < 10 mL/ min/1.73 m²	Liver impairment
Acetaminophen (Tylenol)	No change (interval is q4–6 h)	Every 6 hours	Every 8 hours	Avoid (limited, low-dose therapy is tolerated in hepatic cirrhosis. Maximum dose should be <2 g/day)
Amoxicillin (Trimox, Amoxil)	No change (250–500 mg q8h interval)	Every 12 hours	Every 24 hours	Safe to use with usual dosage
Amoxicillin/ clavulanate (Augmentin) (immediate-release form)	No change (500 mg q12h or 250 mg q8h)	Every 12 hours	Every 24 hours	If history of amoxicillin/ clavulanate-associated hepatic damage then it is contraindicated
Aspirin	No change	No adjustment	avoid	Avoid due to increased risk of bleeding
Azithromycin (Zithromax)	No change (500 mg once, then 250 mg qd×4 days)	No adjustment	No adjustment	Avoid
Clarithromycin (Biaxin)	No change (250–500 mg q12h)	<30: 500 mg once, then 250 mg every 24 hours	Increase interval to every 24 hours or reduce dose by 50%	No adjustment
Clindamycin (Cleocin)	No change (150–450 mg tid)	No adjustment	No adjustment	No adjustment with hepatitis; decrease dose by 50% in cirrhosis
Codeine (with acetaminophen)	No change (60 mg (no. 3) q4–6 h	Administer 50% of dose with same interval (15–30 mg)	Administer 75% of dose with same interval (7.5–15 mg)	Consider decreasing dose in moderate to severe disease or avoid
Diflunisal (Dolobid)	No change (500–1000 mg followed by 250–500 mg q8–12 h; maximum daily dose: 1.5 g)	Best to avoid or decrease dose 50%	Best to avoid or decrease dose 50%	Avoid
Doxycycline (Vibramycin, Doryx)	No change (100 mg q12h on day 1, then 100 mg qd)	No adjustment	No adjustment	Administered cautiously in patients with pre-existing liver disease or biliary obstruction. Reduced dosages may be appropriate, since doxycycline undergoes enterohepatic recycling. Best to give alternative antibiotic
Erythromycin (Eryc, EES)	No change (base: 250–500 mg q6h) (EES: 400 mg)	No adjustment	No adjustment	Avoid with the estolate – may cause hepatotoxicity

(continued)

Table 3.19 *(cont'd)*

Drug	GFR > 50 mL/min/1.73 m²	GFR 10–50 mL/min/1.73 m²	GFR < 10 mL/min/1.73 m²	Liver impairment
Hydrocodone and acetaminophen (Vicodin, Lorcet, Lortab)	One to two tabs q4–6 h	Start conservatively and titrate dosage carefully to desired effect	Start conservatively and titrate dosage carefully to desired effect	Consider decreasing dose and use for 2–3 days or avoid. Avoid chronic use.
Ibuprofen (Advil, Motrin, Nuprin)	No change (OTC: 200 mg q4 to 6 h; max 1200 mg/24 h))	Best to avoid; or reduce dose in significantly impaired renal function; caution advised	Best to avoid; or reduce dose in significantly impaired renal function; caution advised	Avoid in severe hepatic disease (hepatitis and cirrhosis)
Metronidazole (Flagyl)	No change (500 mg q6–8 h interval)	No adjustment	Every 12–24 hours	Reduce dose in severe liver disease because drug can accumulate. No dose adjustment needed with mild liver disease.
Naproxen (Naprosyn) Naproxen sodium (Aleve)	Naprosyn: 250–500 mg bid Aleve: 220 mg q8h	<30: not recommended	Not recommended	Not recommended
Penicillin VK (Pen-V, V-Cillin K, Veetids)	No change (250–500 mg q6h)	No adjustment	No adjustment	Safe to use usual dosage
Tetracycline (Sumycin)	No change (250–500 mg q6h)	Best to avoid and use doxycycline instead	Best to avoid and use doxycycline instead	Avoid

Adapted from: Brockmann, W. & Badr, M. (2007) Chronic kidney disease. Pharmacological considerations for the dentist. *Journal of the American Dental Association*, 141(11):1330–1339; Munar, M.Y. & Singh, H. (2007) Drug dosing adjustments in patients with chronic kidney disease. *American Family Physician*, 75(10):1487–1496.

References

Back, D.J. & Orme, M.L. (1990) Pharmacokinetic drug interactions with oral contraceptives. *Clinical Pharmacokinetics*, 18:472–484.

Brockmann, W. (2010) Chronic kidney disease. Pharmacological considerations for the dentist. *Journal of the American Dental Association*, 141:1330–1339.

Fayans, E.P., Stuart, H.R., Carsten, D. *et al.* (2010). Local anesthetic use in the pregnant and postpartum patient. *Dental Clinicsl of North America*, 54:697–713.

Little, J.W., Falace, D.A., Miller, C.S. *et al.* (2008). Liver disease. In: *Dental Management of the Medically Compromised Patient* (eds Little, J.W., Falace, D.A., Miller, C.S., *et al.*), 7th edn. pp. 140–161. Mosby Elsevier, St. Louis MO.

Lomaestro, B.M. (2009) Do antibiotics interact with combination oral contraceptives? Medscape. Available from www.medscape.com/viewarticle/707926 (accessed 10 December 2011).

Lynch, C., Sinnott, IV J., Holt, D.A. *et al.* (1991) Use of antibiotics during pregnancy. *American Family Physician*, 43:1365–1368.

Mandel, L.A., Wunderink, R.G., Anzueto, A., *et al.* (2007) Infectious Diseases Society of America/American Thoracic Society consensus guidelines on the management of community-acquired pneumonia in adults. *Clinical Infectious Diseases*, 44(Suppl 2): S27–72.

Moore, P.A. (1998) Selecting drugs for the pregnant dental patient. *Journal of the American Dental Association*, 129:1281–1286.

Munckoff, W. (2005) Antibiotics for surgical prophylaxis. *Australian Prescriber*, 28:38–40.

Pamplona, M.C., Muňoz, M.M. & Pérez, M.G.S. (2011) Dental considerations in patients with liver disease. *Journal Clinical and Experimental Dentistry*, 3:e127–134.

Turner, M.D., Singh, F., Glickman, R.S. (2006) Dental management of the gravid patient. *New York State Dental Journal*, 72:22–27.

Additional websites

- http://www.fdalawblog.net/fda_law_blog_hyman_phelps/2009/05/fda-petition-response-reaffirms-fda-orange-book-dosage-form-nomenclature-policy.html).
- http://www.drugguide.com/ddo/ub/view/Davis-Drug-Guide/109514/0/Pediatric_Dosage_Calculations
- USP DI. Drug Information for the Health Care Professional. Volume 1. Thomson Micromedex. 25th edition. 2005 Greenwood Village, CO.

Chapter 4

Formulary sections

I. Antimicrobials, systemic

a. *General considerations*

Q. What is the difference between an antibiotic and chemotherapeutic agent?

A. An antibiotic denotes a substance that is of biological origin; whereas, a chemotherapeutic agent denotes a chemical made synthetically. The term "antimicrobial" agent is an inclusive term referring to either an antibiotic or chemotherapeutic agent.

Q. What factors are important in the choice of a suitable antibiotic for dental infections?

A. Before selecting an antibiotic for the treatment of an infection the dentist must first consider two major factors: the patient and the susceptibility of the bacteria. Factors related to the patient that must be considered when selecting the appropriate antibiotic include:

- history of allergy to antibiotics
- renal and hepatic function
- resistance to infection (e.g., whether a compromised host)
- ability to tolerate oral drugs
- severity of the infection
- age
- if female, whether pregnant, nursing or taking an oral contraceptive.

Q. How long should an antibiotic be prescribed?

A. Duration of therapy depends on the nature of the infection and the response to treatment. Courses should not be unjustifiably prolonged because it is wasteful and may lead to adverse effects including antibiotic resistance. If the patient has not clinically improved by the 3rd day, then the antibiotic should be stopped and another antibiotic started.

Q. What is the difference between bactericidal and bacteriostatic antibiotics?

A. First, antibiotics must enter the bacteria in order for it to be effective. Bactericidal antibiotics work by killing the bacteria as a result of inhibiting bacterial cell wall synthesis or interfering with bacterial DNA. Bacterial cells must be multiplying for a bactericidal antibiotic to be effective. A bacteriostatic antibiotic weakens, disables, and reversibly inhibits the growth and replication of bacteria thereby giving the body's natural defense mechanisms time to become effective in overcoming an infection. If an infection is quiet without multiplying and forming new protein, the bacteriostatic antibiotic will not work.

The Dentist's Drug and Prescription Guide, First Edition. Mea A. Weinberg and Stuart J. Froum.
© 2013 John Wiley & Sons, Inc. Published 2013 by John Wiley & Sons, Inc.

Q. Does it make a difference when choosing the appropriate antibiotic?

A. Yes. In the majority of cases, and particularly in patients whose natural resistance is lowered by disorders of the immune system (e.g., HIV/AIDS, diabetes mellitus), it is *preferable to choose a bactericidal agent resulting in a decrease in the number of bacteria, rather than simply preventing an increase with bacteriostatic agents*. When a bacteriostatic antibiotic is used the duration of therapy must be sufficient to allow cellular and humoral host defense mechanisms to eradicate the bacteria. Bactericidal drugs are effective during the log phase of bacterial growth. If growth is slowed or stopped, then the bactericidal drugs will not have such an effect. As a result, combination therapy with a bactericidal and a bacteriostatic should not be used (Chambers, 2003).

With bacteriostatic antibiotics it is important to maintain minimum inhibitory concentrations of the antibiotic during treatment.

Q. What are the minimum inhibitory concentration (MIC) and minimum bactericidal concentration (MBC) and their importance in choosing an antibiotic?

A. MIC indicates the sensitivity of an antibiotic; it is the lowest concentration of an antibiotic that results in inhibition of visible bacterial growth on a plate or culture. The MBC is the lowest concentration of an antibiotic that kills 99.9% of the original inoculum (pool of bacteria). For an antibiotic to be effective the MIC or MBC must be achieved at the site of the infection. The MIC and MBC are important in laboratories to verify the resistance of bacteria to an antimicrobial agent. In simple terms, the MIC is a basic laboratory measurement of the activity of an antimicrobial agent against a bacteria. The MIC is determined in vitro and uses a standardized inoculum of about 10^5 cells per mL. For example, an MIC_{50} of 16 indicates that this is the concentration ($16\,\mu g/ml$) of antibiotic required to inhibit 50% of the bacterial strains. MIC_{90} of 128 indicates the concentration of antibiotic ($128\,\mu g/ml$) required to inhibit 90% of the bacterial strains.

Q. Can a bacteriostatic antibiotic become bactericidal?

A. Yes. Either increasing the dose of the bacteriostatic antibiotic or combine it with another bacteriostatic antibiotic.

Q. Which bacteria are bacteriostatic and which are bactericidal?

A. *Bacteriostatic*: tetracyclines, macrolides (erythromycin), azilides (azithromycin, clarithromycin), clindamycin
Bactericidal: penicillins, cephalosporins, quinolones, metronidazole

Q. What is the difference between a narrow-spectrum and a broad-spectrum antibiotic?

A. Narrow-spectrum antibiotics are effective against only a limited range or organisms, such as Gram-negative or Gram-positive bacteria. Broad-spectrum antibiotics affect a wider range against Gram-negative and Gram-positive bacteria. *It is recommended to choose a narrow spectrum antibiotic when treating non-life threatening dental infections*. The primary indication for use of broad-spectrum antibiotics coverage is in severe life-threatening dental infections where identification of causative agent is unknown. Every time bacteria are exposed to antibiotics, the opportunity for development of resistant strains is present. If narrow-spectrum antibiotics are used fewer bacteria have the opportunity to become resistant. Also, specific narrow-spectrum antibiotics usually are more effective against specific susceptible bacteria than the broad-spectrum antibiotics. Extended-spectrum antibiotics have bacterial activity in between a narrow and a broad-spectrum agent.

Q. Which antibiotics are considered to be narrow-spectrum and which are broad-spectrum?

A. Narrow-spectrum antibiotics: penicillin VK, erythromycin, azithromycin, clarithromycin, clindamycin.
Extended-spectrum antibiotics: amoxicillin, amoxicillin/clavulanate (Augmentin).
Broad-spectrum antibiotics: tetracyclines (doxycycline, minocycline), ciprofloxacin (Cipro).

Q. How is it determined that an antibiotic is not working after its course?

A. The patient is not clinically responding in about 3 days and the infection is not clearing up. Resistance may develop in which case culture and sensitivity may be necessary. In this case another antibiotic or another antibiotic added should be prescribed. For example, if no clinical improvement is seen in a patient taking penicillin VK in 48 to 72 hours, then metronidazole (both are bactericidal) should be added.

Q. Why is combination antibiotic therapy sometimes better than monodrug therapy?

A. Combination therapy with two or more antibiotics is used in special cases to: prevent the emergence of resistant strains; treat emergency cases during the period when an etiological diagnosis is still in progress; andtake advantage of antibiotic synergism, which is defined when the effects of a combination of antibiotics is greater than the sum of the effects of the individual antibiotics. Sometimes when using combination drugs a lower dose of one or the other can be used.

Q. How do antibiotics get distributed in the body?

A. Through the plasma. Most antibiotics are well distributed in soft tissues.

Q. What adverse effects can occur with antibiotics that you need to warn the patient about and how is it managed?

A. Antibiotics, especially broad-spectrum, alter the microflora of the stomach resulting in diarrhea and fungal infections. To help avoid this problem it is beneficial to consume living organisms referred to as probiotics (Weinberg, 2002).

- **Superinfections**: fungal infections (e.g., vaginal) and infections by other bacteria include enteric rods, pseudomonads, and staphylococci are especially more prone with broad-spectrum antibiotics but can occur with any. The narrow-spectrum antibiotic will not kill as many of the normal microorganisms in the body as the broad spectrum antibiotics. So, it has less ability to cause superinfection. This occurs because the bacteria are targeted which allow for growth of *Candida* sp. To help avoid this it is recommended to all patients, especially females, to either eat yogurt (containing live and active cultures such as Kefir, Dannon or Yoplait). *To prevent antibiotic-related suprainfections about 5 ounces of yogurt should be taken twice daily while on the antibiotic.* An alternative method is to take acidophilus supplementation (capsule), which is available in the alternative therapy section of the store. As long as the product is produced by a reliable manufacturer, most acidophilus supplements are relatively equal, and should not cause unpleasant side effects; some cause slight bloating for the first few days or weeks of taking the product, but this does not usually last. *Lactobacillus acidophilus* is one of the bacteria found in these supplements, but the term acidophilus usually refers to a combination of *L. acidophilus* with other beneficial bacteria.
- **Gastrointestinal problems** (nausea, vomiting, and diarrhea): To help avoid antibiotic-related diarrhea it is recommended to all patients to eat yogurt (containing live and active cultures such as Kefir, Dannon or Yoplait). *Approximately 4 to 8 ounces of yogurt should be taken twice daily while on the antibiotic. Yogurt should be taken at least 2 hours before or 2 hours after the antibiotic.* However, antibiotic-associated diarrhea that is constant and watery/bloody diarrhea (new onset of >3 partially formed or watery stools per 24 hour period) can be caused by toxins released from *Clostridium difficile* resulting in pseudomembranous colitis or *C. difficile*-associated diarrhea. *C. difficile* is the leading known cause of nosocomial intestinal infections (McFarland *et al.*, 1994). If this happens the patient should discontinue the antibiotic and call emergency services. The patient should not take antidiarrheal medications because it is advantageous to eliminate the bacterial toxins. *Pseudomembranous colitis symptoms could appear after a few doses or from 2 to 9 days or even months after the start of antibiotic therapy; it could happen at any time while taking the antibiotic.* Unless it is known that the patient has a proclivity toward pseudomembranous colitis, it is not known if the patient will develop it. In reality, any antibiotic can cause pseudomembranous colitis. Any antibiotic can cause pseudomembranous colitis, but if used appropriately there are fewer incidences.
- **Antibiotic resistance**: The narrow-spectrum antibiotic will cause less resistance of the bacteria as it will deal with only specific bacteria. This is the reason for initially choosing a narrow-spectrum antibiotic. Antibiotic resistance is an increasing problem worldwide.
- **Allergic reactions**: Allergic reaction ranging from a mild rash to wheezing and anaphylaxis. The antibiotic should be discontinued immediately.
- **Photosensitivity**: exaggerated sunburn when taking doxycycline. Avoid sunlight.

Q. How long after an antibiotic is taken can an allergic reaction occur?

A. Allergic reactions are classified based on the time of onset. Type I acute (anaphylactic) reactions can occur within minutes of taking the antibiotic and can be life-threatening. Accelerated reactions can occur between 30 minutes and 72 hours and are usually not life-threatening. Delayed allergic reactions can be seen up to 2 or more days later.

Q. What conditions may increase the risk of infection with antibiotic-resistant bacteria?

A. Indiscriminant use of antibiotics; recent (within 6 weeks) use of antibiotics for other conditions; previous antibiotic treatment that was not successful; and being in close contact with someone who recently was treated with an antibiotic. Patient must be compliant (adherent) with dosage regimen and avoid missing doses.

Q. What is the definition and symptoms of gastrointestinal distress?

A. Gastrointestinal distress is a term used to describe a variety of symptoms that arise from disturbances in the stomach/lower intestinal tract. Symptoms include nausea, vomiting, cramping and diarrhea. Most of the time GI symptoms are caused by the irritative properties of the antibiotic and can be minimized by taking it with food.

Q. What is the cause of gastrointestinal distress while taking antibiotics?

A. Gastrointestinal disturbances occur due to an alteration in the normal GI flora.

Q. Can combination antibiotics use used in dentistry?

A. Yes. Because multiple pathogens not just one type are present in a dental infection. Two of the same category of antibiotics can be used. For example, you can prescribe two bactericidal antibiotics but not a bactericidal and a bacteriostatic. Often amoxicillin and metronidazole are prescribed for aggressive periodontitis. Both are bactericidal antibiotics and the combination of metronidazole with penicillin VK or amoxicillin increases the bacterial susceptibility.

Q. Is the mouth sterile?

A. No. There are many bacteria present in the oral cavity: both beneficial and pathogenic (disease producing). It is clear that anaerobic bacteria both facultative and obligate are involved in the two major oral diseases, dental caries and periodontitis.

Q. Which oral bacteria are facultative (can live with or without oxygen) anaerobes?

A. Gram-positive facultative cocci: *Streptococcus sanguis, S. mitis, S. salvarius, Staphylococcus aureus*.
Gram-positive facultative rods: *Actinomyces* (including *A. viscosus, A. naeslundii*).
Gram-negative facultative rods: *Eikenella corrodens, Capnocytophaga* spp., *Aggregatibacter actinomycetemcomitans* (formerly *Actinobacillus actinomycetemcomitans*).

Q. Which oral bacteria are obligate or strict anaerobes?

A. Gram-positive obligate anaerobic coccus: *Peptostreptococcus* spp.
Gram-positive obligate anaerobic rods: *Eubacterium* spp.
Gram-negative obligate anaerobic rods: *Porphyromonus gingivalis, Prevotella intermedia, Tannerlla forsynthensis* (formerly *Bacteroides forsythus*), *Fusobacterium nucleatum*.
Gram-negative anaerobic spirochete: *Treponema* spp.

Q. Which bacteria are obligate aerobes?

A. Obligate aerobic: *Mycobacterium tuberculosis, Pseudomonas aeruginosa*.

Q. How is an antibiotic chosen for prophylaxis?

A. The choice of the antibiotic for prophylaxis is based on several factors. The antibiotic should be active against the bacteria most likely to cause an infection related to the dental procedure. Second, an antibiotic must be chosen that the patient is not allergic to or interacts with the patient's other medications.

b. Antibiotics

Beta-lactam antibiotics

Q. What is the mechanism of action of the penicillins?

A. Penicillins cause bacterial lysis (breaking up) by interfering with the synthesis of peptidoglycan that is necessary for the formation of the bacterial cell wall. This results in the lysis of the cell wall and death to the bacteria. Therefore, penicillin is most active against rapidly dividing bacteria and has no effect on nonmultiplying organisms.

Q. What is the spectrum of bacterial activity of penicillin?

A. Even though narrow-spectrum penicillin VK (penicillin V potassium) inhibits both Gram-negative and Gram-positive organisms, the cell wall of Gram-negative bacteria is more complex, therefore these bacteria are more resistant to the lytic effects of penicillin. Some bacteria effective against penicillin include:
Gram-positive coccus: *Streptococcus* spp. (penicillin is the traditional drug of choice for treatment of streptococcal infections)
Gram-negative anaerobes associated with dental infections: *Fusobacterium*, peptostreptoccci, spirochetes, *Actinomyces*, and some *Bacteroides*.
Spirochetes (*T. pallidum*)

Q. Why is penicillin G never prescribed in dentistry?

A. Penicillin G is completely destroyed by acid in the stomach so that it is only available for parenteral administration.

Q. How is penicillin made?

A. An antibiotic is a natural substance produced by a microorganism that will kill or stop growth of another microorganism. Penicillin, discovered by Alexander Fleming in 1929 is made by the mold *Penicillium chrysogenum*. The mold forms the beta-lactam ring. Amoxicillin and ampicillin are considered to be semisynthetic antibiotics, consisting of a mixture of natural and synthetic substances; a substance produced by a microorganisms that is subsequently chemically modified to achieve desired properties. Some "antibiotics" such as fluoroquinolones are totally synthetically produced and are not really considered to be antibiotics by the true definition.

Q. What does the "V' in penicillin V stand for?

A. Penicillin V is also known as phenoxymethyl penicillin and is the orally active form of penicillin (penicillin G is not orally active). The "V" stands for the Latin word *vesco/vescor* meaning "eat". Sometimes it is written penicillin VK where the "K" stands for potassium.

Q. What is amoxicillin?

A. Amoxicillin is a semisynthetic analog of penicillin with a broader spectrum of antibacterial activity.

Q. What are other drug names for amoxicillin?

A. Amoxil, Trimox

Q. What is the spectrum of bacterial activity of amoxicillin?

A. Amoxicillin is an extended-spectrum analog of penicillin VK. However, it has limited activity against streptococci or oral anaerobes compared to penicillin VK. It is a broader spectrum against bacteria not in the oral cavity (e.g., *Haemophilus influenzae, Streptococcus pneumoniae, Escherichia coli, Salmonella*). Thus, it is not any more effective in oral odontogenic/periodontal infections than penicillin VK and actually since it is a broad-spectrum antibiotic it can cause many more adverse effects including superinfection. *Penicillin VK is the drug of choice for odontogenic infections because of its superior bioavailability.*

Q. What is the difference between penicillin and amoxicillin?

A. Amoxicillin has a broader spectrum of bacterial activity and it is completely absorbed (about 90% of an oral dose is absorbed) so that there is less gastrointestinal distress (e.g., diarrhea) because it does not stay in the intestine that long and it produces higher plasma and tissue concentrations. Also, absorption is not affected by food.

Q. How are the penicillins excreted?

A. Penicillin is actively excreted via the kidneys in the urine and about 80% of a penicillin dose is cleared from the body within 3–4 hours of administration.

Q. Can penicillin be given to a patient with renal impairment?

A. Yes, since penicillin is excreted by the kidneys, renal impairment may lead to high concentrations, and neurotoxicity (damage to nervous tissue) can develop from high concentrations in the cerebrospinal fluid. A reduction of dosing *interval*, not dosage is necessary if glomerular filtration rate (GFR) is 10–50: Administer q8–12h. If GFR is <10 mL/min: Administer q12–16h.

Q. What are the adverse effects of penicillins?

A. Hypersensitivity (anaphylactic reaction), gastrointestinal distress, nausea, vomiting, suprainfections (fungal infections), and *Clostridium difficile*-associated diarrhea (CDAD), which has been reported with use of nearly all antibacterial agents and not just penicillins.

Q. Why are individuals allergic to penicillin?

A. Approximately 5% of individuals are hypersensitive to penicillins. The breakdown products of the penicillin molecule act as the sensitizing agent for allergic reactions (Montgomery & Droeger, 1984). If the reaction is mild (rash) the penicillin should be discontinued and an antihistamine such as diphenhydramine (Benadryl) may be administered orally. This does not necessarily occur in a patient with a previous history of a reaction to penicillin. For more severe anaphylactic reaction emergency services should be contacted (Fairbanks, 2007).

Q. Is the incidence of developing a hypersensitive reaction to penicillin and amoxicillin the same?

A. No. Almost 7% of individuals can develop a rash-type reaction to aminopenicillins (e.g., amoxicillin) than do the other penicillins (Fairbanks, 2007).

Q. If someone is allergic to penicillin VK is he/she also allergic to amoxicillin and ampicillin?

A. Yes. The penicillin nucleus is the same of all penicillins including amoxicillin and ampicillin.

Q. What is the treatment of *Clostridium difficile*-associated diarrhea?

A. Metronidazole or oral vancomycin is effective in 80% of cases. The remaining 20% of patients will have more episodes of diarrhea or colitis up to 3 to 28 days after the antibiotic has been discontinued (Kekety *et al.*, 1989). The patient can have repeated episodes of the disease for several years thereafter (Kekety & Shah, 1993).

Q. What drug interactions occur with the penicillins?

- Probenecid (anti-gout medication): Decreases renal tubular secretion of penicillin leading to higher and more prolonged serum concentrations.
- Bacteriostatic antibiotics (e.g., tetracyclines, erythromycins): Penicillin, a bactericidal antibiotic, requires the bacteria to be multiplying. If a bacteriostatic antibiotic, which stops multiplication of the bacteria, is taken concomitantly with penicillin, the penicillin will not be effective. To manage this interaction wait a few hours before taking one or the other antibiotic.
- Oral contraceptives: penicillins interfere with oral contraceptive efficacy.

Q. Can penicillin and amoxicillin be prescribed to a woman taking an oral contraceptive?

A. Some studies have shown that some antibiotics such as penicillin VK and amoxicillin can interfere with oral contraceptive efficacy. It is best to ask a woman if she is taking an oral contraceptive before prescribing antibiotics and to explain to either practice abstinence or choose another method of birth control.

Q. Can bacteria become resistant to penicillin?

A. Yes. Certain Gram-negative bacteria produce and secrete enzymes called beta-lactamases which break down the beta-lactam ring on the penicillin (including amoxicillin) and cephalosporin molecule. Penicillinase, a type of beta-lactamase specially breaks down the beta-lactam ring on the penicillin molecule rendering the penicillin or amoxicillin inactive resulting in treatment failure.

Q. What can be given to a patient if penicillin or amoxicillin does not work?

A. Penicillins can be destroyed by beta-lactamases (penicillinases) produced by certain resistant bacteria. The enzyme attaches to the beta-lactam ring and breaks it up. This renders the penicillin ineffective and is a reason for the patient not getting clinically better. To prevent this type of resistance from occurring, Augmentin, a combination of amoxicillin and clavulanate, is prescribed (the generic is usually prescribed). Clavulanate is an inert ingredient that also has a beta-lactam ring similar to penicillin, which strongly irreversibly binds to the penicillinase blocking the actions of penicillinase from breaking down the amoxicillin molecule and restoring the antimicrobial activity to amoxicillin. It is an acid (clavulanic acid) and can cause gastrointestinal irritation (e.g., nausea, vomiting, and diarrhea). It is usually prescribed in refractory cases when absolutely no other antibiotic has been clinically successful.

Q. How can the gastrointestinal adverse effects be minimized when taking amoxicillin and clavulanic acid?

A. It is recommended to take amoxicillin/clavulanic acid with meals and lactobacillus preparations such as Lactinex, acidophilus or yogurt with active cultures, which should be taken 2 hours before or 2 hours after the antibiotic.

Q. Does penicillin VK have a wide margin of safety?

A. Yes, penicillin has a very wide margin of safety. It is ideal to select a drug that has a wide margin of safety. This means that a drug's usual effective dose is not toxic and if a little more of the drug is given it still is not toxic. This is in contrast to antibiotics called aminoglycosides, which are not used in dental infections and have a narrow margin of safety so that even usual doses can be toxic.

Q. What is the usual dose of penicillin VK?

A. *Supplied*:
Tablet: 250, 500 mg
Dose: Loading dose (LD): 1000 mg (two 500 mg tablet) stat on day 1, followed by 500 mg (one 500 mg tablet) q6h after the LD, up to day 7 to 10.

Q. What is the usual dose of amoxicillin trihydrate?

A. Amoxicillin is supplied as capsules, oral suspension and chewable tablets.
Supplied:
Tablet: 500 mg, 875 mg
Chewable tablet: 125 mg, 400 mg
Capsule: 250 mg, 500 mg
Oral suspension: 125 mg/5 mL, 250 mg/5 mL, 400 mg/5 mL
Dose: LD: 1000 mg (two 500 mg capsules) stat, followed by 500 mg (one 500 mg capsule) q8h × 7 days.

Q. Why is the dosing interval of amoxicillin q8h and penicillin q6h?

A. The half-life ($t_{1/2}$) of amoxicillin is 1–1.3 hours and of penicillin 30 minutes. Dosing is less frequent with amoxicillin that has a longer $t_{1/2}$ and stays in the body longer than penicillin with a shorter half-life.

Q. What is the adult dosing for amoxicillin chewable tablet?

A. A loading dose of 1000 mg on day 1 is acceptable followed by 250–500 mg three times a day (every 8 hours) after the LD up to day 7 to 10.

Q. What is the usual dose of amoxicillin/clavulanate?

A. *Supplied*: (all tabs have 125 mg clavulanic acid)
Tablet: 250 mg, 500 mg, 875 mg
Chewable tablet: 125 mg, 200 mg, 400 mg chewable tab.
Dose: (can give a LD of 1000 mg) 250 to 500 mg q8h depending upon the severity of the infection. When writing the prescription only the strength (500 mg) needs to be designated because all dosage forms come with 125 mg clavulanate.

Q. Are two tablets of 250 mg amoxicillin/clavulanate equivalent to one 500 mg tablet?

A. No. Two amoxicillin/clavulanate 250 mg tablets are not equivalent to one 500 mg tablet and should not be substituted for one 500 mg tablet.

Cephalosporins

Q. Why are cephalosporins not a drug of choice in dental infections?

A. Cephalosporins are structurally related to penicillins with a similar mechanism of action. However, because most cephalosporins are poorly absorbed orally and display poor permeability into bacteria, routine use for dental infections is precluded. Additionally, cephalosporins' broader spectrum does not provide any advantage over penicillin V against principal odontogenic pathogens.

Q. Why is a cephalosporin indicated for total joint replacement prophylaxis?

A. Cephalosporins have very good bone penetration and increased activity against *Staphylococcus aureus*. Cephalexin is the first drug of choice along with amoxicillin for antibiotic prophylaxis for total joint replacement.

Q. Can a cephalosporin be given to a patient allergic to penicillin?

A. No. Cephalosporins should not be prescribed to patients allergic to penicillin since there is a 10% cross-reactivity with the cephalosporins. Penicillins share a common beta-lactam ring (Herbert *et al.*, 2000).

Erythromycins

Erythromycin

Q. Erythromycins belong to which classification of drugs?

A. Macrolides

Q. How is erythromycin produced?

A. Erythromycin is produced from a bacterial strain of *Streptomyces erythreus*. It is very difficult to produce erythromycin synthetically.

Q. What is the mechanism of action of erythromycins?

A. Erythromycins are bacteriostatic antibiotics that inhibit bacterial protein synthesis by binding to the 50S subunit of bacterial ribosomes.

Q. What is the spectrum of activity of erythromycins?

A. Erythromycins are primarily active against Gram-positive facultative anaerobic and strict anaerobic bacteria.

Q. Are erythromycins bacteriostatic or bactericidal?

A. Erythromycin is usually bacteriostatic especially at standard low doses (e.g., doses prescribed in dentistry; about 1500 mg) and bactericidal at high doses (e.g., intravenous) (Engelkirk & Duben-Engelkirk, 2010).

Q. What is the spectrum of microbial activity of erythromycins?

A. Most erythromycins are primarily effective against Gram-positive bacteria and some Gram-negative.

Q. Does bacterial resistance develop to erythromycin?

A. Yes. Bacteria can become resistant especially group A streptococci. Most Gram-negative bacteria are resistant to macrolides. Also, cross resistance can occur between erythromycin and clindamycin.

Q. Can an individual be allergic to erythromycins?

A. Yes. Allergic reactions, ranging from mild skin reactions to anaphylaxis can occur with erythromycins. If an allergic reaction occurs the drug should be discontinued and management of the reaction either with an antihistamine such as diphenhydramine (Benadryl) for mild reactions to epinephrine and calling for emergency services for severe anaphylactic reactions.

Q. Is there crossover allergy between penicillins and erythromycins?

A. No. If an individual is allergic to penicillin any erythromycin is acceptable to prescribe without any crossover allergenicity.

Q. What are the different kinds of macrolides?

A. Erythromycin base (Ery-Tab; Eryc, E-Mycin), erythromycin ethyl succinate (EES), and erythromycin stearate (Erythrocin). The different salts of erythromycin have been developed in order to compensate for the poor bioavailability (absorption). The base and stearate forms are acid-labile (susceptible to breakdown and inactivation by acid in the stomach) so in order for it to be protected from stomach acid it is formulated as filmtabs (enteric coating). The ethylsuccinate form is absorbed first and then hydrolyzed in the blood to free erythromycin.

Q. Why is erythromycin not considered a preferred antibiotic in anaerobic odontogenic infections?

A. Erythromycin is usually bacteriostatic and resistance can develop very rapidly. Since erythromycins are bacteriostatic, the MIC must be maintained by diligently following dosage regimen and not missing doses. Additionally, since erythromycin does not penetrate the cell wall of Gram-negative bacteria, the antibiotic will be ineffective because it needs to enter the bacteria to have an effect.

Q. What are some precautions used when prescribing erythromycins?

A. Gastrointestinal distress is a cause for most patients not following the entire course of therapy. Also, all members of the erythromycins prolong the electrocardiographic QT-interval resulting in the development of ventricular arrhythmias, which can be fatal, including torsade de pointes. Erythromycins should be used with caution in patients with cardiac arrhythmias, uncorrected hypokalemia and with other drugs that are used in the management of arrhythmias that could prolong the QT-interval including quinidine, sotalol or procainamide (Fairbanks, 2007). Caution should be used in patients with severe liver disease because of high risk of hepatotoxicity.

Q. Why is nausea a common adverse effect of erythromycins?

Q. Are there any drug interactions with erythromycins?

A. Yes. Erythromycins are metabolized in the liver via cytochrome P450 enzymes to form a stable metabolite complex that inhibits the metabolism of other drugs that are metabolized by these enzymes including cholesterol lowering drugs: lovastatin (Mevacor), simvastatin (Zocor), and atorvastatin (Lipitor), cyclosporine (anti-organ rejection drug), theophylline (anti-asthma drug), and sildenafil (Viagra) (Fairbanks, 2007).

Azithromycin and clarithromycin

Q. What are azithromycin and clarithromycin?

A. Both are classified as azalides, which are 2nd generation macrolides. Azithromycin is a macrolide derivative and the first of the 15-membered ring azalide class of antimicrobials. Although its mechanism of action and susceptibility to resistance are similar to those of the macrolide antibiotics, azithromycin's extended spectrum of activity includes Gram-positive and Gram-negative organisms. Azithromycin is stable at gastric pH and has a bioavailability of about 37% following oral administration. Although its serum concentrations are typically low, the drug concentrates to a high degree in tissues, including periodontal tissues. Azithromycin is cleared primarily by the biliary and fecal routes; its serum half-life is in excess of 60 hours. Azithromycin and clarithromycin are more completely absorbed than erythromycin with less gastrointestinal distress. The brand name of azithromycin is Zithromax and clarithromycin is Biaxin (Ballow & Amsden, 1992).

Q. What are advantages to prescribing azithromycin or clarithromycin?

A. Azithromycin and clarithromycin are more acid-stable than erythromycin, which means that they are not broken down in the acidity of the stomach before they reach the intestines where absorption occurs. There are few bacteria in the stomach because the high acidity inhibits bacterial growth. Both azalides have structural modifications, which result in better gastrointestinal tolerability and tissue penetration than erythromycin.

Additionally, azithromycin concentrates higher in host (phagocytes) cells (e.g., polymorphonuclear leukocytes or PMNs) and in the periodontal tissues (gingiva) (Sefton *et al.*, 1996). Because of its high concentration in PMNs, azithromycin is actively transported to the site of infection. During active phagocytosis, azithromycin is released in the tissues. Azithromycin has a post-antibiotic effect which means that it concentrates in the gingiva (about 50 times higher in the tissues than plasma) for days after the antibiotic is stopped providing microbial inhibition after the drug concentration has decreased below the MIC. This is a good feature when prescribing for aggressive periodontitis where the bacteria have been found in the gingival connective tissue. This high tissue concentration has been thought to overcome the high incidence of resistance seen with certain bacteria (Sefton *et al.*, 1996).

Q. Is azithromycin adequate to prescribe in oral infections?

A. Yes. Azithromycin has activity against many Gram-positive and Gram-negative bacteria and anaerobic bacteria and in a good choice for mild infections when the patient is allergic to penicillin.

Q. What precautions should be followed when prescribing azithromycin or clarithromycin?

A. Azithromycin or clarithromycin should not be prescribed to patients with severe liver disease (e.g., hepatic failure, cirrhosis), severe kidney disease (e.g., renal failure, pyelonephritis, glomerulonephritis), severe cardiovascular disease, pregnancy, breastfeeding and myasthenia gravis).

Q. What is the usual dose of azithromycin?

A. *Supplied*:
Capsule: 250 mg
Tablet: 250 mg, 500 mg, 600 mg
Dose: Since azithromycin has a long $t_{1/2}$ of 60–70 hours the dose is only once a day. LD: 500 mg on day 1, then 250 mg for 4 days.

Q. Is there an oral suspension available?

A. Yes. Oral Suspension: 100 mg/5 mL (15 mL); 200 mg/5 mL (15 mL, 22.5 mL, 30 mL); Also available in single dose packet: 1 gram (1000 mg). For the single dose packet the entire contents of the packet is mixed with 2 ounces (60 mL) of water and drink the entire contents. Then add 2 oz more and mix and drink to make sure the entire dose was taken. It can be taken with or without food. Do not use packet for children. The single dose packet administers only 1000 mg or 1 g of azithromycin.

Q. Can I prescribe a Z-Pak?

A. Yes. The 250 mg tablets are dispensed in blister packages of six and commonly referred to as a Z-Pak (Zithromax), whereas the 500 mg tablets are available in a blister pack of three tablets, or Tri-Pak, which has a 3-day supply.

Q. When would I prescribe clarithromycin versus azithromycin?

A. Both clarithromycin and azithromycin can be prescribed when a patient is allergic to penicillin. Compared with clarithromycin, azithromycin has increased activity against Gram-negative bacilli. So, essentially, either one can be prescribed for dental infections. The bioavailability of clarithromycin is more than twice that of erythromycin and azithromycin is 1.5 times that of erythromycin. Azithromycin has a longer half-life than clarithromycin so the dosing interval is less. As mentioned in an earlier question, azithromycin also has a better uptake from the circulation into intracellular compartments (better tissue and cells penetration) followed by a slow release. For example, if azithromycin is prescribed for 5 days, it still has active therapeutic levels in the body at day 10. Thus, azithromycin may be more superior to clarithromycin.

Q. What is the usual dose of clarithromycin?

A. *Supplied*:
Tablet: 250 mg, 500 mg
Extended-release tablet: Biaxin XL 500 mg
Granules for oral suspension: Biaxin®: 125 mg/5 mL, 250 mg/5 mL
Dose: Since the $t^{1/2}$ is 3 to 7 hours dosing is 250–500 mg q12h. The extended-release formulation is given two 500 mg extended release tablets once daily.

Q. Are azithromycin and clarithromycin more expensive than erythromycin?

A. The brand names are more expensive, but there is less frequent dosing because of its long half-life (less frequent dosing), post-antibiotic effect and better tolerability, which may make them a better choice than erythromycin. With these advantages it is not necessary to prescribe a macrolide.

Q. What are some common adverse effects of azithromycin and clarithromycin?

A. Common adverse effects include diarrhea, nausea, vomiting, dyspepsia, rash, pruritus, and abdominal pain.

Q. Are there a lot of drug interactions with azithromycin and clarithromycin?

A. Clarithromycin and erythromycin are metabolized by the cytochrome P450 system in the liver resulting in many drug interactions. Clarithromycin is a CYP3A4 substrate (metabolized by this isoenzyme) and a strong inhibitor of 3A4. See Chapter 5 for more detailed information about drug interactions. However, azithromycin is unlikely to interact with drugs metabolized via the hepatic cytochrome P450 enzyme system, and few interactions have been reported clinically (Shakeri-Nejad & Stahlmann, 2006).

Q. What are some drug interactions with azithromycin?

A. See Table 5.5.

Q. Is there a potential interaction of azithromycin with warfarin?

A. Yes. In 2009, the FDA revised the label for azithromycin warning of a potential interaction with warfarin resulting in elevated international normalized ratio (INR) values. There is a risk that the patient can become over-anticoagulated. If azithromycin is given then patient should be monitored or treatment modified. Consult with the patient's physician (Waknine, 2009; Glasheen *et al.*, 2005; Schrader *et al.*, 2004).

Lincomycins

Q. What is the mechanism of action of clindamycin?

A. Clindamycin is bacteriostatic at low doses but can be bactericidal at usual doses (600 mg) and extended-interval dosing (Klepser *et al.*, 1997). It inhibits bacterial protein synthesis by binding to the 50S ribosomal subunit.

Q. What is the spectrum of activity of clindamycin?

A. Clindamycin is a narrow-spectrum antibiotic effective against most Gram-positive organisms including, group A streptococci, staphylococci and pneumococci. Gram-negative aerobic microbes are resistant because clindamycin is poorly permeable to the outer membrane, but most anaerobes (*Prevotella*, *Peptostreptococcus*, *Fusobacterium*) are sensitive.

Q. Is clindamycin a good choice for odontogenic infections?

A. Yes. Clindamycin is superior to other antibiotics against anaerobes (chronic infection) making it a good choice in anaerobic infections especially if refractory to other antibiotics. It shows good distribution in soft tissues as well as penetration into bone. Clindamycin also shows high plasma concentrations.

Q. What are some common adverse effects of clindamycin?

A. Diarrhea, nausea, vomiting, abdominal pain, and rash. Serious reactions include clostridium difficile-associated diarrhea, Stevens Johnson syndrome, granulocytopenia (low concentration of white blood cells) and esophagitis.

Q. Is clindamycin the only antibiotic that causes *Clostridium difficile* colitis or pseudomembranous colitis?

A. No. Almost any antibiotic can cause pseudomembranous colitis, especially if two or more antibiotics are used together. Clindamycin was the first antibiotic reported to cause pseudomembranous colitis and that is why it is always associated with this condition.

Q. Is clindamycin contraindicated in any patients?

A. Yes. Precautions/contraindications in patients with inflammatory bowel disease, ulcerative colitis, and pseudomem-branous colitis.

Q. If a patient is allergic to erythromycin can clindamycin be prescribed?

A. Yes. The mechanism of action of both antibiotics is relatively the same but they are two different antibiotics.

Q. What is the dose of clindamycin?

A. *Supplied*:
Capsule: 75 mg, 150 mg, 300 mg
Oral solution: 75 mg/5 mL (note that this is a solution, not a suspension as most other antibiotics)
Dose: LD: 600 mg stat, followed by 150–450 mg q6h–8 h.

Metronidazole

Q. What is the spectrum of antibacterial action for metronidazole?

A. Metronidazole is effective against Gram-negative obligate (strict) anaerobes such as *Prevotella intermedia*, *Porphyomonas gingivalis*, *Bacteroides*, *Fusobacterium*.

Q. What is the mechanism of action of metronidazole?

A. Metronidazole is taken up into the bacteria where it produces toxic products which accumulate in the anaerobes and interacts with DNA to cause a loss of the helical structure.

Q. Does metronidazole concentrate in the gingival crevicular fluid (GCF)?

A. Gingival crevicular fluid (GCF) or crevicular fluid is a serum transudate that originates in the gingival connective tissue. Irritation and inflammation of the gingival tissue increase the flow of GCF from the connective tissue into the gingival crevice. Metronidazole concentrates equally in the crevicular fluid and serum as well as in the gingival tissue.

Q. Can metronidazole be used in the management of chronic periodontitis?

A. Loesche & Grossman (2001) have shown in numerous studies documented that metronidazole plus scaling and root planing is statistically better than a placebo plus scaling and root planing. However, the majority of clinical studies have reported that the use of metronidazole or tetracycline or any systemic antibiotic in the treatment of chronic periodontitis cannot be justified unless it is refractory periodontitis where conventional therapy (the patient has attempted to maintain meticulous oral hygiene and regular maintenance or recare visits) has been unsuccessful (Vergani *et al.*, 2004).

Q. Why is metronidazole not recommended for the treatment of odontogenic infections?

A. Metronidazole alone is mainly effective against Gram-negative anaerobic rods and is not effective against *Streptococcus viridans*, which is primarily isolated in odontogenic infections. However, when used together with amoxicillin there is an additive effectiveness against Gram-negative anaerobic rods.

Q. Is bacterial resistance to metronidazole common?

A. No. Metronidazole resistance is relatively uncommon.

Q. Does the ingestion of alcohol cause adverse effects when taking metronidazole?

A. Yes. Ingestion of alcohol when taking metronidazole and for 1 week after metronidazole is stopped can result in a disulfiram-like reaction. Disulfiram (Antabuse) is a medication used to wean individuals off alcohol. Chronic alcoholics are treated with disulfiram. If alcohol is ingested while on disulfiram an acute psychoses (hallucinations) and confusion, abdominal cramps, nausea, facial flushing and a headache can occur. This is a similar reaction with metronidazole.

Q. Can alcohol-containing mouthrinses be used while taking metronidazole?

A. No. Any product containing alcohol is contraindicated. This includes alcohol-containing mouthrinses, foods with alcohol and skin-to-skin contact with perfumes.

Q. How long after finishing the course of metronidazole can alcohol be started?

A. About 3 days after the metronidazole is finished.

Q. What is a commonly encountered oral adverse effect of metronidazole?

A. Metallic taste.

Q. Is there an interaction if metronidazole is taken with warfarin (Coumadin; an anticoagulant)?

A. Yes. Metronidazole can decrease the metabolism of warfarin resulting in bleeding. Dosage reduction of warfarin is necessary. Warfarin is metabolized by the cytochrome 2 C and 3A4 and metronidazole are potent inhibitors of CYP2C and 3A4 resulting in decreased metabolism of warfarin (Hersh, 1999). Consultation with the patient's physician is necessary.

Q. What is the dose of metronidazole?

A. *Supplied*:
Tablet: 250 mg, 500 mg
Capsule: 375 mg
Dose: 500 mg q6–8 h × 7–14 days. For severe infections give a loading dose of 1000 mg on day 1 followed by 500 mg q6–8 hours after the LD on day 1 up to 5 to 7 or 10 days if needed.

Tetracyclines

Q. What is the microbial spectrum of activity of the tetracyclines?

A. Effect against many Gram-positive and Gram-negative bacteria.

Q. What is the mechanism of action of the tetracyclines?

A. Tetracyclines are broad-spectrum bacteriostatic antibiotics that inhibit bacterial protein synthesis by binding to the 30S ribosomal subunit.

Q. What are doxycycline and minocycline?

A. Doxycycline and minocycline are semisynthetic members of the tetracycline group that are classified as longer acting tetracyclines with greater half-lives than the parent compound tetracycline HCl.

Q. Is doxycycline the same drug used in the treatment of acne?

A. No. Doxycycline is available in two different salts: hydrate, and monohydrate which is the form prescribed for acne.

Q. Why should doxycycline versus tetracycline be prescribed?

A. Doxycycline has a longer half-life so that dosing is much less frequent than with tetracycline which increases patient adherence.

Q. Why have tetracycline and its analogs, doxycycline and minocycline gained so much attention and popularity in the last two decades?

A. Tetracycline concentrations were found to be higher in GCF than in serum. When tetracycline is administered orally, high levels are found in the gingival crevice or periodontal pocket where it is desirable to have the antibiotic when treating periodontal diseases.

Q. Why is tetracycline prescribed for periodontal diseases?

A. A unique mechanism of action of the tetracyclines is inhibition of the synthesis and release of collagenase (anticollagenase) from human polymorphonuclear leukocytes (PMNs). This collagenase is destructive and breaks down collagen present in the periodontium (gingiva, bone, periodontal ligament). Doxycycline has the greatest anticollagenase activity. A subantimicrobial dose (20 mg) of doxycycline is used in the management of generalized chronic periodontitis in conjunction with scaling and root planing. It is prescribed to take one tablet twice a day (q12h) for up to 9 months. The brand name for doxycycline 20 mg is Periostat.

Q. Do the same adverse effects, precautions and contraindications follow with a subantimicrobial dose of doxycycline 20 mg?

A. Yes. It is still a tetracycline so it is contraindicated in pregnant women and children less than 8 years of age. Follow the same instructions to the patient as with antibiotic strength dose of doxycycline.

Q. Can doxycycline be taken at bedtime?

A. Doxycycline should not be taken at bedtime. Numerous reports have documented an increased incidence of esophageal erosions (ulcers). It is best to tell the patient to drink a full glass of water and not to lie down directly afterward (Segelnick & Weinberg, 2008).

Q. Can dairy products, iron and antacids be taken together with tetracycline?

A. Not at the same time. Divalent or trivalent cations including antacids containing aluminum (Amphojel), aluminum and magnesium combinations (Gelusil, Maalox, Mylanta), calcium including antacids (Tums, Citracal, Caltrate, Os-Cal) and dairy products (milk), iron and magnesium (Milk of Magnesia) reduce the absorption of tetracycline when taken concurrently by forming insoluble complexes or chelates with tetracycline resulting in a reduction of the amount of tetracycline. Note: the amount of tetracycline is reduced not the time of absorption. The tetracycline that is not absorbed into the bloodstream is eliminated in the feces. To manage this interaction, wait 1 hour before or 2 hours after taking the dairy product before tetracycline is taken.

Q. Can food and dairy products be taken with doxycycline?

A. It depends on the brand of doxycycline. With most brands there is only about a 30% decrease in bioavailability (absorption). The effects of dairy products, including milk, on doxycycline absorption are less than observed with other tetracycline derivatives, including tetracycline and minocycline.

Q. Can antacids and iron be taken with doxycycline?

A. No. Antacids, zinc and iron should not be taken at the same time of doxycycline, minocycline or tetracycline. Antacids (containing calcium, aluminum, magnesium) and iron markedly reduce absorption of the amount of tetracycline. Space the antacid apart about 1 hour or 2 hours after taking doxycycline.

Q. Why is it contraindicated to prescribe tetracyclines, including doxycycline and minocycline to a pregnant woman and children less than 8 years of age (children that do not have all permanent teeth)?

A. Tetracyclines are readily deposited into bone and teeth during calcification which can cause a yellow-gray-brown discoloration/fluorescence and can inhibit bone growth. The color of staining actually is dependent on which tetracycline was used, dosage and the length of time used. The tetracycline binds or chelates to calcium ions present on the hydroxy-apatite crystals in the dentin forming a stable calcium orthophosphate complex (ADA, 2010).

Q. Can individuals taking tetracycline be exposed to sunlight?

A. Photosensitivity or a phototoxic reaction can occur when taking any tetracycline, especially doxycycline. Phototoxic reactions occur due to the damaging effects of light-activated compounds on cell membranes and DNA.

Q. Is dizziness an adverse effect of tetracycline?

A. Yes, especially with doxycycline (Segelnick & Weinberg, 2010). Care must be taken not to fall when taking doxycycline.

Q. Is there a problem if an expired tetracycline product is systemically taken?

A. Yes. Expired tetracyclines can become nephrotoxic at a pH less than 2 due to the formation of anhydro-4-epitetracy-cline, which can cause acquired Fanconi syndrome – a disorder with clinical features of polyuria, polydipsia and dehydration (Ubara *et al.*, 2005; Fathallah-Shaykh, 2011).

Q. What is the dose of doxycycline?

A. *Supplied*: 50 mg, 100 mg capsule; 20 mg, 50 mg, 100 mg tablet. LD: 100 mg q12h on first day, followed by a maintenance dose of 100 mg once daily.

Fluoroquinolones

Q. What are fluoroquinolones?

A. Fluoroquinolones are not really considered to be antibiotics because they are entirely synthetic, but they are still classified as broad-spectrum antibiotics.

Q. What is the mechanism of action of fluoroquinolones?

A. Fluoroquinolones are bactericidal and block bacterial nucleic acid synthesis by inhibiting DNA gyrase.

Q. What is the microbial spectrum of activity of fluoroquinolones?

A. They are broad-spectrum drugs active against aerobic Gram-negative bacteria and many Gram-positive microorganisms. Anaerobes are usually resistant.

Q. If a patient is allergic to penicillin can a fluoroquinolone be prescribed?

A. Yes.

Q. Is there cross-resistance between a fluoroquinolone and other antibiotics such as penicillins?

A. No. Since fluoroquinolones have a different mechanism of action bacteria resistant to other antibiotics may be susceptible to fluoroquinolones.

Q. Why are fluoroquinolones useful for the treatment of pneumonia?

A. Because tissue and fluid concentrations exceed the serum drug concentration.

Q. When are fluoroquinolones prescribed in dentistry?

A. Fluoroquinolones are prescribed in dentistry if a patient is allergic to penicillin and/or has substantial gastrointestinal upset with erythromycins and clindamycin.

Q. What are some common fluoroquinolones used in dentistry?

A. Ciprofloxacin (Cipro) and levofloxacin (Levaquin)

Q. What are the adverse effects of fluoroquinolones?

A. Nausea, vomiting, diarrhea, headache, dizziness, phototoxicity (exaggerated sun reaction when exposed to the sun), insomnia, abnormal liver function tests, tendonitis and Achilles tendon rupture (especially in children and the elderly). Do not prescribe in patients younger than 18 years of age.

Q. Can fluoroquinolones be prescribed in pregnant patients?

A. Ciprofloxacin and levofloxacin are assigned a pregnancy category C. It is recommended not to prescribe either drug to pregnant or nursing women.

Q. Is there a **Black Box Warning** with fluoroquinolones?

A. Yes there are two **Black Box Warning**s.

1. March 2011; fluoroquinolone antibiotics including levofloxacin (Levaquin) can exacerbate muscle weakness in persons with myasthenia gravis. Fluoroquinolones have neuromuscular blocking activity.
2. July 2008; fluoroquinolone antibiotics [ciprofloxacin (Cipro), levofloxacin (Levaquin)] have an increased risk of tendonitis and tendon rupture that could cause permanent injury. This risk is further increased in patients over 60 years of age, in patients taking corticosteroid drugs, and in patients with kidney, heart or lung transplants.

Q. Does pseudomembranous colitis occur with fluoroquinolones?

A. Yes. There is a high association between fluoroquinolones and *Clostridium difficile*.

Q. Should fluoroquinolones be prescribed to a patient who is athletic and does a lot of running?

A. No. Fluoroquinolones can cause tendonitis and tendon rupture. The patient should be informed about this adverse effect and stop running while taking the medication.

Q. Can divalent and trivalent cations be taken concurrently with fluoroquinolone?

A. No. Similar to tetracyclines, divalent and trivalent cations [e.g., antacids containing aluminum and magnesium alone or in combination, iron and calcium (calcium supplements such as Caltrate, Citracal, Os-Cal, Tums) or dairy products] form insoluble complexes in the gut if they are taken concurrently with fluoroquinolones resulting in lower amounts of the antibiotic being absorbed. Management of this drug interaction involves spacing the antibiotic apart from the divalent or trivalent cation product for about 1 or 2 hours.

Q. Can a fluoroquinolone be prescribed to someone taking warfarin?

A. There is a drug interaction between levofloxacin and warfarin which may cause the patient to be over-anticoagulated with elevated INR values. If a fluoroquinolone is prescribed to a patient taking warfarin, the frequency of INR monitoring needs to be increased. Consult with the patient's physician.

Q. What is the dosing for ciprofloxacin?

A. *Supplied*:
Tablet: 250 mg, 500 mg
Dose: 250–500 mg every 12 hours for 7–10 days.
Renal dosing: CrCL > 30: no changes
CrCL 5–30: 250 mg every 12 h or 250–500 mg every 18 to 24 hours

Q. What is the dosing for levofloxacin

A. *Supplied*:
Tablet: 250 mg, 500 mg 750 mg
Dose: 500 mg every 24 hours for 7–10 days
Renal dosing: CrCL > 50: no change
CrCL 20–49: 500 mg once, then 250 mg every 24 hours
CrCL 10–19 & <10: 500 mg once, then 250 mg every 48 hours

c. Specific instructions for taking antibiotics

Q. Does dosing "every 6 hour interval" for penicillin need to be strictly followed?

A. Bactericidal agents such as penicillins that inhibit bacterial cell wall synthesis, *do not* require constant blood levels to be maintained because at or above the minimal lethal concentration for susceptible bacteria, permanent damage to the cell wall occurs in growing bacteria resulting in the lysis (break down) of bacterial cells. Thus, pulse dosing, where the dose is given as four doses in 24 hours, is adequate to be taken as "every 6 hours while awake." The patient does not need to follow the "every 6 hours, day and night" schedule and get up in the middle of the night. The dosing for bacteriostatic agents does need to be exactly followed as "every 6 hours." The same follows for amoxicillin.

Q. Does the dosing interval need to be strictly followed for bacteriostatic antibiotics?

A. Yes. In contrast to bactericidal antibiotics, bacteriostatic antibiotics require constant blood levels, which need to be above the MIC for the pathogen be maintained. That means that the patient must follow the prescribed dosing interval strictly even if it means getting up in the middle of the night. Prescribing azalides such as azithromycin or clarithromycin is best to prescribe for the easiest dosing interval.

Q. If a patient is taking a bacteriostatic antibiotic such as azithromycin for a medical condition and a bactericidal antibiotic needs to be given (e.g., amoxicillin for antibiotic prophylaxis or bactericidal doses of clindamycin) how far apart should the antibiotics be given?

A. Allow at least a 6 hour interval between the bacteriostatic antibiotic and the bactericidal drug because if the two were given together a drug/drug interaction occurs whereby the bactericidal drug will not be effective because it requires active, multiplying bacteria (Ganda, 2008).

Q. Which antibiotics can cause dysgeusia (taste disturbances)?

A. Patients with dysgeusia have an alteration in the four taste sensations including excessively sweet, bitter, salty or metallic taste while eating. Some antibiotics that can cause dysgeusia are metronidazole, tetracycline and clarithromycin.

Q. How antibiotic-associated diarrhea best prevented?

A. To help prevent diarrhea resulting from antibiotic it is recommended that patients eat 4 ounces of yogurt containing "Live and Active Cultures" such as Dannon Activia, Yoplait, or Kefir twice a day while taking the antibiotic. It has been suggested to take the yogurt at least 2 hours before or 2 hours after the antibiotic.

Q. What is recommended to do if the patient has developed diarrhea?

A. First confirm that the patient does not have pseudomembranous colitis. If this is negative it is recommended to take 4 ounces of yogurt containing probiotic *Lactobacillus casei* twice a day.

Q. What should the patient be warned about pseudomembranous colitis?

A. If the patient experiences a watery or bloody diarrhea in addition to fever and abdominal cramps the antibiotic should be immediately stopped and medical attention sought. Dehydration, low blood pressure and low levels of potassium can occur due to significant loss of fluids and electrolytes due to diarrhea. Symptoms are caused by the bacterium *Clostridium difficile* releasing a powerful toxin. If it is truly pseudomembranous colitis it is life-threatening. The patient should not take an antidiarrheal medication such as Lomotil or Imodium because the objective of treatment is to rid the body of the toxins and antidiarrheal medications would only reduce the chances of eliminating of the toxins. Treatment involves discontinuing the offending antibiotic which may be enough to stop the diarrhea. If it continues then administering by mouth metronidazole or vancomycin is indicated. Signs and symptoms usually begin to improve within a few days.

Q. Should caution be used when prescribing antibiotics to women on oral contraceptives?

A. It is still a controversial issue. All women of child-bearing age should be asked if she is taking an oral contraceptive before prescribing an antibiotic. Even though there are limited cases reports regarding this interaction it is still considered to be a potential drug interaction. Ethinyl estradiol, an estrogen present in oral contraceptives, is only about 40% absorbed systemically in an inactive form. The remainder undergoes extensive first-pass metabolism. Inactive ethinyl estradiol becomes active in the gut by bacterial gut flora, which releases active ethinylestradiol. The active ethinylestradiol is then reabsorbed in the small intestine. Thus, there is a concern when taking antibiotics, especially broad-spectrum, because bacteria are needed to activate ethinylestradiol for the oral contraceptive to be effective. Antibiotics destroy the bacteria which dihyrolyze sulfate and glucuronide conjugates (metabolites of ethinylestradiol) (Gibson & McGowan, 1994). Thus, the enterohepatic recirculation of ethinylestradiol that usually occurs does not. There are conflicting reports on which antibiotics are the offending agents. Additionally, drug interactions may be more common with the low-dose estrogen oral contraceptives (Gibson & McGowan, 1994). However, The American College of Obstetricians and Gynecologists concluded that tetracycline, doxycycline, ampicillin and metronidazole do not affect oral contraceptive levels (Lomaestro, 2009; Archer & Archer, 2002). However, this activation by bacterial gut flora does not occur with progestins, the other component of oral contraceptives. The first reported published link between oral contraceptives and antibiotics occurred with rifampin, an antituberculosis drug in 1971 (Gibson & McGowan, 1994). Since it cannot be predicted which women will be at greater risk for this drug interaction, it has been suggested that women use an additional contraceptive method while taking the antibiotic and for at least 1 week after completing the antibiotic (Osborne, 2004). It is plausible that some women may have low levels of ethinyl estradiol due to differences in the pharmacokinetics of the drug which would result in oral contraceptive failure when taking antibiotics (Bauer & Wolf, 2005).

In 2004, The World Health Organization (WHO) reported that there have been uncertainties that broad-spectrum antibiotics may lower oral contraceptive effectiveness; however, pregnancy rates are similar in women taking oral contraceptives concurrently with antibiotics or without antibiotics (WHO, 2004).

Q. What are specific instructions to the patient on how to take antibiotics?

A. Table 4.1 reviews patient counseling on how to take antibiotics?

II.   Antimicrobials, local

a.   *Chlorhexidine gluconate*

Q. What is the difference between first generation and second generation oral rinses?

A. First generation mouth rinses have a high substantivity whereby the agent binds to oral structures and slowly is released over time and remains active. Chlorhexidine gluconate is an example of a first generation mouth rinse. The extending binding to oral soft tissues and tooth structure and slow release reduces bacterial recolonization for approximately 8 to 12 hours afterward. Second generation agents have low substantivity and are not as therapeutically effective as first generation agents. Examples of second generation agents include: Listerine, Scope, and Cepacol.

Q. What is the alcohol content of chlorhexidine gluconate?

A. Chlorhexidine gluconate 0.12% contains 11.6% alcohol. The alcohol present in oral rinses is ethyl alcohol. Isopropyl alcohol is present in the skin cleanser.

Table 4.1   Patient counseling on how to take antibiotics.

Antibiotic	Patient instructions	Common adverse effects
Amoxicillin (Amoxil, Trimox)	Taken without regards to meals (with or without food), Advise patient to take with some kind of probiotic (e.g., yogurt, or acidophilus supplement) to help prevent superinfections and gastrointestinal distress	Gastrointestinal distress (water diarrhea could be pseudomembranous colitis), allergic reactions (e.g., rash, difficulty breathing, swelling of your face, lips, tongue, or throat), black hairy tongue. Do not take concurrently with a bacteriostatic antibiotic (wait a few hours in between)
Amoxicillin/clavulanate (Augmentin)	Because potassium clavulanate is an acid (also referred as clavulanic acid) it is best to take with food to avoid gastrointestinal distress. Advise patient to take with some kind of probiotic (e.g., yogurt, or acidophilus supplement)	Most common adverse effect is diarrhea (water diarrhea could be pseudomembranous colitis), allergic reactions (e.g., rash; difficulty breathing; swelling of your face, lips, tongue, or throat), black hairy tongue. Do not take concurrently with a bacteriostatic antibiotic.
Azithromycin (Zithromax)	Food delays absorption of azithromycin capsules, however tablets may be taken without regard to food. Take capsules with a full glass of water on an empty stomach (1 hour before or 2 hours after meals) for best absorption. Oral suspension (single dose packet) can be taken without regards to meals.	Diarrhea, nausea, and abdominal pain. Most of these events are mild or moderate in severity. Azithromycin is unlikely to interact with drugs metabolized via the hepatic cytochrome P450 enzyme system, and few interactions have been reported clinically. Do not take antacids that contain aluminum or magnesium within 2 hours before or after you take azithromycin. These antacids can cause decreased absorption of azithromycin.
Ciprofloxacin (Cipro)	Can be take with food to minimize stomach upset.	Stay out of the sun; photosensitivity reaction. Avoid caffeine. Do not take concurrently with di-and trivalent cations (e.g., antacids, iron, calcium, zinc). Interaction with warfarin. Report any tendon pain or inflammation
Clarithromycin (Biaxin)	Acid stable and is well absorbed from the gastrointestinal tract, irrespective of the presence of food.	Fewer gastrointestinal adverse effects than erythromycin. The most frequently side effects with clarithromycin are diarrhea, nausea, abnormal taste, dyspepsia, abdominal discomfort, and headache Because clarithromycin is metabolized by hepatic cytochrome P450 microsomal enzymes, it, like erythromycin, has the potential to interact with other drugs. However, clarithromycin is less potent P450 inhibitor than erythromycin
Clindamycin (Cleocin)	Take with a full glass of water. Given without regard to meals (food may delay, but not decrease, absorption).	Nausea, diarrhea, skin rashes, pseudomembranous colitis, allergic reactions

(continued)

Table 4.1   *(cont'd)*

Antibiotic	Patient instructions	Common adverse effects
Doxycycline (Vibramycin, Doryx)	Take with a full glass of water (to prevent esophageal ulceration) on an empty stomach (1 hour before or 2 hours after meals). It can be taken with food if GI upset occurs.	Causes less alterations of intestinal flora than the other tetracyclines. Esophageal erosions and dizziness. Can cause sore throat. Binds to calcium in teeth and bones which may cause discoloration of teeth in children <8 years of age. Alright to give in renal impairment. Do not take concurrently with antacids containing di- or trivalent cations, bismuth salts, iron, or zinc salts since these products causes a reduction in absorption of doxycycline. Do not prescribe to pregnant women. Do not take concurrently with bactericidal antibiotics such as penicillins which may decrease antibiotic activity.
Erythromycin (Eryc, EES.)	Take with a full glass of water on an empty stomach (1 hour before or 2 hours after meals) for best absorption.	Gastrointestinal and are dose-related. They include nausea, vomiting, abdominal pain, diarrhea and anorexia. Onset of pseudomembranous colitis symptoms may occur during or after antibacterial treatment. Symptoms of hepatitis, hepatic dysfunction and/or abnormal liver function test results may occur. Erythromycin has been associated with QT prolongation and ventricular arrhythmias, including ventricular tachycardia and torsades de pointes. Allergic reactions with rash and eosinophilia can occur rarely. A less well-known but nonetheless significant adverse reaction to erythromycin, especially after intravenous administration, is ototoxicity, manifest as tinnitus and/or deafness. Erythromycin inhibits CYP3A4 enzymes resulting in many drug interactions and reducing metabolism of the following drugs: triazolam, warfarin, and cyclosporine.
Metronidazole (Flagyl)	Given without regard to meals. However, taken with meals may minimize gastrointestinal distress	Diarrhea, loss of appetite, nausea, abdominal cramps, vomiting, metallic taste, dry mouth; alcohol and warfarin (increase anticoagulation effect) interactions
Penicillin VK	Take with a full glass of water on an empty stomach (1 hour before or 2 hours after meals) for best absorption.	In excessive doses, seizures are common. Do not take concurrently with a bacteriostatic antibiotic.
Tetracycline (Sumycin)	Take with a full glass of water (to prevent esophageal ulceration) on an empty stomach (1 hour before or 2 hours after meals). It can be taken with food if GI upset occurs.	Nausea, diarrhea, esophageal erosions, dizziness (doxycycline), photosensitivity. Do not take concurrently with antacids containing di- or trivalent cations, bismuth salts, iron, or zinc salts since these products causes a reduction in absorption of tetracycline. Do not prescribe to pregnant women. Do not take concurrently with bactericidal antibiotics such as penicillins.

Medical Economics Staff. 2000.

Q. Is chlorhexidine gluconate 0.12% available alcohol-free?

A. Yes. GUM® chlorhexidine gluconate oral rinse 0.12%.

Q. What is the alcohol content of Listerine?

A. Listerine: 26.9% and Listerine Cool Mint or Freshburst: 21.6%

Q. What type of alcohol is present in oral rinses?

A. Ethanol.

Q. Does the alcohol in mouth rinses cause dry mouth?

A. Yes. The alcohol is a drying agent and can cause xerostomia.

Q. What is the mechanism of action of chlorhexidine?

A. Chlorhexidine is a cationic (positive charged) bisbiguanide. Chlorhexidine binds to the negative charged bacterial cell surface causing a disruption of the cytoplasmic membrane allowing for the chlorhexidine to enter the bacterial cytoplasm and kill the bacteria.

Q. What is the spectrum of antibacterial activity?

A. Chlorhexidine is active against Gram-positive and Gram-negative, facultative aerobic and anaerobic bacteria.

Q. What are the indications for chlorhexidine?

A. Chlorhexidine gluconate 0.12% is a prescription medication for gingivitis, not periodontitis.

Q. How should the patient use chlorhexidine?

A. Rinse bid with 15 mL of solution which is measured in the cap of the bottle. Rinse for 30 seconds and expectorate. The patient should not eat or drink for at least 30 minutes after rinsing.

Q. How is a prescription for chlorhexidine written?

A. See Figure 4.1.

Q. Can fluoride-containing toothpaste be used directly before or after rinsing with chlorhexidine?

A. No. Fluoride toothpaste that contains sodium lauryl sulfate should be spaced at least 30 minutes apart before using chlorhexidine. The positively charged chlorhexidine causes it to bind to the negatively charged sodium lauryl sulfate (a detergent) causing inactivation.

Q. What are some adverse effects of chlorhexidine that I should warn the patient?

A. Brown staining of dorsum of tongue, teeth, and restorations, increased supragingival calculus formation, and temporary alteration in taste perception.

Rx chlorhexidine gluconate oral rinse
Disp: 1 bottle
Sig: Rinse with 15 mL (capful) of solution for 30 seconds, twice a day. The solution should be swished through the mouth and then expectorate. Do not swallow.

Figure 4.1   How to write a prescription for chlorhexidine.

Q. What can be done to minimize the brown staining?

A. The patient should routinely brush and floss. If this is inadequate interproximal staining may be removed when the patient returns to the office, though staining of restorations may be permanent.

Q. Is recommending a "natural" mouthrinse acceptable?

A. A 2008 study found that a herbal mouthrinse may provide oral health benefits by inhibiting the growth of periodontal and cariogenic pathogens but more clinical studies are required (Haffajje *et al.*, 2008).

b. Other mouthrinses and periodontal health products

Q. Is Scope clinically effective as an antimicrobial mouthrinse?

A. Quaternary ammonium compounds (e.g., Scope, Cepacol) bind to oral tissues but substantivity is only about 3 hours. There is inconclusive data as an antiplaque/antigingivitis rinse. The active ingredient in these rinses is cetylpyridinium chloride.

Q. Is the use of iodine efficacious?

A. Povidone/iodine has been advocated as a topical antiseptic that has been used as an irrigant in periodontal pockets. Povidone/iodine 7.5–10% (Betadine) is a combination of polyvinylpyrrolidone and iodine and is used as a surgical scrub and for the prevention of skin infections. Mixed results have been published concerning the reduction of periodontal pathogens with povidone iodine. Some clinical studies have shown that irrigation with povidone iodine in conjunction with mechanical debridement may improve the percent of total microbial counts (Hoang *et al.*, 2003). Other studies have shown no additional benefit when compared with ultrasonic debridement or scaling and root planing (Leonhardt *et al.*, 2007). A main disadvantage is staining of clothes and tissues and irritation.

Q. Is it safe to recommend hydrogen peroxide rinses?

A. 3% hydrogen peroxide has been used as an oxygenating rinse for inflamed oral tissues. Hydrogen peroxide liberates gaseous oxygen providing a cleansing action and effervescence for oral wounds. It also has been used as an antimicrobial agent (rinse or irrigant diluted with water). However, antiplaque/antigingivitis claims are not well supported. Hydrogen peroxide may cause irritation and delayed wound healing so it is not advocated to be used as an oral antimicrobial agent. When hydrogen peroxide is used undiluted it causes burning of the oral mucosa.

Q. Is Gly-Oxide recommended for oral wounds?

A. Gly-Oxide is approved as a temporary debriding agent in the oral cavity. It is composed of peroxide. It is an oxygenating agents whereby oxygen is released providing a cleansing action and gentle effervescence for oral wounds.

Q. Are there any new oral health products on the market besides mouthrinses?

A. Yes. GUM® PerioBalance® is promoted as being a daily dental probiotic. It is available over-the-counter (OTC) as lozenges. The active ingredient is *Lactobacillus reuteri* Prodentis, which functions to keep the oral environment balanced with "good bacteria" resulting in a significant reduction (42%) in moderate-severe plaque by 28 days. Directions say to take one lozenge daily after brushing and flossing. The lozenge should dissolve in the mouth for at least 10 minutes, allowing the active ingredient bacteria to be ingested. There should be no brushing or rinsing immediately after using the lozenge. Also, if you miss a day, don't take two to make up for the missed day. Just start again the following day with one.

Q. Are there any new over-the-counter mouthrinses on the market?

A. Yes. GUM® PerioShield™ Oral Health Rinse has as its active ingredient, delmopinol 0.2%. The mechanism of action of PerioShield is to slow the formation of new plaque biofilm by inhibiting the ability of bacteria to produce polysaccharides which bacteria use to multiply. By interfering with biofilm formation, the plaque deposit becomes loosely adherent to the tooth making it easier to remove.

Q. What is the indication of use for PerioShield?

A. PreShield is indicated in patients with gingivitis as an adjunct to tooth brushing and flossing.

Q. What is delmopinol?

A. Delmopinol is a morpholinoethanol derivative antiplaque surface-active agent that adsorbs on to saliva-coated hydroxyapatite resulting in a reduction of plaque formation.

Q. How much alcohol does PerioShield™ contain?

A. PerioShield contains 1.5% alcohol.

Q. What are some adverse effects of PerioShield?

A. Adverse effects of PerioShield include tingling of the tongue and possible changes to taste perception which have been reported to be reduced over the first 10 days of treatment.

III.   Controlled-release drug delivery

Q. What does controlled-release drug delivery mean?

A. When a drug is released from a device beyond 24 hours. For example, doxycycline in Atridox is reportedly released for a period of 21 days (American Academy of Periodontology, 2006).

Q. What is some controlled-release drug delivery systems used in the treatment of periodontal disease?

A. Atridox®, Arestin® and PerioChip®. All products are bioabsorbable and do not need to be removed.

Q. What are the major ingredients in Arestin, Atridox and PerioChip?

A. Arestin: 1 mg minocycline hydrochloride microspheres; Atridox: 10% (42.5) doxycycline hyclate in a gel formulation; and PerioChip: 2.5 mg chlorhexidine gluconate.

Q. When is it indicated to use one of these products?

A. As an adjunct to scaling and root planing for the reduction of pocket depth, gain of clinical attachment and reduction of bleeding in patients with localized chronic periodontitis with recurrent pockets of ≥5 mm that continue to bleed on probing.

Q. Can Atridox and Arestin be administered to a patient who is pregnant?

A. No. Since these products are analogs of tetracycline the same contraindications/precaution used with systemic tetracycline must be followed with locally applied tetracyclines.

Q. How many applications must be done with Arestin?

A. Administration of Arestin does not require local anesthesia. Up to three treatments, at 3-month intervals are recommended. No periodontal packing is required after application.

Q. What are important post-application patient instructions?

A. Avoid toothbrushing and flossing for 7 days.

Q. Does Arestin, Atridox or PerioChip need to be refrigerated?

A. No. Arestin, Atridox and PerioChip do not need to be refrigerated; they should be stored at room temperature.

IV.　Antivirals/antifungal agents

a.　Antiviral agents

Q. For which common oral conditions is antiviral therapy appropriate?

A. Herpes simplex virus (HSV) infections.

Q. What is the incidence of herpes infection?

A. Herpes simplex virus (type 1, herpes-1or HSV-1) causes about 80% of cases of oral herpes infections and 20% of genital lesions. Adolescents, about 30 to 40% of genital herpes is caused by HSV-1. About 80% of genital herpes is due to HSV-2 and 20% of oral lesions (Sharma & Dronen, 2011).

Q. What are the different types of oral herpes infections?

A. The first infection with HSV-1 usually causes primary herpetic gingivostomatitis and is most common in children under 5 years of age. Prodromal symptoms include fatigue, malaise, anorexia, muscle aches, irritability, fever and chills. A few days later, vesicles appear which rupture leaving painful ulcers. The gingiva, lips, palate, buccal mucosa and throat are also affected. Eating and drinking is difficult and they quickly become dehydrated. Signs and symptoms of dehydration usually warrant going to a hospital's emergency department, especially in infants under 6 weeks of age. After the primary infection or exposure to herpes virus, individuals can develop recurrent herpes simplex virus infections. This infection which occurs around the vermillion boarder of the lips and in the mouth is referred to as recurrent herpes labialis, cold sores or fever blisters. Lesions develop from stress, sunlight, fever, trauma (e.g., after a dental procedure) or in immunocompromised patients. Cold sores or herpes labialis is caused by the HSV-1 strain. Even though the preference of HSV-2 strain is for the genital region it is less often transmitted to the oral region. Both are contagious when the virus is producing and shedding.

Q. What is the management of primary herpetic gingivostomatitis?

A. Fluids, bed rest, acetaminophen or ibuprofen (aspirin is contraindicated in viral infections in children because of the risk of developing Reye's syndrome), and topical application of a local anesthetic containing lidocaine or benzocaine such as: Anbesol, Orabase with benzocaine 20%, Zilactin L, and Xylocaine 2% viscous. Do not give ibuprofen to children that are asthmatic or have a hypersensitivity to aspirin. Topical antiviral medications are generally not highly effective.

Q. What is herpes labialis?

A. Herpes labialis (known as fever blisters or cold sores) occurs after an individual has had a first experience with herpes simplex infection. HSV-1, a DNA virus, causes primarily oral lesions with a small percent of genital lesions. HSV-2 causes primarily genital lesions and a small percent of oral lesions.

Typically an individual will have prodromal symptoms of pain, tingling, burning or itching before eruption of the lesions. Healing of ulcers occurs over a few weeks. Herpes labialis presents at the commissure of the lips.

Q. Can herpes occur intraorally?

A. Yes. Herpes infection can occur anywhere intraorally. Sometimes after a dental procedure is completed the patient will have intraoral lesions on the attached gingival due to stress or trauma.

Table 4.2   Antiviral agents.

Drug	Supplied	Dosing
Acyclovir (Zovirax)	Tabs: 400, 800 mg; Caps: 200 mg Cream or ointment: 5% (15 g tube) Suspension: 40 mg/mL	Apply thin layers of ointment with a finger cot or latex glove to affected area every 3 hours up to 6 times a day for 7 days. Take 200–400 mg po 5 times a day. (administer within 1 to 2 hours of prodromal symptoms such as tingling, itching, burning, pain, or lesion
Penciclovir (Denavir)	Cream 1% (2 g tube)	Apply five times a day at first sign of cold sore. Use until lesion is healed
Famciclovir (Famvir)	Tabs: 125, 250, 500 mg	1500 mg as a single dose or 500 mg every 12 hours (recurrent infection) (administer within 1 to 2 hours of prodromal symptoms)
Valacyclovir (Valtrex) Docosanol (Abreva)	Tabs: 500 mg, 1000 mg Cream: 10% (OTC)	2 g twice a day at a 12 hour interval for one day only Apply 5 times a day at first sign of cold sore. Use until lesion is healed.

Medical Economics Staff. 2000.

Q. How should herpes labialis be managed?

A. Intraoral herpes infections should be treated with antiviral agents and palliative care. The mechanism of action of the antiviral drugs is to inhibit viral DNA synthesis/replication. Unfortunately, HSV remains latent in sensory ganglia so that there is a high incidence of recurrence or relapse even after the lesions are treated. The goal of using antiviral drugs is to shorten the clinical course, prevent complications, prevent future recurrences, and decrease transmission. Antiviral agents are listed in Table 4.2.

A. See Table 4.2.

Q. Should antibiotics be used in the management of recurrent herpes labialis?

A. No. Antibiotics further suppress the immune system and could prolong the duration of the infection.

Q. Why is it important to administer acyclovir early?

A. Acyclovir binds viral DNA polymerase, ending viral replication. Its mechanism of action necessitates early administration, because replication may end as soon as 48 hours after a recurrence (Emmert, 2000). Acyclovir reduces the pain and duration of symptomatic lesions.

Q. Can acyclovir be prescribed to children?

A. Acyclovir is recommended in individuals older than 12 years of age.

Q. What are some other features of acyclovir?

A. It is a safe and well-tolerated drug with only about 15 to 30% bioavailability after oral administration. Its half life is 2.5 hours and adjustment is necessary in renal impairment. It has a pregnancy category of C.

Q. When should systemic acyclovir with or without topical agents be prescribed?

A. Systemic acyclovir is widely used as an off-label use in the treatment of recurrent herpes labialis which means that it is used in the treatment but it is not FDA-approved. Administering systemic antiviral medications such as acyclovir can reduce the duration of pain, decrease the size and duration of lesions and may decrease the recurrence rate (but this controversial). Additionally, systemic antiviral drugs can be prescribed:

Table 4.3   Active ingredients in OTC topical anesthetics.

Benzocaine: Anbesol, Orabase with benzocaine 20%
Benzyl alcohol: Zilactin
Camphor and phenol: Campho-phenique, Blistex, Carmex, ChapStick Medicated
Lidocaine: Zilactin L

1. Oral lesions are severe and secondarily infected or may become infected
2. Systemic involvement (e.g., fever)
3. Immunocompromised patients (e.g., HIV/AIDS)

Q. Is there systemic absorption after taking acyclovir cream?

A. Yes, but it is minimal in adults. The systemic absorption of acyclovir following topical administration of cream has not been documented in patients <18 years of age.

Q. Does acyclovir come in an oral suspension?

A. Yes. It can be prescribed for intraoral herpes infection. Acyclovir oral suspension; 200 mg per 5 mL. So, if the dose is 200 mg then only 5 mL needs to be taken. One teaspoonful equal 5 mL. This medicine should be shake well before use and taken with water. It does not require refrigeration. Acyclovir can be taken with or without food. The suspension should be taken with plenty of water (www.drugs.com/pro/zovirax-cream.html).

Q. What other systemic agents are FDA-approved for the management of recurrent herpes labialis?

A. Valacyclovir, the prodrug of acyclovir (valacyclovir is rapidly converted to acyclovir before having any antiviral effects), is FDA-approved for use in recurrent herpes labialis in patients ≥12 years of age. The efficacy of Valtrex initiated after the development of clinical signs of a cold sore (e.g., papule, vesicle, or ulcer) has not been established. Although it is more expensive than acyclovir it has a more convenient dosing (Sharma & Dronen, 2011).

Q. What agent is FDA-approved in immunocompromised patients?

A. The oral prodrug of penciclovir, famciclovir is FDA-approved for RHL in immunosuppressed patients; it demonstrates efficacy in addition to a more convenient dosing regimen. It should not be used in patients under 18 years of age.

Q. What should be done if it is too late after the first symptoms appear to apply an antiviral agent?

A. Apply a topical anesthetic agent containing benzocaine such as: Anbesol, Orabase with benzocaine 20%, or lidocaine such as Zilactin L. Patients who are allergic to *para*-aminobenzoic acid (PABA) may also be allergic to benzocaine and tetracaine, so it is best to recommend Zilactin L.

Q. What is the active ingredient in OTC topical anesthetics used in the management of oral ulcer pain?

A. See Table 4.3.

Q. Are there any reported clinical toxicity related to topical local anesthetics?

A. Yes. Topical anesthetics including lidocaine and benzocaine can cause seizures, bradycardia and methemoglobinemia. Methemoglobinemia is a condition characterized by high levels of methemoglobinemia, an oxidized metabolite of hemoglobin, in the blood. The main problem is that methemoglobin does not bind to oxygen, as does hemoglobin, which leads to an anemia. Symptoms include bluish coloring of the skin, headache, fatigue, and shortness of breath. Mild cases can go unrecognized. Treatment of severe methemoglobinemia is with methylene blue, or ascorbic acid is useful.

Q. Which is the most recommended systemic antiviral agent for the treatment of oral herpes?

A. Acyclovir (Zovirax) is the most commonly prescribed antiviral agent for the management of herpes labialis. Famciclovir (Famvir) and valacyclovir (Valtrex) are also just as effective with convenient dosing but are often more expensive than acyclovir. Both also have higher bioavailability than acyclovir.

Q. Are there any reactions to applying topical acyclovir?

A. Yes. It can be very painful.

Q. What are adverse effects of systemic acyclovir?

A. Headache, seizure, nausea, vomiting, diarrhea, skin rash.

Q. Which antiviral drug is available OTC?

A. Docosanol (Abreva). Abreva prevents viral entry and replication at the cellular level.

Q. What are the instructions on how to apply Abreva?

A. Apply a thin layer of medication to completely cover the area of the cold sore or the area of tingling/itching/redness/swelling and rub in gently, usually five times a day every 3–4 hours.

Q. Should a patient with active herpes labialis be treated in the dental chair?

A. No. The viral lesions are highly infectious during the first 2 days of appearance of the vesicles, the crusted lesions also have high viral titers and infectious during this time.

Q. What are potential adverse effects of systemic acyclovir?

A. Some adverse effects of systemic acyclovir include nausea, vomiting, itching, hypotension, diarrhea, dizziness, fever, and renal failure.

b.   Antifungal agents

Q. What types of oral fungal infections do dentist encounter?

A. Oral candidiasis involving the oropharyngeal area.

1. Acute pseudomembranous candidiasis also referred to as oral thrush.
2. Chronic atrophic candidiasis is known as denture sore mouth.
3. Angular cheilosis or angular cheilitis.

Q. What is oral thrush?

A. Oral thrush usually develops suddenly rather than taking a long time (chronic). Oral thrush causes slightly raised, creamy white, curd-like patches on the oral soft tissues or on the tongue. The affected site may bleed if the lesion is wiped. The lesions can spread to the esophagus.

Q. What are some causes of oral thrush?

A. Corticosteroids (asthmatics that use a corticosteroid inhaler must rinse the mouth and brush teeth after every use of the inhaler), antibiotics (due to suppression of normal bacterial flora), diabetes, HIV infection, cancer, dry mouth, oral contraceptives (due to increased estrogen levels).

Q. What is chronic atrophic candidiasis?

A. Chronic atrophic candidiasis is known as denture sore mouth. The lesion characteristically appears as a reddish outline on mucosal tissue seen under a denture. Usually it occurs when a denture is not removed for daily cleansing by the patient.

Q. What is angular cheilitis?

A. Angular cheilitis or angular cheilosis features sore red splits at each side of the mouth (commissures of the lip). Angular cheilitis used to be thought to be caused by vitamin B deficiency but it is actually due to a fungal infection (candida). It is seen in patients without teeth or with ill-fitting dentures that have a loss of vertical dimension causing accumulation of saliva at the commissures of the lip (increased moisture).

Q. What treatment is there for angular cheilitis?

A. Elimination of the moisture should be the first step. Application of an antifungal topical ointment or cream is recommended. See Table 4.4.

Q. How is oral candidiasis treated?

A. The first step is to correct predisposing factors if possible. It is easier to treat oral thrush in healthy patients than immunocompromised patients. Antifungal agents must be taken for about 2 days after oral lesions disappear to avoid recurrence of lesions. Treatment usually lasts for 7 to 14 days. For the treatment of oral fungal infections there are choices of different formulations including: suspension, troche/pastille, creams and ointment, or vaginal tablets (used as a lozenge). See Table 4.4.

Q. Why prescribe a cream or ointment?

A. An ointment is a semisolid emulsion or suspension that is viscous and greasy. A cream is a semisolid emulsion that is viscous and non-greasy to mildly greasy but not as thick as an ointment. The cream or ointment is applied by the patient inside of the denture and on the palate. This procedure will help the antifungal ointment/cream to stay in contact with the lesion.

Q. Can all formulations be given to patients with a high-risk for dental caries?

A. No. The suspension and troches/pastille formulations contain sugar (sucrose) and should not be given to patients with high-risk caries because these formulations remain the mouth for prolonged periods of time. The oral suspension also contains saccharin sodium. Have the patient suck on vaginal tablets such as nystatin vaginal tablets.

Q. What is Oravig?

A. Oravig is miconazole buccal tablets 50 mg. It is the first product available as a once-daily dosing for oral thrush. It is also orally dissolving.

Q. How is Oravig applied?

A. Oravig is supplied as a 50 mg tablet. The tablet is flat on one side (marked with the letter "L") and a rounded side. The rounded side is applied to the gingiva in the depressed area above the lateral incisor. Once in place, use slight pressure on the outside of the lip for 30 seconds. The tablet will slowly dissolve throughout the day. It is used only once a day. Use alternating sides each time (www.oravig.com).

Q. What is Mycostatin?

A. Mycostatin is the brand name for nystatin. It is suitable to prescribe nystatin, the generic substitute. When prescribing for an oral fungal lesion the oral suspension can be prescribed for the patient to swish in the mouth and then swallow.

Table 4.4 Topical antifungal agents Prescription.

Drug	Prescription
Clotrimazole (Mycelex) Supplied: troche 10 mg, cream 2% (Lotrimin), vaginal suppositories (100 and 200 mg)	*For denture sore mouth or oral thrush* Rx clortrimazole troche 10 mg Disp: #60 troches Sig: Dissolve in the mouth slowly (over 15 to 30 minutes) one lozenge five times a day (every 3 hours) for 14 days. (Note: remove dentures if necessary) *For angular cheilitis or denture sore mouth (on inside lining of denture)* Rx clotrimazole cream 1% is available OTC without a prescription
Miconazole (Monistat) Supplied: cream 2%, ointment 2%, solution, powder, spray, buccal 50 mg tablet (Oravig)	Rx Oravig 50 mg tablet Disp: #14 buccal tabs Sig: Apply one buccal tablet to the gum region once daily for 14 consecutive days. (Note: The tablet is flat on one side (marked with the letter "L") and a rounded side. The rounded side is applied to the gingiva in the depressed area above the lateral incisor. Once in place, use slight pressure on the outside of the lip for 30 seconds. The tablet will slowly dissolve throughout the day. It is used only once a day. Use alternating sides each time.) (www.oravig.com)
Nytatin (Mycostatin) Supplied: oral suspension (100 000 USP Nystatin U/mL, ready to use suspension in 2 fl oz (60 mL) bottles with 0.5 mL, 1 mL, 1.5 mL, 2 mL calibrated dropper), pastilles (lozenge), vaginal tabs, cream, ointment, powder	For denture oral mouth or oral thrush Rx nystatin oral suspension 100 000 units/mL Disp: 1 bottle Sig: Take 1 to 2 mL dropped into the mouth and held for some time before swallowing. Note: This dose may be increased to 4 mL to 6 mL (400 000 to 600 000 units) four times daily for more severe infections. In infants and children the dosage is 2 mL four times a day. Shake the bottle well before each use. Dentures should be removed before using the suspension. The liquid is directly measured and used with the dropper. Place half of the dose in each side of the mouth and hold it there or swish it around for a few minutes before swallowing. It can also be spit out. Do not eat or drink for 30 after using the oral suspension. Rx nystatin pastille 200 000 units Disp: #60 pastilles Sig: Remove the dentures. Dissolve slowly and completely in the mouth one pastille five times a day for 14 days. (This can take up to 15 to 30 minutes. Do not chew or swallow pastilles whole. Continue to use pastilles for at least 48 hours after symptoms disappear. Store in the refrigerator.) *For angular cheilitis or denture sore mouth (on inside of denture)* Rx nystatin ointment Disp: 30 gm tube Sig: Apply to affected area two times daily. Rx nystatin cream Disp: 30 g tube Sig: Apply to affected area two times daily.

Medical Economics Staff. 2000.

The oral suspension contains 100 000 units of nystatin per mL The inactive ingredients include artificial flavoring, FD&C yellow #10, alcohol, sucrose, purified water, glycerin, sodium citrate, magnesium aluminum silicate, saccharin sodium, xanthan gum, benzaldehyde, edetate calcium disodium, polysorbate 80, methylparaben and propylparaben. The bottles come in 24, 48 and 100 mL volumes.

Q. What are some common adverse effects of oral nystatin?

A. Diarrhea, nausea, vomiting and rash.

Q. What are some prescriptions for antifungal drugs that can be prescribed to patients?

A. For a patient with denture sore mouth a recommendation would be to prescribe nystatin oral suspension, nystatin pastille, or clotrimazole troche if there are no contraindications (e.g., high risk for caries) and then to prescribe an ointment to be applied to the denture base and placed in the mouth. See Table 4.4.

Q. Which antifungal agent should be used initially in the treatment of oral candidiasis?

A. Clotrimazole troches or nystatin oral suspension, pastilles or vaginal tablets should be used before an azole such as fluconazole (Diflucan) because these agents are as effects and less expensive than the azoles.

Q. When should a systemic antifungal drug be used to treat oral candidiasis?

A. Systemic antifungal agents should be prescribed in severe cases that do not respond to topical treatment for at least 7 days or if relapse occurs after topical treatment, especially in immunocompromised patients.

Q. What systemic antifungal drug can be prescribed to the above patient?

A. Ketoconazole (Nizoral) or fluconazole (Diflucan) tablets. With ketoconazole it is important to monitor liver function because hepatotoxicity is one of the adverse effects. Fluconazole is probably more recommended.

Q. What is the adult dose for fluconazole for oropharyngeal candidiasis?

A. Supplied: 50 mg, 100 mg, 150 mg and 200 mg. Prescription: (loading dose) 200 mg on the first day, followed by 100 mg once daily for 14 days.

Q. Should the dosage interval be adjusted for fluconazole in renal impairment?

A. No. Fluconazole is eliminated by renal excretion an unchanged drug. There is no need to adjust the dosage or dosing interval in patients with renal impairment.

Q. What is the FDA pregnancy category of fluconazole?

A. The FDA pregnancy category of fluconazole is C.

Q. Are there any drug interactions with fluconazole?

A. Yes. There are many drug interactions. Fluconazole is a potent inhibitor of cytochrome (CYP) P450 isoenyzmes and a moderate inhibitor of CYP3A4. The follow drugs interact with fluconazole: warfarin, oral hypoglycemics, phenytoin, cyclosporine, nonsteroidal anti-inflammatory drugs (ibuprofen), oral contraceptives, calcium channel blockers, azithromycin, carbamazepine, celecoxib (Celebrex), "statin" drugs for cholesterol lowering [simvastatin (Zocor), rosuvastatin (Crestor), lovastatin (Mevacor), pravastatin (Pravachol)], and losartan (Cozaar).

Q. Besides management of oral fungal infections what else should be emphasized with the patient?

A. Maintenance of good oral hygiene. Inform the patient the importance of taking out his/her denture at night and cleaning it.

V.   Prescribing for pain control

a.   *General considerations*

A. Pain is classified as acute (short duration, easily diagnosed with a predictable prognosis, and treatment successful with analgesics) or chronic (pain lasting a long time – months to years, difficult to localize origin of pain, and treatment involves many disciplines). Dental pain is acute and nociceptive (nociceptors or nerves that sense tissue damage – not caused by injury in the nervous system.). Severity of pain is classified as mild, moderate and severe.

Q. What are the different classifications of analgesics?

A.

• Aspirin
• Acetaminophen
• Nonsteroidal anti-inflammatory drugs (NSAIDs): nonselective and selective
• Narcotics (opioids).

Q. What is the safest analgesic for pregnant patients?

A. Acetaminophen (Tylenol).

Q. What should be reviewed before prescribing an analgesic?

A. The patient's medical history/condition, vital signs, status of liver and kidneys, medication use and assessment of the severity of pain.

b.   *Aspirin*

Q. What is the classification of aspirin?

A. Aspirin is a salicylate and not a NSAID like ibuprofen. It acts peripherally and not centrally in the central nervous system (CNS).

Q. Why is aspirin's analgesic mechanism of action?

A. Aspirin acts peripherally not centrally by inhibiting the formation of prostaglandins by blocking the cyclo-oxygenase (COX) enzymes at the receptors for pain, which is the source of the pain (due to inflammation).

Q. What is low-dose aspirin?

A. Low-dose aspirin is only used in the prevention of heart attack and strokes in certain susceptible people. It is not used as an analgesic or for the reduction of inflammation. It is discussed in detail in Chapter 7.

Q. Why does aspirin cause an increased bleeding time?

A. It is dose dependent so the larger the dose the higher the incidence of an increased bleeding time. In the gastrointestinal tract and blood, aspirin breaks down into salicylate (salicylic acid) and acetic acid. The acetic acid irreversibly binds to COX-1 within the platelets, preventing the formation of thromboxane A_2 (a potent vasoconstrictor and induces platelet aggregation), resulting in a decrease in the ability to form clots and increase bleeding time. Since platelets are nonnucleated cells and incapable of synthesizing new COX enzymes, the effect lasts for the life of the platelet which is about 7 days at which time new platelets are formed. The salicylate portion has the analgesic and anti-inflammatory actions. A dose of aspirin as small as 40 mg will prolong the bleeding time for up to 5 days (Page, 2005).

Q. What are cyclo-oxygenase enzymes?

A. Cyclooxygenase enzymes are endogenous enzymes normally found in most body cells and is responsible for tissue homeostasis. There are essentially two types of cyclooxygenase isoenzymes; COX-1 and COX-2. COX-1 is considered to be the "housekeeping or protective" enzyme responsible for tissue homeostasis and serves to protect the gastric mucosa in the gastrointestinal tract, uterus, maintain renal blood flow, and maintains normal platelet function. On the contrary, COX-2 is produced by cells only in the presence of inflammation and is found in low amounts in the tissues (Awtry & Loscalzo, 2000).

Q. What is the mechanism of action of anti-inflammatory drugs?

A. Anti-inflammatory drugs including aspirin and NSAIDs reduce inflammation which is caused by COX-2 by inhibiting the cyclooxygenase enzymes. However, the drug is not selective to only inhibiting COX-2 but it also inhibits the protective COX-1 causing adverse effects of these drugs (e.g., bleeding).

Q. What is the mechanism of aspirin's effect on gastrointestinal bleeding?

A. Gastrointestinal bleeding is due to a combination of a local irritating effect of aspirin on the gastric mucosa due to particles of undissolved aspirin, aspirin's antiplatelet aggregation effect and inhibition of protective function of the prostaglandins, specifically cyclooxygenase-1 (Cowan, 1992). Aspirin-induced gastrointestinal toxicity is dose-dependent in the range of 30 to 1300 mg per day (Patrono *et al.*, 2004).

Q. What is Reye's syndrome?

A. Reye's syndrome is a rare but serious sequela of influenza, chickenpox and other viral infections usually in children. Symptoms include repetitive vomiting, lethargy, headache and fever. Damage to the brain and liver occurs at later stages organ failure and death. The cause is unknown. Aspirin has been implicated in causing Reye's syndrome in children with a viral infection. Aspirin should not be given to children with a suspected viral infection.

Q. Should aspirin be stopped before extractions, scaling and root planing or periodontal surgery?

A. It is conclusive from many clinical studies that patients taking aspirin to prevent blood clot formation should continue to take the aspirin during surgical procedures because there is an increased risk for emboli formation. In most cases, bleeding can be controlled by local means.

Q. If a patient is taking regular aspirin or low-dose aspirin does INR (international normalized ratio) values need to be determined before dental procedures that cause bleeding?

A. No. INR values only need to be known for anticoagulants such as warfarin (Coumadin). Aspirin is an antiplatelet drug, not an anticoagulant.

Q. What are some adverse effects of aspirin?

A. Gastrointestinal irritation, gastrointestinal ulceration, increased bleeding time, tinnitus (ringing in the ears), hypoglycemic effect (aspirin should not be used in diabetics).

Q. How much blood loss occurs during periodontal surgery?

A. A 2012 clinical study confirms previous studies that blood loss during periodontal surgery is minimal. In fact, the amount of blood lost during open flap debridement and regenerative periodontal surgery is approximately 6.0 to 145.1 mL (overall mean of 59.47 ± 38.2 mL) and is much less than blood loss during maxillofacial surgery. Patients taking 100 mg/day of aspirin had a mean blood loss of 43.26 ± 31.5 mL which was not clinical or statistically different from patients who did not take aspirin (Zigdon *et al.*, 2012).

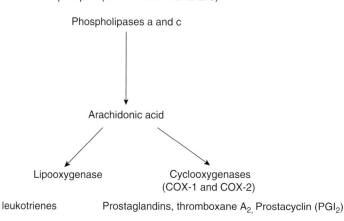

Trauma to blood vessel (platelet) wall causes:

Phospholipids (bound in cell membrane)

Phospholipases a and c

Arachidonic acid

Lipooxygenase   Cyclooxygenases
                       (COX-1 and COX-2)

leukotrienes   Prostaglandins, thromboxane A_2, Prostacyclin (PGI_2)

(involved in allergic reactions)

Figure 4.2   The sequence of prostaglandin synthesis.

c.   *Nonsteroidal anti-inflammatory drugs (NSAIDs)*

Q. What are the indications for use of NSAIDs?

A. NSAIDs indications are as an analgesic (for mild to moderate pain), an anti-inflammatory, and an antipyretic (fever reducer).

Q. What is the mechanism of action of NSAIDs?

A. NSAIDs have a similar mechanism of action as aspirin. NSAIDs inhibit prostaglandin synthesis by blocking the COX enzymes in the arachidonic acid pathway. Prostaglandins are fatty acids found in most tissues and organs in the body. They are produced in the cell membrane of platelets, endothelium, uterine and mast cells. Prostaglandin (PG) E_2 is a mediator of inflammation in diseases such as rheumatoid arthritis and periodontal diseases. When released from the damaged cell membrane during mechanical/tissue trauma (e.g., dental surgery) prostaglandins act locally with a short half-life of about 5 minutes (Schwartz, 2006). Some actions of prostaglandins include aggregation of platelets, control blood pressure, modulate inflammation, increase glomerular filtration rate, increase uterine contraction and cause fever. Prostaglandins are metabolized into many pro-inflammatory substances that cause pain and fever. COX-2 plays a role in inflammatory conditions. The anti-inflammatory action of NSAIDs is probably due to the inhibition of COX-2. However, it is not selective in inhibiting COX-2 and also inhibits the protective actions of COX-1 leading to the many adverse effects including, ulcers, bleeding, and gastrointestinal distress. NSAIDs than inhibit both COX-1 and COX-2 are called nonselective NSAIDs and the prototype is ibuprofen. Celebrex is a selective COX-2 NSAID because it only inhibits COX-2 and not COX-1 (Figure 4.2).

Q. What are the different kinds of nonselective NSAIDs used in dentistry?

A. See Table 4.5.

Q. Are there differences between NSAIDs?

A. Yes. NSAIDs differ in their potency and duration of action. However, there is no evidence that any one NSAID is more effective than another. If two people take an identical drug and dose, their individual response may be considerably different. It is sometimes necessary to try one drug for a week, and then try a different one to find the optimal combination

Table 4.5   Common nonsteroidal anti-inflammatory drugs (NSAIDs).

Drug	Supplied/dosage	OTC/Rx	Onset/duration of effect
Diflunisal (Dolobid)	Supplied: 250 mg, 500 mg tablets Dose: 1000 mg followed by 500 mg q8–12 h with meals. (Maximum 1500 mg/day)	Rx	Onset: 1 h Duration: 12 h
Etodolac (Lodine)	Supplied: 400 mg, 500 mg tablets; 200 mg, 300 mg capsules Dose: 200–400 mg q6–8 h with meals. (Maximum 1200 mg/day)	Rx	Onset: 30 minutes Duration: 4–12 h
Ibuprofen (Advil, Nuprin, Motrin)	Supplied: tablets: 400 mg, 600 mg, and 800 mg tablets Dose: 400 mg q4h with meals. 600 mg q6h with meals (Maximum: 2,400 mg/day)	Rx; OTC 200 mg	Onset: 1 hour Duration: 6–8 h
Ketorolac tromethamine (oral: Toradol nasal spray: Sprix)	Supplied: Tablets: 10 mg nasal spray: 15.75/spray Dose: Oral: 10 mg q4–6 h (Maximum: 40 mg/day). Short term use only (≤5 days) Nasal spray: 18–65 years of age: 1 spray in each nostril ≥ 65 years old: 1 spray in one nostril	Rx for both tablets and nasal spray	Onset: Oral- 30–60 minutes Nasal spray-within 20 minutes. Maximum concentration in blood is 30 to 45 minutes. Duration: Oral- 6–8 hours Nasal spray- 6–8 hours
Naproxen sodium (Aleve, Anaprox)	Supplied: Aleve: 220 mg Anaprox: 275 mg tablets Anaprox Dose: Anaprox: 275–550 mg q12h or 500 mg initially, then 275 mg q6–8 h Aleve Dose: 1 tab q8–12 h (maximum 1,375 mg/day)	Rx; OTC: Aleve 220 mg	Onset: 30 minutes Duration: 7–12 h
Naproxen (Naprosyn)	Supplied: 250, 375, 500 mg tablets Dose: Initial dose 500 mg followed by 250 mg q12h Maximum: 1250 mg/day	Rx	Onset: 30 minutes Duration: 7–12 h

Medical Economics Staff. 2000.

of these factors. Lower doses of NSAIDs, as recommended for use with nonprescription NSAIDs, are adequate to relieve pain in most people. To fully treat inflammation, a higher dose of the NSAID must be taken on a regular basis for several weeks before the full anti-inflammatory benefit is realized.

If the initial dose of NSAIDs does not improve symptoms, either recommend increasing the dose gradually or switching to another NSAID. If the patient is taking one NSAID a second NSAID should not be taken at the same time. This is a synergistic type of drug interaction where the effect of two or more drugs when taken together is greater than if given separately.

Q. What is Toradol and can it be prescribed to a dental patient after surgery?

A. The generic name for Toradol is ketorolac and it is a nonsteroidal anti-inflammatory drug which has been found to be as effective as 6–12 mg of morphine making it more potent than other NSAIDs. It has been prescribed as an alternative to narcotics for postextraction acute pain control (Abbas *et al.*, 2004; Fricke *et al.*, 1993; Walton *et al.*, 1993).

Q. Is there a **Black Box Warning** for ketorolac?

A. Yes. The black box warning is that ketorolac is indicated for moderate to severe pain that requires analgesic action on an opioid level. As with any NSAID, there is serious gastrointestinal bleeding and ulcer formation and is contraindicated in patients with active peptic ulcer disease (PUD). As with any NSAID, there are increased cardiovascular thrombotic events, such as heart attack and stroke. Ketorolac is contraindicated in patients with advanced kidney impairment. Ketorolac should *not* be prescribed to patients already taking aspirin or another NSAID. Dosage adjustment is necessary in patients >65 years of age (www.rxlist.com).

Q. Is there a NSAID that is administered as a nasal spray?

A. Yes. Ketorolac (Sprix®). Sprix has the same precautions and contraindications as oral ketorolac. It is indicated for moderate to severe pain as an alternative to narcotics. In patients ≥18 and <65 years of age the dose is one spray in each nostril q6–8 hours and in patients ≥65 years of age the dose is only one spray in one nostril q6–8 hours. Each bottle contains eight doses or a 1 day supply. Sprix should only be used for not more than 5 days (www.sprix.com).

Q. What is the average onset of analgesic action of Sprix®?

A. Intranasal ketorolac has a quick onset of analgesia with an onset of analgesia in 20 minutes and peak or profound analgesia reached in 30 to 60 minutes (McAleer *et al.*, 2007).

Q. Can Sprix® be administered prophylactically?

A. A clinical study was conducted with administration of intranasal ketorolac 30 minutes before an endodontic procedure. Results showed that intranasal ketorolac given prophylactically provided better pain relief before and after the procedure than a placebo (Turner *et al.*, 2011).

Q. Can Sprix be prescribed as a dental analgesic?

A. Yes. It is indicated in adult patients for the short term (up to 5 days) management of moderate to moderately severe pain that requires analgesia at the opioid level. One study was published using Sprix for pain secondary to third molar impaction surgery (Grant & Mehlisch, 2010).

Q. What is the prescription for Sprix for a 30 year-old patient?

A. See Table 4.6.

Q. What are some common adverse effects of Sprix?

A. Some common adverse effects of Sprix include dizziness, eye tearing, stuffy or runny nose and throat irritation.

Table 4.6   Prescription for Sprix for a 30-year-old patient.

Rx Sprix nasal spray Disp: # 5 bottles (1 box) Sig: One spray in each nostril q6–8 hours.

Unopened bottle should be refrigerated; once opened a bottle can be kept at room temperature and thrown away after 24 hours.

Q. How come ibuprofen and naproxen sodium are OTC medications?

A. The FDA ruled that ibuprofen 200 mg and Aleve 220 mg pain relief dose was safe for self-care. But the higher anti-inflammatory doses were ruled unsafe for self-care.

Q. Are OTC analgesics as effective as the prescription strength NSAIDs?

A. OTC medicines are intended for use for short periods of time and are usually intended for self-care, while prescription NSAIDs can be for long-term or chronic use when directed by a physician. OTC NSAIDs are usually used at a lower dose than prescription NSAIDs and are intended for self-limiting conditions, and are not intended to be used for long durations.

Q. Which NSAID has a longer-lasting analgesic effect?

A. Naproxen has a longer-lasting effect than most other NSAIDs.

Q. Can Celebrex be used for dental pain?

A. Yes, but it does not replace nonselective NSAIDs for short-term acute dental pain. It is not any more effective than ibuprofen and it is more expensive. Celebrex (celecoxib) is a selective COX-2 inhibitor only inhibiting COX-2 and not affecting COX-1 and the associated adverse effects. Celebrex is also associated with significantly greater number of thrombotic cardiovascular events than the other NSAIDs. There is a **Black Box Warning** stating that there "may be an increased risk of serious and potentially fatal cardiovascular thrombotic events, myocardial infarction (heart attack) and stroke; risk may increase with duration of use; possible increase risk if cardiovascular disease or with cardiovascular disease risk factors" (Jeske, 2002).

Q. Is there a difference between naproxen sodium and naproxen?

A. Sodium, a salt, is formulated with naproxen to increase the rate of absorption to reach therapeutic blood levels faster.

Q. When should an NSAID be recommended or prescribed?

A. In patients with mild to moderate pain. NSAIDs are indicated as an analgesic, anti-inflammatory and antipyretic.

Q. Why do individuals act differently to different NSAIDs?

A. Yes. Each NSAID causes a varying degree of COX-1/COX-2 inhibition. Although, there is no evidence than any one NSAID is more effective than another some are more potent than others. For example, ibuprofen may vary in effectiveness because of alterations in metabolism associated with a P450 cytochrome polymorphism, a genetic alteration (CYP2C9). If a patient does not respond to one NSAID at the maximum therapeutic level, another NSAID should be prescribed because patients may vary in their analgesic response to the different NSAIDs.

Q. How long does it take for an NSAID to take effect?

A. It takes about 30–60 minutes for a profound analgesic effect of an NSAID.

Q. What are aspirin's and NSAIDs ceiling effect of analgesia?

A. Aspirin and NSAIDs display a ceiling effect whereby the dose beyond maximum recommended dose does not provide more analgesic effect but rather can increase the incidence of adverse effects. For example, doses above 1000 mg every 6 hours do not provide significantly greater analgesia than 650 mg every 4 hours. The duration of analgesia may be greater with 1000 mg but the amount of analgesia is not increased. If the ceiling analgesic dose of ibuprofen is 1000 mg and the pain is not relieved with that dose, then a different more potent analgesic should be prescribed (Schwartz, 2006).

Q. Can a patient with asthma or aspirin sensitivity take an NSAID?

A. NSAIDs are contraindicated in patients who have experienced bronchospasm, angioedema or allergic reactions to aspirin or other NSAIDs. Many individuals with asthma also have sensitivity to drugs such as NSAIDs and aspirin that can precipitate an asthmatic attack. A condition called Samter's triad has clinical features including asthma, aspirin sensitivity and nasal polyps. These patients react to aspirin and NSAIDs and cannot take them. The reason for this reaction is most likely when NSAIDs or aspirin inhibits the COX enzymes in the arachidonic acid cascade it causes a shutdown to the other pathway whereby leukotrienes are produced which are involved in an asthmatic/allergic response.

Q. Are there any precautions when prescribing or recommending NSAIDs to a hypertensive patient taking antihypertensive medications?

A. Yes. All NSAIDs in doses adequate to reduce inflammation and pain can increase blood pressure in both normotensive and hypertensive individuals. The average rise in blood pressure is 3/2 mmHg but varies considerably. In addition, NSAID use may reduce the effect of all antihypertensive drugs including diuretics (e.g., hydrochlorothiazide), beta-blockers (e.g., propranolol, atenolol, metoprolol, acebutolol, timolol, nadolol), angiotensin-converting enzyme (ACE) inhibitors (e.g., enalopril, lisinopril, ramipril, quinapril, and captopril) except calcium channel blockers (e.g., diltiazem, verapamil, nifedipine, felodipine, nicardipine, amlodipine). This effect is most likely dose-dependent which means that the higher the dose taken the more hypertensive effect is seen. It is recommended not to take NSAIDs for more than 5 days if patients are taking antihypertensive drugs (except calcium channel blockers) (Warner & Mitchell, 2008; Groaver *et al.*, 2005). Aspirin, but not low-dose aspirin, has the same effect on blood pressure (Bautista & Vera, 2010; Zanchetti *et al.*, 2002).

Q. What is the mechanism of the hypotensive effect of NSAIDs?

A. It involves inhibition of COX-2 in the kidneys, which causes vasoconstriction and reduces sodium excretion and increases intravascular volume.

Q. What happens when NSAIDs are prescribed to a patient taking ACE inhibitors?

A. Administration of NSAIDs and ACE inhibitors in combination may cause acute renal failure and serious hyperkalemia (increased potassium blood levels) in patients with severe heart failure, pre-existing renal disease, or hypovolemic states. Patients need to be closely monitored concerning their renal function and serum potassium levels.

Q. What are the different adverse effects of NSAIDs?

A. Gastrointestinal distress, platelet function inhibition, renal dysfunction (decrease blood flow), and peptic ulcers.

Q. Does enteric-coated aspirin or NSAIDs or buffered aspirin reduce the gastrointestinal toxicity and cause less GI tract bleeding?

A. Not really. It should not be assumed that enteric-coated or buffered tablets are less likely to cause GI tract bleeding than taking tablets that are not specially formulated (Patrono *et al.*, 2004).

Q. Why do NSAIDs cause kidney damage?

A. NSAIDs cause a reduction in blood flow to the kidneys, interstitial nephritis, and papillary necrosis, especially in high-risk patients which decreased renal blood perfusion. In patients taking high doses of NSAIDs, renal failure can occur. By reducing the blood flow to the kidneys they work more slowly so that fluid builds up causing high blood pressure. Fluid retention is the most common NSAID-related renal complication that can occur in any healthy individual even without renal insufficiency. It is only clinically detectable in <5% of patients and is reversible when the NSAID is discontinued. The patient should be warned about this effect (Katz, 2002).

Renal failure can occur in people taking NSAIDs in large amounts and for long periods of time. NSAIDs can induce two different forms of acute kidney injury: hemodynamically mediated; and acute interstitial nephritis, which is often accompanied by the nephrotic syndrome. The former and perhaps the latter are directly related to the reduction in prostaglandin synthesis induced by the NSAID. Acute kidney injury can occur with any NSAID. Although renal prostaglandins are primarily vasodilators, they do not play a major role in the regulation of renal hemodynamics in normal subjects, since the basal rate of prostaglandin synthesis is relatively low. By contrast, the release of these hormones (particularly prostacyclin and PGE_2) is increased by underlying glomerular disease, renal insufficiency, hypercalcemia, and the vasoconstrictors angiotensin II and norepinephrine. The secretion of the latter hormones is increased in states of effective volume depletion, such as heart failure, cirrhosis, and true volume depletion due to gastrointestinal or renal salt and water losses. In these settings, vasodilator prostaglandins act to preserve renal blood flow and glomerular filtration rate by relaxing preglomerular resistance. This is particularly important with effective volume depletion, in which the prostaglandins antagonize the vasoconstrictor effects of angiotensin II and norepinephrine. In glomerular disease, however, the increase in prostaglandin production seems to maintain the glomerular filtration rate in the presence of an often marked reduction in glomerular capillary permeability.

Q. Do NSAIDs have a long lasting effect on bleeding?

A. No. NSAIDs do not cause bleeding but rather make the bleeding worse. NSAIDs prolong bleeding time but do not alter blood clotting or platelet count. NSAIDs reversibly inhibit COX-1 mediated platelet granule release and prevent thromboxane A_2 synthesis. The effect on platelets is temporary and platelet function returns to normal in about 1 day after discontinuing the NSAID.

Q. Does NSAIDs have the same antiplatelet effect as aspirin?

A. Yes, NSAIDs inhibit platelet aggregation through a similar mechanism to aspirin but, NSAIDs reversibly bind to the COX on platelet membranes so the antiplatelet effect does not last as long as with aspirin and is not indication for prophylaxis against strokes as is aspirin.

Q. Are there any thrombotic cardiovascular events associated with NSAIDs?

A. Yes. Cardiovascular risk needs to be addressed before prescribing any NSAID. There are risks of thrombotic reactions (heart attack and stroke) that can lead to death. The chances are increased with longer use of NSAIDs and in patients who have preexisting heart disease. NSAIDs should not be prescribed before or after coronary artery bypass graft (CABG) (www. Fda.gov/downloads/Drugs/DrugSafety/ucm085911.pdf). Celebrex and nonselective NSAIDs have a **Black Box Warning** that states that there "may be an increased risk of serious and potentially fatal cardiovascular thrombotic events, myocardial infarction (heart attack) and stroke; risk may increase with duration of use; possible increase risk if cardiovascular disease or cardiovascular disease risk factors are present." A recent article reported that there are many theories about why NSAIDs increase the cardiovascular risk and more research is needed (Elliott, 2010). Other cardiovascular adverse effects include increased blood pressure, angina and tachycardia. For nonselective NSAIDs, the risk of thrombotic cardiovascular events is also present. According to a recent article, nonselective NSAIDs are also not safe in cardiovascular patients and that cardiovascular risk is not clearly associated only with COX-2 inhibitors (Celebrex). The least harmful of the NSAIDs is naproxen (Trelle *et al.*, 2011).

Also, there is a **Black Box Warning** for all NSAIDs for gastrointestinal bleeding, ulceration and stomach or intestine perforation, which can be fatal; may occur at any time during use without warning; elderly patients are at greater risk for serious gastrointestinal events.

Q. Are there any contraindications with Celebrex?

A. Celebrex is contraindicated in patients hypersensitive to Celebrex and allergic to sulfa/sulfa drugs such as sulfonamides (e.g., Bactrim).

Q. Should an NSAID be discontinued before doing dental surgery?

A. No. In fact ibuprofen can be taken one hour before surgery to help reduce postoperative pain.

Q. If a patient is taking an NSAID does INR (international normalized ratio) values need to be determined before dental procedures that cause bleeding?

A. No. INR valves only need to be known for anticoagulants such as warfarin (Coumadin). Non-steroidal anti-inflammatory drugs affect the platelets and are not an anticoagulant.

Q. Is there a concern with bleeding during a dental procedure in a patient taking an NSAID?

A. Not significantly. Aspirin is the only analgesic that significantly prolongs bleeding time because aspirin's antiplatelet action is irreversible while NSAID's antiplatelet action is mild and reversible when the drug is eliminated from the body (NSAIDs bind weakly and reversibly to platelet cyclooxygenases).

Q. Are there any precautions/contraindications for NSAID use?

Yes. The major contraindications to NSAIDs include stomach problems (e.g., peptic ulcer disease), aspirin allergy (or sensitivity), bleeding problems (gastrointestinal bleeding), pregnancy, hepatic and renal disease, gastroesophageal reflux disease (GERD), chronic indigestion, cardiovascular disease, hypertension, antihypertensive drugs (except calcium channel blockers) and fluid retention.

Q. Can an NSAID be prescribed to someone who is anemic?

A. Yes, as long as the anemia is not due to bleeding from the gastrointestinal tract.

Q. Why are there so many dosages available with NSAIDs?

A. Because NSAIDs are indicated for pain relief and for anti-inflammatory effects and higher doses are usually needed for anti-inflammatory action.

Q. What is the maximum dose of ibuprofen?

A. The maximum dose of ibuprofen is 2,400 mg in 24 hours.

Q. How should the patient be instructed to take ibuprofen?

A. Take with a full glass of water with meals and not on an empty stomach.

d.   Acetaminophen

Q. What is the generic name for Tylenol?

A. Acetaminophen or *N*-acetyl-*p*-aminophenol (APAP) in the US and paracetamol in other countries.

Q. What are the indications for the use of acetaminophen?

A. Mild to moderate dental pain and antipyretic. Acetaminophen has little peripheral anti-inflammatory activity and does not inhibit platelet aggregation as does aspirin and NSAIDs.

Q. What is the mechanism of action of acetaminophen?

A. The analgesic effect is not clearly defined but acetaminophen acts centrally rather than peripherally at the nerve endings and produces its analgesic and antipyretic effect by inhibiting PGE_2 via selectively inhibiting COX-2 enzymes which are responsible for the formation of prostaglandins (Aronoff *et al.*, 2006). Because of CNS activity, acetaminophen's peripherally anti-inflammatory activity is limited.

New insights into the mechanism of action of acetaminophen: Its clinical pharmacologic characteristics reflect its inhibition of the two PGH_2 synthases. However, acetaminophen blocks this enzyme at its peroxidase catalytic rather than at the COX site. Therefore, the acetaminophen-mediated inhibition is sensitive to changes in the tissue peroxide levels; higher concentrations of peroxide in activated leukocytes and platelets block the effect of acetaminophen on inflammation and platelet thrombosis. Acetaminophen then is able to inhibit prostaglandins in the CNS, thus providing relief of pain and fever.

Q. Is there a **Black Box Warning** for acetaminophen?

A. Yes. In an attempt to reduce the risk of acetaminophen toxicity in the United States, many pharmaceutical/federal changes have been introduced since 2009. On 10 January 2011, the FDA notified healthcare professionals of a Black Box Warning for the potential for severe liver injury and a Warning highlighting the potential for allergic reactions (swelling of the face, mouth, and throat, difficulty breathing, itching or rash) will be added to the label of all prescription drug products that contain acetaminophen.

Additionally, In June 2009, the FDA recommended changing the maximum amount of over-the-counter acetaminophen in any single dose to 325 mg. The reason for this was that severe liver damage and even death can occur due to lack of consumer awareness. (www.guideline.gov/content.aspx?id=10222). The panel also recommended that the maximum single adult dose be lowered to 650 mg instead of 1000 mg and to lower the maximum daily dose for acetaminophen below its current 4000 mg. The maximum dose daily dose for extra strength Tylenol was lowered from eight pills totaling 4 g (4000 mg) to six pills totaling 3000 mg. The patient must keep in mind about other products containing acetaminophen.

In January 2011 the FDA asked manufacturers of prescription acetaminophen/narcotic combination products to limit the amount of acetaminophen to 325 mg per unit dose. Johnson & Johnson, manufacturers of Tylenol already have voluntarily announced lower dosing instructions for Tylenol. As of the printing of this book, this recommendation has not yet been applied.

Q. Does acetaminophen affect bleeding?

A. No. Acetaminophen is not an antithrombotic agent as is aspirin or NSAIDs. It is safe to give to patients with or a previous history of gastric bleeding or ulcers.

Q. Why is there concern about using too much acetaminophen?

A. Yes. Acetaminophen overdose can result in severe hepatic necrosis leading to acute liver failure and even death. Currently, the maximum amount of acetaminophen for an adult is not more than 4 g/day but there is ongoing debate to reduce the maximum amount to 3 g/day. The dose for children (<50 kg or 110 lbs.) is 6 mg/kg to 12 mg/kg every 4 hours. The FDA revised OTC labeling as of 29 April 2010. Currently, the container must say "liver warning" with a risk of developing liver damage if taken more than the maximum number of daily doses or if taken with other medications containing acetaminophen or drinks 3 or more alcoholic beverages a day while taking acetaminophen. Not more than one product containing acetaminophen should be taken. Many OTC cold and cough medications also contain acetaminophen. It is important to warn the patient about the additive effect of acetaminophen from additional medications including alcohol.

Q. Is there a ceiling analgesic effect for acetaminophen?

A. Yes. As with NSAIDs, acetaminophen has a ceiling analgesic effect. Doses above 1000 mg every 6 hours do not provide significantly greater analgesia than 650 mg every 4 hours and could only cause more adverse effects including liver toxicity.

Q. What is the mechanism for liver toxicity?

A. With normal dosing, the majority of acetaminophen is metabolized in the liver to water soluble sulfate and glucuronide conjugates which are eventually eliminated in the urine via the kidneys. A small percentage of acetaminophen also conjugates to *N*-acetyl-benzoquinoneimine (NAPQI), a potentially toxic metabolite that is excreted without consequences, which is further metabolized in the liver by glutathione. However, in an acute overdose this pathway becomes dominant and acetaminophen-induced hepatotoxicity (liver failure) occurs when all stores of glutathione are depleted; NAPQI then binds to liver cells causing liver necrosis. Alcohol and individuals with liver disease due to alcohol are contraindicated with acetaminophen because alcohol increases levels of NAPQI (http://www.medscape.com/viewarticle/410911_2). Hepatotoxicity is a leading cause of acute liver failure (ALF). Merely taking two Extra Strength Tylenol tablets more than four times a day can cause an overdose and only takes a few days of exceeding the recommended daily dose to cause liver damage. Caution must be discussed with the patient including the use of other OTC products that also contain acetaminophen.

Q. Can repeated doses of slightly too much acetaminophen be toxic?

A. Yes. A clinical study in the United Kingdom reported that individuals who took repeated (more than a single dose at one time) doses of acetaminophen actually had "damage build up" resulting in more liver damage and requiring kidney dialysis. Repeated doses can also be more fatal than taking a single massive overdose. Additionally, when patients were asked why they repeadly took more than the recommended dose of acetaminophen the answer was that they wanted more pain relief (Barclay, 2011).

Q. Why are single low doses of acetaminophen not hepatotoxic?

A. Low doses of acetaminophen are not damaging because of the "threshold phenomenon". Toxicity to the liver does not occur until the glutathione content of the liver is depleted. If there is an adequate amount of glutathione, the threshold is not exceeded and there will not be any hepatotoxicity. This process whereby more active metabolites are formed is referred to as bioactivation (Fujimoto, 1979). However, in an acute overdose or if the maximum daily dose is exceeded over a long time, metabolism by conjugation becomes saturated, and excess acetaminophen is metabolized to NAPQ1, which is responsible for hepatocellular injury, death and liver necrosis (Farrell *et al.*, 2012).

Q. Do liver enzymes get elevated while taking acetaminophen?

A. Yes. A study reported that an individual taking 4 g of acetaminophen a day for 14 days had elevated plasma alanine aminotransferase.

Q. What other condition can happen with acute liver disease?

A. The liver produces blood clotting factors so when there is liver disease the INR (international normalized ratio) is increased resulting in decrease clotting.

Q. What are the adverse effects of acetaminophen?

A. Hepatotoxicity (either chronic use or acute overdose), less gastrointestinal distress and no platelet effect.

Q. What is the antidote for acetaminophen overdose?

A. *n*-Acetylcysteine (Mucomyst) must be administered within 12 hours of acetaminophen ingestion.

Q. Is acetaminophen as irritating to the stomach as aspirin and NSAIDs?

A. No. it does not cause gastric irritation or ulcerations.

Q. In 2011 was there a drug recall for Tylenol®?

A. Yes. On 15 August 2011, there was a recall of certain lots of Tylenol Cold Multi-Symptom Nighttime Repaid Release Gelcaps. On 28 June 2011, there was a recall of one lot of Tylenol Extra Strength Caplets (due to an odor). On 29 March 2011, there was a recall of some slots of Tylenol 8 Hour, Tylenol Arthritis Pain, Tylenol Sinus, Benadryl, Rolaids, and Sudafed PE products.

Q. What are the different strengths of acetaminophen?

A. Regular strength: 325 mg
Extra strength (rapid release): 500 mg
Arthritis Pain: 650 mg
Tylenol 8 hour: 650 mg

Q. What is the usual dose for acetaminophen?

A. Regular strength: two tablets every 4 to 6 hours but not for more than 10 days. Maximum of 12 tablets in 24 hours.
   Extra strength: two tablets, caplets or gelcaps every 4 to 6 hours but not for more than 10 days. Maximum of eight caplets in 24 hours.
   Arthritis Pain: two gelcaps every 8 hours but not for more than 10 days. Maximum of six gelcaps in 24 hours.
   Tylenol 8 hour: two caplets every 8 hours but not for more than 10 days. Maximum of six caplets in 24 hours.

Q. What is the duration of action of a regular dose of acetaminophen?

A. About 4 hours.

Q. Does acetaminophen have a ceiling analgesic effect?

A. Yes. Acetaminophen as well as NSAIDs has a ceiling analgesic effect where doses above 1000 mg every 6 hours do not provide any greater analgesic effect than 650 mg every 4 hours. The duration of analgesia may be prolonged but the amount of analgesia is not increased.

Q. Is there a drug interaction between acetaminophen and warfarin?

A. Yes. In patients taking warfarin, the administration of acetaminophen elevates the INR resulting in bleeding. If acetaminophen needs to be administered it should be the lowest dose and for the shortest time. This interaction is proposed to be caused by inhibition of warfarin metabolism via hepatic cytochrome P450 enzymes (Bell, 1998; Hylek *et al.*, 1998).

e.   *Narcotic (opioid) analgesics*

Q. What are opioids?

A. Opioid analgesics are the narcotic analgesics obtained from the opium poppy plant. More than 20 different alkaloids are obtained from the unripe seed of the opium poppy plant. The analgesic properties of opium have been known for hundreds of years. The narcotics obtained from raw opium (also called the opiates, opioids, or opiate narcotics) include morphine, codeine, hydrochlorides of opium alkaloids, and camphorated tincture of opium.

Q. What are the different classifications of narcotic analgesics?

A. Narcotic classification is based on duration of action and potency:
Short-acting: Morphine (prototype), hydromorphone, oxycodone, hydrocodone, codeine, meperidine, fentanyl. Long-acting: methadone, levorphanol, oxymorphone

Q. Which opioid analgesics are natural, semisynthetic and synthetic?

A. Natural: morphine and codeine;
Semisynthetic: hydrocodone, oxycodone, hydromorphone
Synthetic: meperidine, fentanyl, methadone.

Q. What are the differences in potencies of the opioids?

A. Strong potency: morphine, methadone, meperidine, oxycodone, hydrocodone.
Moderate potency: codeine.

Q. Do narcotic analgesics have a ceiling effect as does aspirin and NSAIDs?

A. No. Because there is a not maximum dose after which there is no more analgesic effect, all narcotics can supposedly provide the same amount of analgesia if administered in the same dosages and the analgesic response continues to improve as the dose is increased. The problem is that more of a narcotic is taken increasing the risk for adverse effects and overdose (Cooper, 1993).

Since there is no ceiling effect for opioids, dosage requirements vary widely among patients and opioids must be titrated to an acceptable level of analgesia or until side effects occur. Essentially, the dose has to be increased until pain relief is obtained. A dosage increase of 10% to 20% during the first few days is appropriate with opioids. Elderly patients or those with comorbidities, such as pulmonary or CNS diseases, may require lower starting dosages. In addition, longer duration of analgesia has been reported for older patients, who commonly experience prolonged elimination of opioids (Zichterman, 2007).

Q. Does tolerance develop to opioids?

A. Yes. Tolerance occurs when a constant opioid dosage produces a decreasing therapeutic response. More of the drug is necessary to produce the same effect that was obtained with the smaller dose. With the exception of constipation and miosis (constriction of the pupils), tolerance develops to opioid-induced adverse effects including respiratory depression, sedation and nausea. This means that constipation and visual changes will become bothersome for the patient. Tolerance to analgesic effects may occur within the first week or two of therapy and is usually characterized by a decrease in the duration of analgesia. After this time tolerance to analgesia is relatively uncommon. If a patient has been stabilized on an opioid regimen and a dosage escalation is required, the development of new pathology is the most common cause.

Q. Can a patient develop physical dependence to opioids?

A. Physical dependence is an expected therapeutic drug effect that is characterized by the development of a withdrawal syndrome after therapy is rapidly stopped. Physical dependence may be expected in patients who have taken repeated doses of an opioid for more than two weeks. Withdrawal syndrome may be avoided by tapering doses by 10% to 20% per day.

Q. Is potency of an opioid important?

A. Yes. Potency of individual narcotics is an important factor. When comparing potency of different narcotics it is the amount of drug necessary to produce a therapeutic effect when the two drugs have the same mechanism of action and given the same route of administration. For example, when administered intramuscularly (IM) 120 mg codeine is equal to 10 mg of morphine (the prototype opioid); morphine is much more potent. Also, 30 mg codeine orally is equal to less than 2 mg IM morphine.

For example, 45 mg of codeine produces the same amount of pain relief as 5 mg oxycodone and 7.5 mg of hydrocodone.

Q. Why is morphine not as effective orally as is codeine, hydrocodone and oxycodone?

A. Morphine undergoes extensive first-pass metabolism. Before reaching the systemic circulation and brain it goes to the liver where much is metabolized before it can reach therapeutic blood levels in the blood. Almost 90% of morphine is metabolized in the liver before it gets to the blood.

Q. Why is codeine not adequate for moderate-to-severe dental pain?

A. Codeine is a weak analgesic and should be used only for mild-to-moderate pain. Codeine cannot be used for severe pain because of its lack of potency; a 60-mg dose produces less analgesia than two 325-mg aspirin tablets.

Q. Which are opioids antagonists?

A. Antagonists inhibit the effects of opioids in an overdose. Naloxone (Narcan) is a commonly used antagonist that is administered intramuscularly, intravenously or subcutaneously. Antagonist drugs bind to the receptor but have no therapeutic action, whereas agonists bind to the receptors and have a therapeutic effect.

Q. When should a narcotic analgesic be prescribed?

A. For moderate to severe pain. A narcotic should never be prescribed alone unless it is in combination with a non-narcotic such as acetaminophen or ibuprofen. Both the nonopioid plus the opioid have a greater synergistic analgesic effect.

Q. What does codeine get metabolized to?

A. Codeine is a prodrug. Codeine is different from the other opioids in that needs to be metabolized to morphine via the cytochrome P450 (CYP2D6) enzymes in the liver which is the active form for an analgesic effect. A problem with effective analgesic effect occurs if a patient is taking a drug that inhibits the CYP2D6 enzyme (e.g., a phenothiazine, haloperidol, fluoxetine, or paroxetine) thereby inhibiting the metabolism of codeine resulting in a reduced analgesic efficacy. Additionally, up to 10% of the population lack the CYP2D6 enzyme and may not achieve analgesia with codeine-containing products.

Q. Why is codeine alone not used for pain management?

A. About 10% of Caucasians are deficient in the cytochrome (CYP2D6) enzymes that metabolize codeine, resulting in lack of efficacy so that codeine alone is a relatively poor analgesic.

Q. What is the minimum dose of codeine that is an effect analgesic dose when used in a combination non-narcotic?

A. 30 mg but 60 mg is recommended as the initial dose. Codeine is not needed for mild pain, only moderate pain. Thus, a minimum of 60 mg is probably required for pain relief. A 60-mg dose of codeine produces less analgesia than two 325-mg aspirin tablets. That is why it is used in combination with a non-narcotic.

Q. Does codeine doses need to be adjusted in liver and renal impairment?

A. Yes. Codeine is excreted in the urine via the kidneys and is not recommended in patients with severe renal impairment.

Q. What are the different formulation and doses of codeine available?

A. Codeine phosphate is usually given in combination with acetaminophen as follows:
Tylenol # 1 (7.5 mg codeine/300 mg acetaminophen)
Tylenol # 2 (15 mg codeine/300 mg acetaminophen)
Tylenol # 3 (30 mg codeine/300 mg acetaminophen)
Tylenol # 4 (60 mg codeine/300 mg acetaminophen)

Q. What is the usual dose of codeine/acetaminophen?

A. 30–60 mg (acetaminophen #3 or #4); Even though # 3 is mostly prescribed (one to two tabs q4–6 h for dental pain. Maximum dose is 12 tabs over 24 hours). It makes more sense to prescribe two tablets rather than one because two tablets equal 60 mg codeine and 600 mg acetaminophen. If Tylenol # 4 were prescribed there is 60 mg of codeine but only 300 mg acetaminophen and it is best to have 600 mg acetaminophen which will provide most of the analgesic effect.

Q. What are other narcotic/non-narcotic combinations?

A. A combination of 400 ibuprofen and 15 mg hydrocodone is a better analgesic choice than 400 mg ibuprofen alone.

Q. When prescribing combination an opioid analgesic is the amount of acetaminophen as important as if it were used alone and not in combination with an opioid?

A. Yes. Remember that the maximum amount of acetaminophen is 4 g/day or 4000 mg/day. For example, Vicodin ES contains 7.5 mg of hydrocodone and 750 mg of acetaminophen. So, five tablets of Vicodin ES provide the maximum amount of acetaminophen per day and 37.5 mg of hydrocodone. On the other hand, Vicodin has 5 mg hydrocodone and

500 mg acetaminophen. So, eight tablets are the maximum amount of acetaminophen to be taken in 24 hours and 40 mg of hydrocodone. The patient can take 6 tablets of Vicodin HP (10 mg hydrocodone/600 mg acetaminophen) which will provide the maximum of 3960 mg of acetaminophen and 60 mg of hydrocodone. Therefore, it is best to prescribe Vicodin HP for moderate to severe pain (see Table 4.7).

Q. Is hydrocodone available alone and not in combination with a non-narcotic?

A. No. Compared to codeine hydrocodone gives more pain relief with a longer duration of action. Hydrocodone is a prodrug, as is codeine, metabolized via CYP2D6 cytochromes to hydromorphone, the active metabolite.

Q. Is there any concern about overdosing on combination opioid/acetaminophen?

A. Absolutely. Titrating (continuously adjusting the drug dosage) the dose of an opioid is difficult due to the acetaminophen (non-opioid) component of the combination drug. Most hydrocodone combination agents contain a minimum of 500 mg of acetaminophen. At these dosages, the maximum 4 g dose of acetaminophen is reached after ingestion of eight tablets. When taken as usually prescribed at one or two tablets every 4–6 hours, the daily dose of acetaminophen will exceed the maximum of 4 g, which may result in liver toxicity. So, care must be taken and patient must be instructed not to take more than the maximum 4 g of acetaminophen.

Q. Does everyone taking an opioid obtain an analgesic response?

A. No. Certain individuals (e.g., Caucasians) have a genetic predisposition whereby codeine and hydrocodone are metabolized poorly. These selective individuals will not develop analgesia in the same way individuals that do not have the inherited gene for cytochrome P450 CYP2D6.

Q. Is Darvon still available?

A. No. On 19 November 2010, the FDA recalled propoxyphene (Darvon) and propoxyphene/acetaminophen (Darvocet). The FDA panel reported that the minimal pain relief benefits provided by the drugs do not outweigh the substantial risk of overdose, suicide and development of fatal heart rhythm abnormalities. Both drugs are not available.

Q. When I write a prescription for Vicodin do I have to write 5 mg hydrocodone/500 mg acetaminophen?

A. No. It is not necessary. Just write for Vicodin or Vicodin ES or Vicodin HP. It is not necessary to write the components.

Q. Can I write for generic Vicodin?

A. Yes.

Q. What is Tramadol (Ultram)?

A. Tramadol is a central synthetic analgesic compound that is not derived from natural sources nor is it chemically related to opiates. Tramadol is a synthetic, centrally acting pain reliever indicated for moderate to moderately severe oral pain. Its analgesic action affects both opioid receptor and serotonin uptake, so it does not act through a narcotic mechanism and is not a nonscheduled drug. The serious adverse effects usually seen with opioids, such as dependence, sedation, respiratory depression and constipation, occur less often with tramadol. Even though there is a low rate of abuse, practitioners should be cautious when prescribing this drug for patients recovering from substance abuse disorders. It is contraindicated in patients with a previous history of seizures. There is also a lack of sedation which is advantageous if taken on the same day as the surgical procedure. Dose of tramadol (Ultram) is: supplied: 50 mg tablet: 1–2 tabs q4–6 h for dental pain. (max: 400 mg/d) or 37.5 mg tramadol/325 mg acetaminophen (Ultracet): 2 tabs q4–6 h. Ultracet is tramadol plus acetaminophen. It is supplied as tablets and orally disintegrating tablets.

Table 4.7 Narcotic/non-narcotic combination products.

Hydrocodone/acetaminophen combinations	Brand name & narcotic schedule	Dosage
2.5 mg hydrocodone bitartrate/500 mg acetaminophen	Lortab 2.5/500 C-III	1 tab q4h
5 mg hydrocodone bitartrate/500 mg acetaminophen	Vicodin C-III	1 tab q4h
	Lortab 5/500 C-III	
	Lorcet HD	
7.5 mg hydrocodone bitartrate/325 mg acetaminophen	Narco 7.5/325 C-III	1 tab q4h
7.5 hydrocodone bitartrate/750 mg acetaminophen	Vicodin ES C-III	1 tab q4h
7.5 mg hydrocodone bitartrate/500 mg acetaminophen	Lortab 7.5/500 C-III	1 tab q4h
7.5 mg hydrocodone bitartrate/650 mg acetaminophen	Lorcet Plus	1 tab q4h
10 mg hydrocodone bitartrate/325 mg acetaminophen	Narco 10/325 C-III	1 tab q4h
10 mg hydrocodone bitartrate/660 mg acetaminophen	Vicodin HP C-III	1 tab q4h
10 mg hydrocodone bitartrate/500 mg acetaminophen	Lortab 10/500 C-III	1 tab q4h
7.5 mg hydrocodone/ 200 mg ibuprofen	Vicoprofen C-III	1 tab q4h
Oxycodone/acetaminophen combinations		
1.5 mg oxycodone HCl/ 325 mg acetaminophen	Percocet C-II (must indicate the strength prescribed)	1 tab q6h
5 mg oxycodone HCl/ 325 mg acetaminophen		
7.5 mg oxycodone HCl/ 325 mg acetaminophen		
10 mg oxycodone HCl/ 325 mg acetaminophen		
7.5 mg oxycodone HCl/ 500 mg acetaminophen		
10 oxycodone HCl/ 650 mg acetaminophen		
5 mg oxycodone HCl/500 mg acetaminophen	Tylox C-II	1 tab q6h
5 mg oxycodone HCl/400 mg ibuprofen	Combunox C-II	1 tab q4h
4.5 mg oxycodone HCl/0.38 mg aspirin	Percodan C-II	1 tab q4h
16 mg dihydrocodeine/325 mg aspirin	Synalgos DC C-III	1 tab q4h
Controlled-release tablets: 10 mg, 15 mg, 20 mg, 30 mg, 40 mg, 60 mg, 80 mg, 160 mg (60, 80 and 160 mg are used in opioid-tolerant patients only	OxyContin C-II	Not recommended for dental pain. OxyContin (oxycodone HCl) is only indicated for postoperative use if the patient is already receiving the drug prior to surgery or if the postoperative pain is expected to be moderate to severe and persist for an extended period of time; around the clock dosing. (http://www.rxlist.com/oxycontin-drug.htm)
Centrally acting analgesics		
50 mg tramadol	Ultram C-IV	should be started at 25 mg/day qam and titrated in 25 mg increments as separate doses every 3 days to reach 100 mg/day (25 mg qid). Thereafter the total daily dose may be increased by 50 mg as tolerated every 3 days to reach 200 mg/day (50 mg qid). After titration, 50 to 100 mg can be administered as needed for pain relief every 4 to 6 hours not to exceed 400 mg/day. (http://www.rxlist.com/ultram-drug.htm)
37.5 mg tramadol/325 mg acetaminophen	Ultracet C-IV	
Other analgesics		
12.5 mg pentazocine/650 mg acetaminophen	Talwin compound C-IV	

Medical Economics Staff. 2000.

There are conflicting reports if tramadol is indicated for management of acute dental pain in dentistry; used more for chronic pain. If use of NSAIDs or narcotics is contraindicated then it is a plausible alternative analgesic. The dose of tramadol is one tab q4–6h and for tramadol/acetaminophen two tabs q4–6h for dental pain. In patients with creatinine clearances of <30 mL/min, the recommended dose and dosing interval is 2 tabs q12h. *On 25 May 2010, the FDA warned healthcare professionals about the risk of suicide for patients who are addiction-prone, taking tranquilizers or antidepressant drugs and also warns of the risk of overdose.*

Q. Can Talwin be used for the management of dental pain?

A. Talwin (pentazocine) has been used in the management of acute dental pain. However, there are some adverse effects such as psychotic events (hallucinations) that may preclude its use. The incidence of abuse is relatively low (Swift & Hargreaves, 1993). Also, it when discontinued there is withdrawal. Therefore, Talwin is not an analgesic of choice for dental pain.

Q. Can I prescribe meperidine (Demerol) for dental pain?

A. It is not such a good drug for dental pain because it undergoes extensive first-pass metabolism reducing the amount of active drug to produce an analgesic response and it has a short duration of action so that constant dosing would be necessary.

Q. How many days should a narcotic be prescribed for a patient to take?

A. Not for more than 2–3 days. After that the patient should take a non-narcotic analgesic.

Q. What is oxycodone?

A. Oxycodone, unlike codeine, is a very potent analgesic with fewer severe adverse effects such as histamine release and nausea. Oxycodone, a prodrug is metabolized by CYP2D6 to an active metabolite, oxymorphone. However, unlike codeine and hydrocodone, oxycodone is itself a potent analgesic. It is unknown whether oxymorphone significantly contributes to the analgesic activity of oxycodone. Patients with CYP2D6 deficiencies who do not respond well to codeine or hydrocodone may achieve more pain relief from using oxycodone. Oxycodone is available in combination with non-opioids or alone. In the elderly and in patients with renal impairment less dosage adjustment is needed.

Q. How is a prescription for codeine, hydrocodone/acetaminophen combination drugs written since they are schedule III narcotics?

A. Schedule III drugs can be written and renewed not more than 5 refills for up to 6 months or ordered over the phone. The prescription is valid only up to 30 days from the date of issue.

Q. How does physical dependence develop with long-term narcotic use?

A. With long-term narcotic use liver enzymes enhance the metabolism of the narcotic thus, requiring more drug to be stratified (tolerance develops).

Q. When are narcotic analgesics appropriate to prescribe?

A. In patient with moderate to severe dental pain such as surgical removal of impacted wisdom teeth.

Q. For which type of patients should narcotics be avoided?

A. Patients taking antipsychotics or CNS depressants, acute alcoholism; patients addicted to narcotics, respiratory insufficiency or depression, bronchial asthma, advanced emphysema, heart failure secondary to chronic lung disease, cardiac arrhythmias, known hypersensitivity, and pregnant women (Category C drugs). Precautions should be used in the elderly and in patients with undiagnosed abdominal pain, liver disease, and a history of addiction to the opioids, hypoxia, supraventricular tachycardia, prostatic hypertrophy, and renal or hepatic impairment. The obese must be monitored closely for respiratory depression while taking the narcotic analgesics. For a complete list of narcotic–drug interactions see Table 5.6.

Patient with: severe asthma, aspirin sensitivity, gastrointestinal ulcers, gastrointestinal bleeding, anticoagulant therapy.

Q. Is it alright to prescribe codeine, hydrocodone or oxycodone to patients taking fluoxetine (Prozac) and paroxetine (Paxil)?

A. No. Drugs that are inhibitors of CYP450 2D6 may interfere with the analgesic effect of codeine. The mechanism is decreased in vivo conversion of codeine to morphine, a metabolic reaction mediated by CYP450 2D6. Fluoxetine (Prozac) and paroxetine (Paxil) are selective serotonin reuptake inhibitors (SSRIs) and there is a definitive drug–drug interaction with codeine and its derivatives. These drugs can delay the metabolism of codeine resulting in less of an analgesic response because codeine and its derivatives require metabolism to be effective. These two drugs should not be taken concurrently. There seems to be documented response with only these two SSRIs.

Q. What is the difference in the narcotic prescribed?

A. Codeine alone has not been found as effective as other common analgesics (acetaminophen and NSAIDs) for relief of dental pain. Oxycodone and hydrocodone are about as effective as codeine. Dihydrocodeine, pentazocine and meperidine show no advantages over codeine orally and can even be less effective. Their effectiveness in combination therapy (combining opioids with acetaminophen and NSAIDs) is better than that in monotherapy. It is all related to the different degrees of potency.

Q. Why is it important to know different potencies of narcotics?

A. The relative potencies of narcotics aid in the decision on which narcotic to prescribe. Ideally, when prescribing a narcotic the most effective analgesic effect for moderate to severe pain has been found to be with 60 mg codeine. So, if a hydrocodone/non-narcotic drug is prescribed a hydrocodone strength equivalent to 60 mg of codeine is ideal:

- 30–60 mg codeine orally is equivalent to 5–10 mg hydrocodone and 5 mg oxycodone.

Q. Why can histamine-like symptoms appear after taking a narcotic?

A. Narcotics bind to histamine receptors causing the release of histamine. This results in symptoms such as itching. This is not a true allergy which would be a reaction due to the drug molecule. A true allergy to opioids is very rare. Rather, itching is just an adverse effect. If the patient reports in the medical history an allergy to codeine it is important to question the patient as to what happened when it was taken. This will sort out if it was a true allergic reaction or merely an adverse effect of the drug. Naturally occurring and semisynthetic compounds are the most potent histamine releasers.

Q. What are other adverse effects of narcotics?

A. Constipation, nausea, vomiting, dizziness, vertigo, sedation, dizziness, pruritus, urine retention, and cardiovascular and respiratory depression. All patients must be aware of these adverse effects. However, the relative risk of opioid-like adverse effects varies with individuals. Remind patients not to drive due to sedation and dizziness.

Q. Why does constipation occur with opioids?

A. Constipation occurs when the sphincters and intestinal wall contract.

Q. Is dose adjustment needed in liver impairment?

A. Yes. The dose is reduced and the dosing interval is increased.

Q. What should be done if a patient says he/she is allergic to codeine?

A. First, the patient should be questioned what happened when the narcotic was taken. A true allergy to opioids is rare. If the patient states itching or stomach problems occurred, the patient is most likely not allergic to opioids. These are adverse effects, not anaphylaxis, relating to the release of histamine and constipation.

Q. Why has there been a lot of media about abuse of OxyContin?

A. First introduced in 1995, OxyContin is a scheduled II controlled substance with an abuse potential similar to morphine. OxyContin has been used inappropriately and is easily abused for its euphoric effect. It is supplied in a controlled (slow) release form of oxycodone. It is not available in combination with a non-narcotic as is Percodan, Percocet or Tylox. It is indicated for moderate to severe pain when continuous, around-the-clock opioid analgesic is need. The reason for causing death is because when used as a recreational drug it is either crushed and snorted or dissolved in water and intravenously injected. When taken in this form it can cause an overdose and death (American Dental Association 2010).

f. *Management plan for acute dental pain*

Q. What features are used to aid in which analgesic should be prescribed to a patient?

A. Patient's medical condition, severity of pain (mild, moderate or severe), medications taken by the patient.

Q. Why is the use of NSAIDs important in dental pain?

A. The major component of dental pain is inflammation and NSAIDs possess anti-inflammatory properties while the opioids do not.

Q. What analgesic is acceptable to use in patients taking blood thinners such as aspirin or warfarin?

A. The only analgesics that can be used are acetaminophen or opioids. NSAIDs taken with blood thinner cause an additive effect and this is contraindicated.

Q. What is the best analgesic for a recovering substance abuser?

A. It is recommended to contact the patient's primary care physician or drug abuse physician. First, it is important to determine if the patient is a former or current substance abuser. In former abuse patients with severe acute dental pain it is advisable not to avoid prescribing opioids because of addiction concerns. If an opioid is prescribed, it is advisable that drug users should be treated with longer-acting opioids and hydrocodone/acetaminophen and not to start with a weaker drug and wait until it fails to prescribe a stronger narcotic. Only prescribe enough to last for a couple of days. Do not give the patient more than six tablets and no refills. The concern with using opioids in former or current substance abusers is the effect of euphoria from the opioid. Another obstacle in treating these patients is that most develop tolerance and physical dependence to the opioid. The patient usually will require a higher dose of the opioid at more frequent intervals to achieve adequate pain relief. To achieve adequate pain relief the doses should be give "around-the-clock" or scheduled rather than on an "as needed" basis. Using "around-the-clock" dosing suppresses the pain better than dosing on an "as needs" basis where the pain may go up and require more medication to control the pain. If there are concerns with prescribing an opioid for moderate to severe pain, an NSAID (dose: 400 to 600 mg) can be taken preoperatively and postoperatively (Denisco *et al.*, 2011; Goureitch & Arnsten, 2005; Prater *et al.*, 2002).

Q. How much of an analgesic should initially be prescribed to any patient?

A. It is always advisable to prescribe the smallest dose that produces an acceptable analgesic response. Overprescribing of narcotics happens when the dentist prescribes in excessive quantities that are needed to relieve dental pain. There is no need to prescribe a narcotic for more than a few days. If severe pain persists afterward then most likely there is either poor healing or an infection which requires the patient to go immediately to the dental office or emergency department (Denisco *et al.*, 2011).

Q. Is it acceptable to take the analgesic just when the patient has pain?

A. No. An analgesic should not be taken on a "prn" basis because therapeutic bloods levels will not be maintained. It is recommended at least for the first few days to take the analgesic on an "around-the-clock" or scheduled basis to provide a fairly consistent level of pain control. The disadvantage of administering analgesics on an "as needed" basis is that pain must be present before it can be managed. Repeated prn dosing may result in high peaks and low levels, causing alternating periods of uncontrolled pain and toxicity as more doses may be used to catch up with the pain.

Q. Why do individuals respond differently to the same drug?

A. Yes. Sometimes drugs especially opioids can cause unpredictable and inconsistent therapeutic effects because everyone differs in the way they metabolize the drug. If one drug does not produce the therapeutic effects anticipated switch to another one. Everyone responds differently.

Q. Is pre-treating with a non-narcotic analgesic before a painful dental procedure to reduce post-surgical pain effective?

A. Yes. The patient should take an NSAID within 2 hours before the dental procedure. Pretreatment with acetaminophen has not been shown to be as effective as pre-treating with an NSAID. It is best and most effective in managing postoperative pain when the NSAID is administered between 30 to 60 minutes before the procedure and after the procedure as well. The reasoning behind this is that trauma caused by tissue manipulation during the dental procedure releases prostaglandins within 2 hours and by having the analgesic already in the blood it prevents the synthesis of inflammatory prostaglandins are quickly released after the surgical insult (Huynh & Yagiela, 2003). Giving analgesics before the procedure delays the onset of postsurgical pain and the severity is much less.

Q. Do pediatric patient require more than the strength of OTC analgesics?

A. Generally pediatric patients do not require prescription strength analgesics. For children:

- ibuprofen oral suspension (100 mg/5 mL) at a dose of 10 mg/kg every 4 hours with a maximum dose of 40 mg/kg/day. (each 5 mL = 1 teaspoonful)
- acetaminophen oral suspension (contains 160 mg acetaminophen/5 mL) (ages 2 to 11) 15 mg/kg every 4 hours. It is recommended to consult with the pediatrician for 2 year olds.

Q. Which analgesic is recommended to start with for dental pain?

A. Generally, if there are no contraindications an NSAID is the first line drug.

Q. Can an NSAID be taken together with acetaminophen?

A. Yes. It is best to take the combination for short-term only. NSAID plus acetaminophen are superior to NSAID alone (Altman, 2004; Hyllested *et al.*, 2002;). Combining acetaminophen and NSAIDs can lead to greater efficacy with fewer adverse effects (Altman, 2004). However, Altman (2002) emphasizes that further clinical studies are needed to determine the clinical safety of acetaminophen/NSAID combination analgesic therapy for common conditions associated with mild-to-moderate pain. So, in the meantime it is recommended to the pain medications as directed to help avoid any potential adverse effects of either medication. There are many products on the market that contain both. For example, Excedrin Migraine contains acetaminophen, aspirin and caffeine (caffeine has been reported to increase the analgesic effect) (Granados-Soto *et al.*, 1993).

Q. When should narcotics be prescribed for acute dental pain?

A. Effective doses of a non-narcotic such as ibuprofen or acetaminophen is more efficacious than a narcotic alone for moderate to severe pain and almost or equally effective as a narcotic/non-narcotic combination product. Remember to advise patients about the many adverse effects of opioids and that a car should not be driven while on an opioid. The general management plan is as follows:

- The ideal non-narcotic to start with is 400–800 mg ibuprofen q4–6 h. Can increase dosage if needed but the maximum dose is 2400 mg/day.
- If an NSAID is contraindicated then acetaminophen 650–1000 mg is recommended. The maximum dosage is 4000 mg (4 g) per day.
- Can use acetaminophen plus an NSAID. This combination produces synergistic actions.
- Acetaminophen or COX-2 inhibitor (Celebrex) recommend in patients at risk of experiencing gastrointestinal distress.
- If this regimen does not provide adequate pain relief then: 650 mg acetaminophen/10 mg hydrocodone q4–6 h (following strictly the q4–6 h and not just as needed) *or* Tylenol # 3 (2 tablets q4–6 h) (following strictly the q4–6 h and not just as needed) OR 7.5 mg hydrocodone/ 200 mg ibuprofen (Vicoprofen) *plus* (if needed) 200–400 mg ibuprofen.
  ○ Should not exceed 360 mg codeine a day
  ○ Caution should be followed because opioids do not have a ceiling effect so when used in combination with acetaminophen increasing the dose for more profound analgesic effect will also increase the dose of acetaminophen which can result in hepatotoxicity.

Q. Can a combination of narcotic and non-narcotic analgesic be prescribed?

A. Yes. NSAIDs have an opioid sparing effect of 20–30%. Combinations of NSAIDs with opioids produce a synergistic effect. Additionally, all analgesics do not work the same way. Most non-narcotics work peripherally, while opioids work centrally on brain receptors. Combining analgesics with different modes and sites of action can increase the analgesic effect and be better tolerated by the patient because lower doses are used (Mehlisch, 2002).

Q. Can taking two different NSAIDs or two different narcotics be more beneficial in reducing pain?

A. No, because with NSAIDs, the maximum pain relief is usually reached with an effective dose of a single NSAID. Taking more than one NSAID only increases the incidence of adverse effects. There will be increased analgesic effect by taking two or more narcotics by also increased adverse effects and the increased analgesic effect could also be achieved with a larger dose of just a single narcotic (Huynh & Yagiela, 2003).

Q. For moderate-to-severe pain is it better to take non-narcotics alone or as a combined tablet with a narcotic or separate non-narcotic and separate narcotic at the same time or a separate non-narcotic plus a combination non-narcotic/narcotic?

A. For all severities of acute pain it is recommended to begin management with ibuprofen or acetaminophen. Always use the lowest possible effective dose to avoid unwanted adverse effects. If either one alone does not provide profound pain relief then for moderate pain relief add to the ibuprofen a non-narcotic/narcotic combination drug such as Tylenol # 4 or 10 mg hydrocodone (Vicodin HP). Remember the maximum amount of ibuprofen for profound pain relief is 2400 mg/day (Mehlisch, 2002).

Q. What is an approach to enhance the analgesic effect of oral drugs?

A. To enhance the analgesic effect it has been recommended to combine two different drugs with different mechanisms of action: for example, ibuprofen and hydrocodone or acetaminophen and codeine.

Q. Can acetaminophen be combined with an NSAID?

A. Yes, but there is not enough literature to show if the combination of acetaminophen plus NSAIDs produces any more pain relief than just taking acetaminophen alone because it is not exactly known if acetaminophen has the same mechanism of action as NSAIDs (Huynh & Yagiela, 2003).

Q. Why is caffeine added to many OTC analgesics?

A. Caffeine does not have any analgesic action but is added to many OTC analgesics to increase the potency of the other ingredients including ibuprofen, acetaminophen and aspirin (Huynh & Yagiela, 2003). Caffeine, a vasoconstrictor, is useful in these OTC analgesics to help relief headaches.

Q. What is the best analgesic for *mild* dental pain (e.g., after scaling and root planing, restorative dentistry)?

- STEP 1: To start: 200–400 mg ibuprofen q4–6 h for dental pain when there are no contraindications such as ulcers, gastric bleeding, anticoagulant therapy, aspirin sensitivity or asthma.
  - The maximum dose of ibuprofen is 800 mg per dose or 2400 mg/day.
- If the patient is hypertensive and taking any antihypertensive drug except for calcium channel blockers then the duration of use should be limited to 5 days.
- If ibuprofen is contraindicated (see the above situations) then recommend 650–1000 mg acetaminophen alone (World Health Organization, 1986). If not enough pain relief with 200–400 mg ibuprofen: a higher dosage can be prescribed; initially prescribe up to 600 mg q4–6 h then reduce to 400 mg as needed.
- Note: if the patient takes Aleve (naproxen sodium 220 mg) then take 2 tabs q8h.

Q. What is the best analgesic for *moderate* dental pain (e.g., periodontal surgery, endodontic therapy)?

- STEP 1: To start: ibuprofen 400–600 mg for the first day, if there are no contraindications such as ulcers, gastric bleeding, aspirin sensitivity, anticoagulant therapy or asthma.
  - The maximum dose of ibuprofen is 800 mg per dose or 2,400 mg/day.
- Reduce dose after the first day to ibuprofen 400 mg.
- If the patient is hypertensive and taking any antihypertensive drug except for calcium channel blockers then the duration of use should be limited to 5 days.
- If ibuprofen is contraindicated (see above situations) then recommend 600–1000 mg acetaminophen plus a narcotic such as codeine (60 mg) or hydrocodone (10 mg) OR 37.5 mg tramadol/325 mg acetaminophen (Ultracet): one
- STEP 2: If inadequate pain relief with ibuprofen: a narcotic/non-narcotic combination is necessary. Choices include *adding* to 400 mg ibuprofen (taken 2 hours before surgery) then:
  - Tylenol # 3 – 2 tabs q4–6 h for dental pain (taking two # 3 is equal to 600 mg acetaminophen and 60 mg codeine) *or*
  - 10 mg hydrocodone/650 mg acetaminophen (Vicodin HP) *or*
  - 7.5 mg hydrocodone/200 mg ibuprofen (Vicoprofen) *or*
  - if NSAIDs are contraindicated just use the recommended narcotic combinations without NSAID.

Q. What is the best analgesic for *severe* dental pain (e.g., extraction of impacted wisdom teeth, extensive periodontal surgery, and acute pulpitis)?

- to start: ibuprofen 400–600 mg then add
  - 10 mg hydrocodone/650 mg acetaminophen (Vicodin HP) *or*
  - 7.5 mg hydrocodone/200 mg ibuprofen (Vicoprofen) *or*
  - 10 mg oxycodone/650 mg acetaminophen (Percocet) (try hydrocodone before prescribing oxycodone)

(Hersh *et al.*, 2011; American Association of Endodontists, 1995).

Q. Does Vicoprofen provide a ceiling analgesic effect for ibuprofen?

A. No. 200 mg of ibuprofen is not enough of a dose of an NSAID to provide a ceiling analgesic effect which is 1000 mg. Vicoprofen is then not considered to be a good choice for moderate to severe pain but is recommended for patients that cannot take acetaminophen either because of liver problems or cannot tolerate it.

Q. Which opioid is safest to prescribe in a patient with renal insufficiency?

A. It is not recommended to prescribe codeine and hydrocodone and oxycodone should be used with caution (reduction in dosage interval).

VI.   Moderate sedation

Q. What is moderate sedation?

A. Moderate sedation is a more up-to-date term for conscious sedation. Moderate sedation is a pharmacologically induced state of depressed consciousness and analgesia where the patient's protective airway reflexes are intact and the patient can ventilate. The patient can respond to physical or verbal stimuli.

Q. Can moderate sedation be performed in the dental office?

A. Yes. Moderate sedation is usually administered in the dental office or hospital.

Q. What is minimal sedation?

A. Minimal sedation is primarily used in the dental office for anxious patients. It is a drug-induced state during which patients respond normally to verbal commands. Ventilatory and cardiovascular functions are not affected (American Academy of Periodontology, 2001).

Q. What does moderate sedation induce?

A. Anti-anxiety, decreased stress response and some degree of amnesia.

Q. Can moderate sedation be achieved by the oral administration of drugs?

A. Yes. Moderate sedation is administered either orally (enteral), intravenously (parenteral) or by inhalation. Combinations enteral and inhalation can be used or inhalation and parenteral.

Q. How should the patient be assessed before any anesthesia is administered?

A. The American Society of Anesthesiologists has a classification of the physical status of patients. Every patient should be given a classification before local or sedative anesthesia is administered. Table 4.8 describes the classification. Patients who are ASA I and ASA II must have vital signs including blood pressure, pulse rate and respiration being monitored at all times. Talking to the patient is important to make sure he/her is responsive to your commands. More extensive monitoring including EKG should be done for ASA III and ASA IV. (American Society of Anesthesiologists, 2007).

Table 4.8   Patient physical status classification.

ASA I	Normal healthy patient
ASA II	Patient with mild systemic disease: type 2 diabetes, hypertension
ASA III	Patient with severe systemic disease: stable angina, type 1 diabetes, chronic obstructive pulmonary disease
ASA IV	Patient with severe systemic disease that is a constant threat to life: heart attack within 6 months, unstable angina, uncontrolled diabetes or uncontrolled epilepsy
ASA V	Moribund patient who is not expected to survive without the operation: patient is not expected to survive 24 hours with or without medical intervention
ASA VI	A declared brain-dead patient whose organs are being removed for donor purposes
E	Emergency operation used to modify any of the above classifications

ASA: the American Society of Anesthesiologists.
E, Emergency.
Adapted from: ASA Physical Status Classification System (www.asahq.org.clinical/physicalstatus.htm).

Q. What are commonly used intravenous agents used for moderate sedation?

A. Propofol, midazolam, fentanyl.

Q. What is EMLA?

A. EMLA is eutectic mixture of local anaesthetics. It is cream that supplied effective topical analgesia to intact skin with an occlusive dressing and placed at least one hour before venipuncture.

a. *Benzodiazepines*

Q. What are some orally administered anti-anxiety drugs used for patients who are anxious about dental treatment?

A. Benzodiazepines (anti-anxiety) are the main drugs used for minimal sedation because they produce sedation, anxiolysis, and amnesia, which are desirable attributes for moderate sedation. There is no respiratory depression like with the opioids. Table 4.9 lists the common benzodiazepines.

Q. What are common adverse effects of benzodiazepines that the patient should be counseled?

A. Sedation (do not drive a car), drowsiness, xerostomia, blurred vision, diarrhea, nausea, decrease respiratory rate.

Q. What is the **Black Box Warning** for midazolam?

A. Midazolam HCl syrup has been associated with respiratory depression and respiratory arrest, especially when used for sedation in noncritical care settings. Midazolam HCl syrup has been associated with reports of respiratory depression, airway obstruction, desaturation, hypoxia, and apnea, most often when used concomitantly with other central nervous system depressants (e.g., opioids). Midazolam HCl syrup should be used only in hospital or ambulatory care settings, including physicians' and dentists' offices, which can provide for continuous cardiac and respiratory monitoring.

Table 4.9   Common benzodiazepines used for minimal sedation/anti-anxiety.

Drug	Dosage
Alprazolam (Xanax)	Anti-anxiety: Adults: 0.25–0.5 mg Child: has not be determined Supplied: tabs: 0.25, 0.5, 1, 2 mg
Clorazepate (Tranxene)	Anti-anxiety: Adults: 7.5–15 mg bid or tid Child: has not be determined Supplied: Tabs: 3.75, 7.5,. 11.25, 15, 22.5 mg Caps: 3.75, 7.5, 15 mg
Diazepam (Valium)	Anti-anxiety: Adults: 2–10 mg bid, tid or qid Child: 0.1–0.5 mg/kg (maximum dose: 10 mg) Supplied: 2,5, 10 mg
Lorazepam (Ativan)	Anti-anxiety: Adults: 1–3 mg bid or tid Child: not determined or not recommended Supplied: Tabs: 0.5, 1, 2 mg Sublingual tabs: 0.5, 1, 2 mg
Midazolam (Versed)	0.5 mg/kg oral (syrup) 0.08 to 0.5 mg/kg intramuscular 0.2 to 0.3 mg/kg intranasal

Q. What conditions are benzodiazepines contraindicated?

A. Narrow angle glaucoma and severe chronic obstructive pulmonary disease.

Q. What are common drug interactions with benzodiazepines?

A. Oral contraceptives (decreased metabolism of diazepam), isoniazid (INH; for tuberculosis) (increases half-life of diazepam), valproic acid (anticonvulsant, bipolar disease) (displaces diazepam from its protein binding sites resulting in increased blood levels).

Q. What are patient instructions for taking a benzodiazepine?

A. Avoid alcohol and other CNS depressants, avoid driving or other similar activities, can cause xerostomia. If given for sedation in the dental office, the patient must be discharged into the care of a competent adult and should be warned about not driving.

Q. Can benzodiazepines be prescribed for pregnant women?

A. All benzodiazepines have a Pregnancy Category of D. Benzodiazepines should not be prescribed to pregnant women.

Q. Which benzodiazepine can be given for anti-anxiety to a child?

A. Young children are more prone and sensitive to the CNS depressive effects. Diazepam dose: 0.1–0.5 mg/kg.

Q. Should the dose of a benzodiazepine be adjusted in the elderly?

A. Yes. For example, the adult dose of alprazolam (Xanax) which is 0.25 mg to 0.5 mg should be cut in half in the elderly.

Q. What is midazolam?

A. Commonly used preanesthesia medication (causes relaxation/sleep and amnesia) with a rapid onset and short duration. It does not cause cardiorespiratory depression. Onset of action is about 10 minutes intranasally. Midazolam should not be taken with some antiviral medications (HIV/AIDS), grapefruit juice, ketoconazole, and itraconazole.

Q. Is a benzodiazepine alright to prescribe to the elderly?

A. Yes, but in the smallest dose necessary to produce a therapeutic response.

b.   Other agents

Q. Why are barbiturates not routinely used?

A. Barbiturates have more of an effect on the heart, CNS, and lungs than the benzodiazepines. Their popularity over the years has been reduced by the benzodiazepines, which have fewer adverse effects. Longer-acting barbiturates such as phenobarbital are usually used as anticonvulsants and shorter-acting barbiturates such as pentobarbital and secobarbital are used as sedative/hypnotics.

Q. What is propofol?

A. Propofol is a very potent sedative/hypnotic nonbarbiturate that is administered intravenously with minimal amnesic and analgesic properties. It readily crosses the blood–brain barrier causing a rapid onset of moderate sedation. Recovery is quick because it is rapidly redistributed from the CNS and undergoes rapid metabolism. Caution should be taken not to use high doses since it may lead to respiratory depression or arrest.

Q. What is fentanyl?

A. Fentanyl, an analgesic, has a quick onset of action (highly lipophilic) and short duration so it is frequently used for intravenous moderate sedation. It is 100 times more potent than morphine. In addition its duration is relatively short compared to other opioids, usually lasting only 30 to 60 minutes. Fentanyl is safe for patients with renal failure.

Q. How is chloral hydrate used in the dental office?

A. Despite being widely used for pediatric sedation, it is not the ideal drug and should be used with caution. Children may manifest accumulation of chloral hydrate metabolites (trichloroethanol), leading to prolonged sedation and even sudden death. Its use has been prohibited in California in pediatric dentistry due to an increased number of deaths. In addition, chloral hydrate can cause gastric irritation. It should not be administered to patients with cardiac, renal or liver problems.

VII. Glucocorticosteroids

Q. What are common indications for the use of glucocorticosteroids in dentistry?

A. Mucocutaneous diseases (e.g., pemphigus, pemphigoid, systemic lupus erythematosus, lichen planus), erythema multiforme, aphthous ulcers (canker sores).

Q. What other conditions are glucocorticoids indicated?

A. Rheumatoid arthritis, severe persistent asthma, vesicular bullous disorders.

a. Topical glucocorticosteroids

Q. How are topical steroids used for oral mucocutaneous/bullous diseases?

A. Topical steroids are used for the treatment of inflammatory conditions of the skin or oral mucosa. Topical steroids do not cure the condition and when therapy is discontinued a rebound effect may occur.

Q. When topical steroids are applied in the mouth is there any systemic absorption?

A. Any topical application of medications causes systemic absorption into the blood but only in negligible amounts.

Q. How are topical steroids applied to oral lesions?

A. Topical steroids are applied to oral lesions by using a finger cot and either dabbing or smoothing on the lesion or a soft acrylic mouth guard is custom made from the patient's models and the steroid is applied to the inside of the splint to allow better contact of the steroid to the lesion.

Q. What is the difference between mineralocorticoids and glucocorticoids?

A. Mineralocorticoids are used to treat patients with hypoadrenalism by increasing kidney sodium retention and potassium loss. The medical use of mineralocorticosteroids is limited. Aldosterone is the most important naturally occurring mineralocorticoid.

Glucocorticoids are anti-inflammatory agents used in the treatment of many medical conditions. This is the steroid that is primarily used in medicine and dentistry.

Q. What is the major natural glucocorticoid produced in the human body?

A. Hydrocortisone (cortisol) is synthesized and released from the adrenal gland (adrenal cortex). Remember the adrenal medulla synthesizes catecholamines such as epinephrine. Cortisol production is controlled by adrenocorticotropic hormone (ACTH). In the healthy individual hydrocortisone levels being to rise between 2 a.m. and 6 a.m. with peak levels occurring between 6 a.m. and 8 a.m. Cortisol levels decrease during the day until midnight when minimal levels occur. Cortisol increased available energy in the form of glucose; causes gluconeogenesis (glucose formation).

Q. What are the synthetically manufactured glucocorticoid steroids?

A. Prednisone, beclomethasone, triamcinolone, dexamethasone.

Q. What is the mechanism of action of the anti-inflammatory actions of glucocorticoids?

A. In general, glucocorticoids support cell membrane integrity which results in suppressing an in increase in vascular permeability and preventing the release of damaging lysosomes from inside the cell and the release of prostaglandins. In addition, there is a suppression of vasodilation.

Q. How are topical steroids classified?

A. Steroids are classified according to potency. Table 4.10 lists different topical steroids used for the management of oral lesions. Group VII have the lowest potency and Group I has the highest potency. Group I steroids are not used in dentistry.

Q. What corticosteroid formulations are used in dentistry for treating aphthous ulcers (canker sores), blistering muco-cutaneous diseases of the oral mucosa including pemphigus, lichen planus, and mucous membrane pemphigoid?

A. Topically applied creams, dental paste and rinses.

Q. Why do some steroids contain fluoride atom added to the steroid molecule?

A. Some preparations of steroids are fluorinated which increases the potency and prolongs the duration of action. Also, the incidence of adverse effects is increased.

Q. How is it decided which steroid preparation to use?

A. Absorption of a steroid depends on the water and lipid solubilities of the drug. Lipid solubility is more important for topical administration where the effect is localized with slow absorption.

Table 4.10   Classification of selective topical steroids used in dentistry.

Lowest potency (does not penetrate mucosa well)
• Hydrocortisone 2.5% cream (various brand names – Cortaid, Cortizone – OTC; 0.5% and 1%)
• Hydrocortisone acetate in Orabase 0.5% (for oral lesions) (Orabase®-HCA. (prescription only)
Low potency
• Dexamethasone Elixir (Decadron) F
Medium potency
• Betamethasone valerate ointment (Valisone)
• Triamcinolone acetonide dental paste 0.1% (Oralone) (Prescription only)
High potency
• Fluocinonide gel (Lidex) F
Highest potency
• Clobetasol propionate gel (generic, Temovate) F

F, fluoride.
Adapted from Ference & Last (2009).

Q. Which preparations are used topically for intraoral lesions?

A. Topical gels, dental paste, ointments and elixirs. Hydrocortisone and triamcinolone are specially formulated in a dental paste (Orabase®) that contains cellulose gum, flavor, pectin, plasticized hydrocarbon gel, preservatives, and tragacanth gum. This product is only available with a prescription. Dexamethasone elixir and clobetasol propionate can be prescribed.

Q. When is it contraindicated to use steroid agents?

A. Topical steroids can cause topical and systemic adverse effects. Contraindications: immunocompromised patient, fungal infection, and herpes infection. Potent topical steroids can cause purpura and ulcerations especially in thin-mucosal areas (Cornell, 1987).

Q. How is a prescription written triamcinolone dental paste?

A. See Table 4.11.

Q. What is Orabase?

A. Orabase is the trade name (Oral Colgate Pharmaceuticals) for dental paste.

Q. How should products with dental paste be applied?

A. Products with dental paste should be "dabbed" or "press" on rather than "rubbed" on because the product will not stay on the oral tissue well if rubbed on. Apply to the affected area two to three times daily after meals or at bedtime.

Q. What is Kenalog in Orabase?

A. Kenalog is the brand name for triamcinolone in dental paste. It is a prescription drug.

Q. How is a prescription for clobetasol propionate written (Table 4.12)?

A. Clobetasol topical exists as multiple brands and/or as a generic drug. Clobetasol topical and Temovate are a few names. Also, this product is not labeled for intraoral use and some pharmacists will not fill this prescription.

Q. How is a prescription for dexamethasone elixir written for an adult (Table 4.13)?

A. Dexamethsone elixir is indicated for intraoral use.

Table 4.11 How the prescription for triamcinolone dental paste is written.

Rx Triamcinolone acetonide dental paste 0.1% Disp: 5 g tube Sig: Apply a thin film by dabbing on affected area up to three times a day, preferably after meals.

Table 4.12 How a prescription for clobetasol propionate is written.

Rx Clobetasol propionate 0.05% ointment Disp: 15 g tube Sig: Apply a thin layer of ointment to affected area six times a day until lesion is gone (treatment should be limited to 2 consecutive weeks and amounts greater than 50 g/week should not be used).

Table 4.13   How a prescription for dexamethasone elixir is written for an adult.

Rx Dexamethasone elixir 0.5 mg/mL
Disp: 8 oz
Sig: Rinse with 1 tsp 4 times a day and then expectorate. Do not swallow.

Table 4.14   How a prescription for Benadryl and Kaopectate is written.

Rx diphenhydramine elixir 4 oz
Kaopectate 4 oz
qs 8 oz
Disp: 8 oz
Sig: Swish with one teaspoonful q2h.
(Note: *qs* is a Latin term meaning quantum sufficient or sufficient quantity which means to make the final product ounces.)

Table 4.15   How a prescription for Xylocaine viscous is written.

Rx lidocaine viscous 2%
Disp: 450 mL bottle
Sig: Swish with one tablespoonful qid.

b.   *Other nonsteroidal topical agents used in the management of oral lesions*

Q. How is a prescription for Benadryl and Kaopectate written (Table 4.14)?

A. Benadryl (diphenhydramine) and Kaopectate is prescribed for aphthous ulcers because it is soothing product. This is a compounding product the pharmacist has to make up.

Q. How is a prescription for Xylocaine viscous written (Table 4.15)?

A. lidocaine (Xylocaine) viscous 2% is a topical anesthetic for relief of intraoral pain or burning.

c.   *Systemic corticosteroids*

Q. When is a systemic corticosteroid prescribed in dentistry?

A. Systemic corticosteroids such as methylprednisolone are indicated for sinus floor elevation surgery to minimize swelling and inflammation.

Q. What are the equivalent doses in milligrams of glucocorticoids?

A. See Table 4.16.

Q. How is systemic glucocorticoid preparations classified?

A. Systemic corticosteroids are classified according to short-acting, intermediate-acting or long-acting. See Table 4.17.

Q. Which systemic corticosteroids are used in dental sinus surgery?

A. Usually methylprednisolone pack (Medrol) or dexamethasone (Decadron). The generic can be prescribed with both medications.

Table 4.16 Equivalent doses in milligrams of glucocorticoids.

Corticoid drug	Equivalent dose (mg)
Cortisone	25
Dexamethasone	0.75
Hydrocortisone	20
Methylprednisolone	4
Prednisone	5
Triamcinolone	4

Table 4.17 Systemic glucocorticosteroids.

Short-acting (8–12 hours)
Cortisone
Hydrocortisone
Intermediate acting (12–36 hours)
Methylprednisolone (Medrol)
Prednisolone
Prednisone
Trimacinolone
Long-acting (36–54 hours)
Betamethasone (Celestone)
Dexamethasone (Decadron)

Q. What are common adverse effects with systemic corticosteroids?

A. Adverse effects are usually rare if used for a short time. Some adverse effects include: peptic ulcers, osteoporosis (usually if chronically taken), sleep problems, nervousness, and diabetes.

Q. Are there any drug interactions with corticosteroids?

A. Yes. Insulin, oral diabetic medications, diuretics, ciclosporin, warfarin, estrogen drugs, and oral contraceptives interact with corticosteroids. Consult with patient's physician before prescribing corticosteroids.

Q. What are patient instructions on how to take corticosteroids?

A. Take with food and a full glass of water or milk to minimize development of ulcers.

References

Abbas, S.M., Kamal, R.S. & Afshan, G. (2004) Effect of ketorolac on postoperative pain relief in dental extraction cases – a comparative study with pethidine. *The Journal of the Pakistan Medical Association*, 54:319–323.

ADA Professional Product Review (Fall/October 2010) *Journal of the American Dental Association*, 5:3–4.

Altman, R.D. (2004) A rationale for combining acetaminophen and NSAIDs for mild-to-moderate pain. *Clinical Experimental Rheumatology*, 22:110–117.

American Academy of Periodontology (2001) In-office use of conscious sedation in periodontics. Academy Report. American Academy of Periodontology *Journal of Periodontology*, 72:968–975.

American Academy of Periodontology (2006) American Academy of Periodontology Statement on Local Delivery of Sustained or Controlled Release Antimicrobials as Adjunctive Therapy in the Treatment of Periodontitis. *Journal of Periodontology*, 77:1458.

American Association of Endodontists (1995) Management of acute pain. *Endodontics Colleagues for Excellence*, Spring/Summer:1–4.

American Society of Anesthesiologists (2007) ASA Physical Status Classification System. Available at (ahttp://www.asahq.org/clinical/physicalstatus.htm (accessed October 3, 2011).

Archer, J.S. & Archer D.F. (2002) Oral contraceptive efficacy and antibiotic interaction: a myth debunked. *Journal of the American Academy of Dermatology*, 46:917–923.

Aronoff, D.M., Oates, J.A. & Boutaudm O. (2006) New insights into the mechanism of action of acetaminophen: its clinical pharmacologic characteristic reflect its inhibition of the two prostaglandin H2 synthases. *Clinical Pharmacology and Therapeutics*, 79:9–19.

Awtry, E.H. & Loscalzo, J. (2000) Aspirin. *Circulation*, 101:1206–1218.

Ballow, C.H. & Amsden, G.W. (1992) Azithromycin: the first azalide antibiotic. *The Annals of Pharmacotherapy*, 26:1253–1261.

Barclay, L. (2011) Acetaminophen: repeated use of slightly too much can be fatal. *British Journal of Pharmacology*, Published online November 22, 2011. Available from www.medscape.com/viewarticle/754104?sssdmh.73674&src=nldne

Bauer, K.L. & Wolf, D. (2005) Do antibiotics interfere with the efficacy of oral contraceptives? *The Journal of Family Practice*, 54:1079–1080.

Bautista, L.E. & Vera, L.M. (2010) Antihypertensive effects of aspirin: what is the evidence? *Current Hypertension Reports*, 12:282–289.

Bell, W.R. (1998) Acetaminophen and warfarin. Undesirable synergy. *Journal of the American Medical Association*, 279:702–703.

Chambers, H.F. (2003) Bactericidal vs. bacteriostatic antibiotic therapy: a clinical mini review. *Clinical Updates in Infectious Diseases*, VI(4):October.

Cooper, S.A. (1993) Narcotic analgesics in dental practice. *Compendium*, 14:1061–1068.

Cornell, R. (1987) Contraindications for using topical steroids. *The Western Journal of Medicine*, 147:459.

Cowan, F.F. (1992) Analgesics. In: *Dental Pharmacology*, 2nd edn (ed. Cowan, F.F.), pp. 164–203. Lea & Febiger,. Philadelphia, PA.

Denisco, R.C., Kenna, G.A., ONeil, M.G. *et al.* (2011) Prevention of prescription opioid abuse. *The role of the dentist. Journal of the American Dental Association*, 142:800–810.

Elliott, W.J. (2010) Do the blood pressure effects of nonsteroidal anti-inflammatory drugs influence cardiovascular morbidity and mortality? *Current Hypertension Reports*, 12:258–266.

Emmert, D.H. (2000) Treatment of common cutaneous herpes simplex virus infections. *American Family Physician*, 61:1697–1604, 1705–1706, 1708.

Engelkirk, .PG., Duben-Engelkirk, J. (2010) Controlling microbial growth in vivo using antimicrobial agents. In: *Burton's Microbiology for the Health Sciences*, 9th edn, Chapter 9. p. 147. Lippincott Williams & Wilkins, Philadelphia, PA.

Fairbanks, D.N.J. (2007) *Pocket Guide to Antimicrobial Therapy in Otolaryngology – Head and Neck Surgery*, 13th edn. American Academy of Otolaryngology – Head & Neck Surgery Foundation, Inc., Alexandria, VA.

Farrell, S.E., Tarabar, A., Burns, M.J., et al. (2012) Acetaminophen toxicity. Medscape Reference. www.emedicine.medscape.com/article/820200-overview#aw2aab6b2b2.

Fathallah-Shaykh, S. (2011) Fanconi syndrome clinical presentation. Available at www.emedicine.medscape.com/article981774-clinical#a0218.

Ference, J.D. & Last, A.R. (2009) Choosing topical corticosteroids. *American Family Physician*, 79:135–140.

Fujimoto, J.M. (1979) Pharmacokinetics and drug metabolism. In: *Practical Drug Therapy* (ed. Wang, R.J.H.), pp. 11–16. J.B. Lippincott Company, Philadelphia.

Ganda, K.M. (2008) Odontogenic infections and antibiotics commonly used in dentistry: assessment, analysis, and associated dental management guidelines. In: *Dentist's Guide to Medical Conditions and Complications* (ed. Ganda, K.) pp. 63–82. Wiley-Blackwell. Ames, IA.

Gibson, J. & McGowan, D.A. (1994) Oral contraceptives and antibiotics: important considerations for dental practices. *British Dental Journal*, 177:419–422.

Glasheen, J.J., Fugit, R.V. & Prochazka, A.V. (2005) The risk of overanticoagulation with antibiotic use in outpatients on stable warfarin regimens. *Journal of General Internal Medicine*, 20: 653–656.

Goureitch, M.N. & Arnsten, J.H. (2005) Medical complications of drug abuse. In: *Substance Abuse. A Comprehensive Textbook* (eds Lowinson, J.H., Ruiz P. & Millman, R.B.) pp. 840–862. Lippincott Williams & Wilkins, Philadelphia, PA.

Granados-Soto, V., López-Muñoz, F.J., Castañeda-Hernández, G., *et al.* (1993) Characterization of the analgesic effects of paracetamol and caffeine in the pain-induced functional impairment model in the rat. *Journal of Pharmacy and Pharmacology.* 45:627–631.

Grant, G.M. & Mehlisch, D.R. (2010) Intranasal ketorolac for pain secondary to third molar implaction surgery: a randomized double-blind, placebo-controlled trail. *Journal of Oral and Maxillofacial Surgery*, 68:1025–1031.

Grover, S.A., Coupal, L. & Zowall, H. (2005) Treating osteoarthritis with cyclo-oxygenase-2-specific inhibitors: what are the benefits of avoiding blood pressure destabilization? *Hypertension*, 45:92.

Haffajee, A.D., Yaskell, T. & Socransky, S.S. (2008) Antimicrobial effectiveness of an herbal mouthrinse compared with an essential oil and a chlorhexidine mouthrinse. *Journal of the American Dental Association*, 139:606–611.

Herbert, M,E., Brewster, G.S. & Lanctot-Herbert, M. (2000) Ten percent of patients who are allergic to penicillin will have serious reactions if exposed to cephalosporins. *Western Journal of Medicine*, 172:341.

Hersh, E.V., Kane, W.T., O'Neil, M.G. *et al.* (2011) Prescribing recommendations for the treatment of acute pain in dentistry. *Compendium*, 32(3):22–31.

Hersh, E.V. (1999) Adverse drug reactions in dental practice: interactions involving antibiotics. *Journal of the American Dental Association*, 130:236–251.

Hoang, T., Jorgensen, M.A.G., Kelm, R.G. *et al.* (2003) Povidone-iodine as a periodontal pocket disinfectant. *Journal of Periodontal Research*, 38:311–317.

Huynh, M.P. & Yagiela, J.A. (2003) Current concepts in acute pain management. *Journal of the California Dental Association*, 31:419–427.

Hylek, E.M., Heiman, H., Skates, S.J. *et al.* (1998) Acetaminophen and other risk factors for excessive warfarin anticoagulation. *Journal of the American Medical Association*, 279:657–662.

Hyllested, M., Jones, S., Pedersen, J.L. & Kehlet, H. (2002) Comparative effect of paracetamol, NSAIDs or their combination in postoperative pain management: a qualitative review. *British Journal of Anaesthesia*, 88:199–214.

Jeske, A.H. (2002) Selecting new drugs for pain control: evidence-based decisions or clinical impressions? *Journal of the American Dental Association*, 133:1052–1056.

Katz, W.A. (2002) Use of nonopioid analgesics and adjunctive agents in the management of pain in rheumatic disease. *Current Opinion in Rheumatology*, 14:63–71.

Kekety, R. & Shah, A.B. (1993) Diagnosis and treatment of *Clostridium difficile* colitis. *Journal of the American Medical Association*, 269:71–75.

Kekety, B., Silva, J., Kauffman, C. *et al.* (1989) Treatment of antibiotic-associated *Clostridum difficle* colitis with oral vancomycin: comparison of two dosage regimens. *American Journal of Medicine*, 86:15–19.

Klepser, M.E., Nicolau, D.P., Quintillian, I R. *et al.* (1997) Bactericidal activity of low-dose clindamycin administered at 8- and 12-hour intervals against *Staphylococcus aureus*, *Streptococcus pneumoniae*, and *Bacteroides fragilis*. *Antimicrobial agents and Chemotherapy*, 41:630–635.

Leonhardt, A., Bergström, C., Krok, L. *et al.* (2007) Microbiological effect of the use of an ultrasonic device and iodine irrigation in patients with severe chronic periodontal disease: a randomized controlled clinical study. *Acta Odontologica Scandinavica*, 65:52–59.

Loesche, W. & Grossman, N. (2001) Periodontal disease as a specific, albeit chronic, infection: diagnosis and treatment. *Clinical Microbiology Reviews*, 414:727–752.

Lomaestro, B.M. (2009) Do antibiotics interact with combination oral contraceptives? Available from Medscape. www.medscape.com/viewarticle/707926.

McAleer, S.D., Majid, O., Venables, E. *et al.* (2007) Pharmacokinetics and safety of ketorolac following single intranasal and intramuscular administration in health volunteers. *Journal of Clinical Pharmacology*, 47:13–18.

McFarland, L.V., Surawicz, C.M., Greenberg, R.N. *et al.* (1994) A randomized placebo-controlled trial of *Saccharomyces boulardii* in combination with standard antibiotics for *Clostridium difficile* disease. *Journal of the American Medical Association*, 271;1913–1918.

Medical Economics Staff (2000) Advice for the patient. *USP DI* Vol 2. Thomson MICRONEDEX, Colorado.

Medve, R.A., Wang, J. & Karim, R. (2011) Tramadol and acetaminophen tablets for dental pain. *Anesthesia Progress*, l58:79–81.

Mehlisch, D.R. (2002) The efficacy of combination analgesic therapy in relieving dental pain. *Journal of the American Dental Association*, 133:861–871.

Messerli, F.H. & Sichrovsky, T. (2005) Does the pro-hypertensive effect of cyclo-oxygenase-2 inhibitors account for the increased risk in cardiovascular disease? *American Journal of Cardiology*, 96:872.

Montgomery, E.H. & Droeger, D.C. (1984) Use of antibiotics in dental practice. *Dental Clinics of North America*, 28:433–453.

Osborne, NG. (2004) Antibiotics and oral contraceptives: potential interactions. *Journal of Gynecologic Surgery*, 18:171–172.

Page, II, R.L. (2005) Weighing the cardiovascular benefits of low-dose aspirin. *Pharmacy Times*. ACPE Program I.D. Number 290-000-05-H01.

Patrono, C., Coller, B., FitzGerald, G.A. *et al.* (2004) Platelet-active drugs: the relationhips among dose, effectiveness, and side effects. The Seventh ACCP Conference on Antithrombotic and Thrombolytic Therapy. *Chest*, 234S–264S.

Prater, C.D., Zylstra, R.G. & Miller, K.E. (2002) Successful pain management for the recovering addicted patient. *Prim Care Companion Journal of Clinical Psychiatry*, 4:125–131.

Schwartz, S.R. (2006) Perioperative pain management. *Oral and Maxillofacial Surgical Clinics of North America*, 18:139–150.

Schrader, S.P., Fermo, J.D. & Dzikowski, A.L. (2004) Azithromycin and warfarin interaction. *Pharmacotherapy*, 24:945–949.

Sefton, A.M., Maskell, J.P., Beighton, D. *et al.* (1996) Azithromycin in the treatment of periodontal disease. Effect on microbial flora. *Journal of Clinical Periodontology*, 23:998–1003.

Segelnick, S.L. & Weinberg, M.A. (2010) Doxycycline-induced dizziness in the dental patient. *New York State Dental Journal*, 76:28–32.

Segelnick, S.L. & Weinberg, M.A. (2008) Recognizing doxycycline-induced esophageal ulcers in dental practice. A case report and review. *Journal of the American Dental Association*, 139:581–585.

Shakeri-Nejad, K. & Stahlmann, R. (2006) Drug interactions during therapy with three major groups of antimicrobial agents. *Expert Opinion on Pharmacotherapy*, 6:639–651.

Sharma,R. & Dronen, S.C. (2011) Herpes simplex in emergency medicine mediation. Available from http://emedicine.medscape.com/article/783113-medication#2 (accessed 11 December 2011).

Swift, J.Q. & Hargreaves, K.M. (1993) Pentazocine analgesia: is there a niche for Talwin Nx? *Compendium*, 14:1048,1050.

Trelle, S., Reichenbach, S.,Wandel, S. *et al.* (2011) Cardiovascular safety of non-steroidal anti-inflammatory drugs: network meta-analysis. *British Medical Journal*, 342:c7086.

Turner CL, Eggleston GW, Lunos S, *et al.* (2011) Sniffing out endodontic pain: use of an intranasal analgesic in a randomized clinical trial. *Journal of Endodontics*, 37:439–444.

Ubara, Y., Tagami, T., Suwabe, T. *et al.* (2005) A patient with symptomatic osteomalacia associated with Fanconi syndrome. *Modern Rheumatology*, 15:207–212.

Vergani, S.A., Silva, E.B., Vinholis, A.H. *et al.* (2004) Systemic use of metronidazole in the treatment of chronic periodontitis: a pilot study using clinical, microbiological, and enzymatic evaluation. *Brazilian Oral Research*, 18:121–127.

Waknine, Y. (2009) FDA Safety Changes: Zantac, Zithromax, Noxafil. Medscape Today. Available from (www.medscape.com/viewarticle/701796 (accessed 11 December 2011).

Walton, G.M., Rood, R.P., Snowdon, A.T. *et al.* (1993) Ketorolac and diclofenac for postoperative pain relief following oral surgery. *British Journal of Oral and Maxillofacial Surgery*, 31:158–160.

Warner, T.D. & Mitchell, J.A. (2008) COX-2 selectivity alone does not define the cardiovascular risks associated with non-steroidal anti-inflammatory drugs. *Lancet*, 371:270.

Weinberg, M.A. (2002) Antimicrobial drugs In: *Oral Pharmacology* (eds Weinberg, M.A., Westphal, C. & Fine, J.B.), pp. 100–135. Pearson Education Inc., New Jersey.

World Health Organization. (1986). *Cancer Pain Relief*. WHO, Geneva.

World Health Organization (2004) *Medical eligibility criteria for contraceptive use*, 3rd edn. Reproductive Health and Research, WHO, Geneva.

Zanchetti, A., Hansson, L., Leonetti, G. *et al.* (2002) Low-dose aspirin does not interfere with the blood pressure-lowering effects of antihypertensive therapy. *Journal of Hypertension*, 20:1015.

Zichterman, A. (2007) Opioid pharmacology and considerations in pain management. *US Pharmacist*. Available from www.uspharmacist (accessed 10 April 2011).

Zigdon, H., Levin, L., Filatov, M. *et al.* (2012) Intraoperative bleeding during open flap debridement and regenerative periodontal surgery. *Journal of Periodontology*, 83:55–60.

Additional websites

http://www.pharmacytimes.com/publications/issue/2009/2009–06/RxFocusDrugInteractions-0609

http://emedicine.medscape.com/article/1049648-overview

http://emedicine.medscape.com/article/783113-overview Herpes Simplex in emergency medicine. Sharma R.

St. Pierre SA, Bartlett BL, Schlosser BJ. Practical management measures for patients with recurrent herpes labialis. http://www.medscape.com/viewarticle/715208

Chapter 5

How to manage potential drug interactions

I. Introduction to drug interactions

Q. What are the different types of drug interactions?

A.
a. Pharmacokinetic drug interactions: A change in the pharmacokinetics of one drug caused by the interacting drug. Examples include: inhibition of absorption, cytochrome (CYP) P450 enzymes, altered renal excretion and altered plasma protein binding.
b. Pharmacodynamic drug interaction: A change in the pharmacodynamics of one drug caused by the interacting drug. There are different types of pharmacodynamic drug interactions:

*   Additive (same response as the sum of the two drugs individually)
*   Synergistic (greater response)
*   Antagonistic (less of a response).

Examples include: additive effects when two or more drugs with similar pharmacodynamic effects are given together resulting in excessive response and possible toxicity; synergistic effects where the effects of two drugs taken together is greater than the sum of their separate effect at the same dose and; antagonistic effects where drugs with opposing therapeutic effects may reduce the response to one or both drugs. For instance, nonsteroidal anti-inflammatory drugs (NSAIDs) that increase blood pressure may inhibit the anti-hypertensive effects of angiotensin-converting enzyme (ACE) inhibitors when given together (Hansten & Horn 2003).

Synergistic drug interaction: The effect of two or more drugs when administered together is greater than if the drugs were given separately; may produce responses equivalent to over dosage. For example, patients with hypertension do not respond adequately with one drug must take combination drugs (Meredith & Elliott 1992).

Q. How are drug–drug/food interactions rated according to how much of an impact it makes?

A. Table 5.1 classifies the rating of drug interactions.

Q. What is the relative importance of drug interactions in dentistry?

A. Many drug interactions are usually harmless or go clinically unnoticed; many of those which are potentially harmful occur in only a small percentage of patients given the interacting drugs. Results of the interaction differ among individuals and may be more serious in one patient than another. The drugs most often involved in serious interactions are those with a small therapeutic index, such as phenytoin and those where the dose must be carefully controlled according to the response, as with anticoagulants, antidiabetics and antihypertensives. The elderly and patients with impaired renal and liver function are especially prone to drug interactions.

The Dentist's Drug and Prescription Guide, First Edition. Mea A. Weinberg and Stuart J. Froum.
© 2013 John Wiley & Sons, Inc. Published 2013 by John Wiley & Sons, Inc.

Table 5.1   Rating of drug interactions.

Severity rating	Documentation rating
Major: Potentially life threatening or causing permanent body damage	Established: Proven with clinical studies to cause an interaction
Moderate: Could change the patient's clinical status and require hospitalization	Probable: Very likely to cause an interaction
Minor: Only mild effects are evident or no clinical changes seen	Suspected: Supposed to cause an interaction, but more clinical studies are required
	Possible: Limited data proven
	Unlikely: Not certain to cause an interaction

Q. When does a drug interaction show clinically?

A. It depends. Factors that must be taken into account include the drugs half-lives, the dosages that are being administered and the mechanism of metabolism. For example, if the offending drug takes a long time to accumulate, the interaction may be delayed several days. However, if the patient is receiving a large dose of the drug, the interaction may occur more rapidly. Also, if the patient is not getting the expected response from the drugs then a drug–drug interaction could be suspected.

Q. Explain the cytochrome P450 enzyme interactions?

A. Few drugs are eliminated from the body unchanged in the urine. Most drugs are metabolized or chemically altered to a less lipid-soluble compound which is more easily eliminated from the body. One way of metabolizing drugs involves alteration of groups on the drug molecule via the cytochrome P450 enzymes. These enzymes are found mostly in the liver, but can also be found in the intestines, lungs, and other organs. Each enzyme is termed an isoenzyme, because each derives from a different gene. There are more than 30 cytochrome P450 enzymes present in human tissue.

Q. How does one drug interact with another drug via the cytochrome P450 enzymes?

A. The *substrate* is a drug that is metabolized by a specific CYP450 isoenzyme. An *inhibitor* is a drug that inhibits or reduces the activity of a specific CYP450 isoenzyme. An *inducer* is a drug that increases the amount and activity of that specific CYP450 isoenzyme.

Q. When does a drug interaction occur via the cytochrome P450 enzymes?

A. Drug interactions can occur when a drug that is metabolized and/or inhibited by these cytochrome enzymes is taken concurrently with a drug that decreases the activity of the same enzyme system (e.g., an inhibitor). The result is often increased concentrations of the substrate. Another scenario is when a substrate that is metabolized by a specific cytochrome enzyme is taken with a drug that increases the activity of that enzyme (e.g., an inducer). The result is often decreased concentrations of the substrate.

Some substrates are also inhibitors for the same enzyme, probably due to competitive inhibition of enzyme activity. Some inhibitors affect more than one isoenzyme and some substrates are metabolized by more than one isoenzyme (Weinberg, 2002).

Q. What are common drug–drug interactions that occur with the cytochrome P450 isoenzymes that are significant in dentistry?

A. Table 5.2 lists common drugs (related to drugs the patient is taking and dental medications prescribed to the patient) that are metabolized (substrate) by specific cytochrome P450 isoenzymes and the drugs that inhibit (inhibitor) or

Table 5.2   Substrates (drugs) metabolized by specific isoenzymes.

Isoenzyme	Drug
CYP1A2	Amitriptyline (Elavil) Clozapine (Clozaril) Haloperidol (Haldol) Imipramine (Tofranil) Fluvoxamine (Luvox) Tacrine (Cognex) Theophylline
CYP2C9	Nonsteroidal anti-inflammatory drugs (NSAIDs) [ibuprofen, naproxen, celecoxib (Celebrex)] Glipizide (Glucotrol) Glyburide (Micronase, DiaBeta) Irbesartan (Avapro) Losartan (Cozaar) Phenytoin (Dilantin) Warfarin (Coumadin)
CYP2C19	Amitriptyline (Elavil) Diazepam (Valium) Imipramine (Tofranil) Lansoprazole (Prevacid) Omeprazole (Prilosec) Pantopropazole (Protonix)
CYP2D6	Amitriptyline (Elavil) Clomipramine (Anafranil) Codeine and its derivatives (oxycodone, hydrocodone) Doxepin (Sinequan) Fluoxetine (Prozac) Haloperidol (Haldol) Imipramine (Tofranil) Lidocaine (local) (Xylocaine) Metoprolol (Lopressor) Nortriptyline (Pamelor) Paroxetine (Paxil) Propranolol (Inderal) Risperidone (Risperdal) Timolol (Blocadren) Tramadol (Ultram) Venlafaxine (Effexor)
CYP2E1	Acetaminophen (Tylenol) Ethanol
CYP3A4	Alprazolam (Xanax) Amitriptyline (Elavil) Amlodipine (Norvasc) Aripiprazole (Abilify) Atorvastatin (Lipitor) Citalopram (Celexa) Clarithromycin (Biaxin) Clomipramine (Anafranil) Clonazepam (Klonopin)

(continued)

Table 5.2   (*cont'd*)

Isoenzyme	Drug
	Cyclosporine
	Diltiazem (Cardizem)
	Erythromycin
	Ethinyl estradiol/progesterone (oral contraceptives)
	Fluoxetine (Prozac)
	Haloperidol (Haldol)
	Hydrocodone (Vicodin with acetaminophen)
	Indinavir (Crixivan)
	Ketoconazole (Nizoral)
	Lidocaine, topical
	Lovastatin (Mevacor)
	Methadone
	Methylprednisone
	Midazolam (Versed)
	Nelfinavir (Viracept)
	Nifedipine (Procardia, Adalat)
	Oxycodone (Percodan with acetaminophen)
	Prednisone
	Ritonavir (Norvir)
	Saquinavir (Invirase)
	Sertraline (Zoloft)
	Theophylline
	Simvastatin (Zocor)
	Sirolimus
	Sertraline (Zoloft)
	Tacrolimus (Prograf)
	Triazolam (Halcion)
	Verapamil (Calan)
	Warfarin (Coumadin)

accelerate (inducer) the specific isoenzyme causing a drug interaction. Please note: only commonly encountered drugs used in dentistry are listed. There are many more drugs involved in the cytochrome P450 isoenzyme metabolism. Please refer to Hersh & Moore, 2004 and Cupp & Tracey, 1998 for more details.

Q. Which are the most abundant cytochrome enzymes in humans?

A. The CYP3A isoenzymes make up about 30% of all cytochromes in the liver.

Q. Why is it important to know about substrates and inhibitors and how are the tables used?

A. Inhibitors are drugs prescribed by the dentist that can interfere with a substrate or a drug already taken by the patient. Tables 5.3 and 5.4 are used to look up a drug that you are prescribing to see if it is an inhibitor or an inducer of an iso-enzyme. If it is found on the table then determine which isoenzyme is affected and then go to Table 5.2 to see if the patient is taking a drug that is metabolized by that isoenzyme.

    If the dentist prescribes a drug that could inhibit the metabolism of the above substrate (look under the correct CYP isoenzyme) then possibly there is a drug interaction that could result in toxicity (elevated plasma levels) of the substrate. It is necessary to check on the list to avoid this problem. For example, if the patient is taking atorvastatin for cholesterol problems and an antibiotic is needed because of a dental infection and the patient is allergic to penicillin, clarithromycin (Biaxin) should not be prescribed because according to the table, clarithromycin is a *potent* inhibitor of atorvastatin,

Table 5.3 Inhibitors (drugs) of specific cytochrome P450 isoenzymes: the drugs listed on the right side inhibit the specific isoenzyme on the left side of the table.

CYP1A2	Ciprofloxacin (Cipro) Fluvoxamine (Luvox) Grapefruit juice
CYP2C9	Fluconazole (Diflucan) Ketoconazole (Nizoral) Metronidazole (Flagyl)
CYP2C19	Fluoxetine (Prozac) Ketoconazole (Diflucan) Sertraline (Zoloft) Ticlopidine (Ticlid)
CYP2D6	Cimetidine (Tagamet) Cocaine Fluoxetine (Prozac) Paroxetine (Paxil) Sertraline (Zoloft)
CYP2E1	Disulfiram (Antabuse)
CYP3A4	Clarithromycin (Biaxin) Erythromycin Grapefruit juice Ketoconazole (Diflucan)

Table 5.4 Inducers (drugs) of the CYP450 isoenzymes.

CYP1A2	Charcoal-broiled meat Smoking
CYP2C9	Rifampin
CYP2C19	No drugs
CYP2D6	No drugs
CYP2E1	Ethanol Isoniazid (INH)
CYP3A4	Carbamazepine (Tegretol) Dexamethasone St. John's wort

Hersh & Moore 2004.

resulting in toxic plasma levels of the statin drug. If it is appropriate prescribe clindamycin or azithromycin (Zithromax). Remember that azithromycin is not metabolized by the CYP isoenyzmes so that there are less drug interactions. Table 5.3 lists common inhibitors of the above substrates.

Q. What could happen if the patient is taking alprazolam (Xanax) for anxiety and is prescribed clarithromycin or erythromycin?

A. Excessive central nervous system (CNS) depression could occur.

II.   Antibiotic drug interactions in dentistry

Q. What are common significant antibiotic drug–drug interactions can be seen in the dental practice?

A. Table 5.5 lists clinically significant drug–drug/food interactions in dentistry.

Table 5.5   Clinically significant antibiotic–drug/food interactions in dentistry.

Drug	Interacting drug	Effect	What to do
Doxycycline (including doxycycline 20 mg and Atridox) Minocycline (including Arestin)	Antacids (magnesium hydroxide/aluminum hydroxide), zinc, iron (ferrous sulfate)	Decreased *amount* of doxycycline and minocycline absorption into the blood	Do not take both drugs at same time. Take these products 2 hours apart from the doxycycline.
	Penicillins	Interferes with bactericidal effect of penicillins	Do not take at same time; take penicillin a few hours before doxycycline.
	Warfarin	Increased anticoagulant effect	Minimal risk; monitor patients for enhanced anticoagulant effects; warfarin dosage may need adjustments.
	Oral contraceptives	May interfere with contraceptive effect; altered enterohepatic recirculation	May not be clinically significant; some sources say to use alternative methods of birth control.
	Phenytoin (Dilantin)	Decreased serum doxycycline levels	Either switch to another antibiotic or monitor.
	Vitamin A or related compounds (e.g., retinoids – isotretinoin (Accutane), acitretin, tretinoin)	Risk of pseudotumor cerebri or benign intra cranial hypertension	Tetracyclines including doxycycline and minocycline are contraindicated; choose another antibiotic
	Methotrexate	Elevated serum methotrexate concentrations	Avoid using doxycycline in patients taking high-dose methotrexate
Tetracycline	Antacids (magnesium hydroxide/aluminum hydroxide), calcium-containing products (including calcium containing foods such as milk), zinc, iron(ferrous sulfate)	Decreased tetracycline absorption into the blood	Do not take concurrently. Space 2 hours apart from these products.

(*continued*)

Table 5.5 *(cont'd)*

Drug	Interacting drug	Effect	What to do
	Warfarin	Possible interaction: increased anticoagulant effect due to decrease production of vitamin K in the gut from inhibition of bacteria that produce the vitamin K.	Minimal risk; monitor patients for enhanced anticoagulant effects.
	Penicillins	Interferes with bactericidal effect of penicillins	Do not take at same time; take penicillin a few hours before tetracycline.
	Digoxin	Digoxin is partially metabolized by bacteria in intestine; increased digoxin blood levels	Either switch antibiotic or monitor for increased serum digoxin levels.
	Oral contraceptives	May interfere with contraceptive effects; altered enterohepatic recirculation	May not be of clinical significance; some sources recommend to use alternative birth control.
	Vitamin A or related compounds (e.g., retinoids – isotretinoin (Accutane), acitretin)	Risk of pseudotumor cerebri or benign intra cranial hypertension	Tetracyclines including doxycycline and minocycline are contraindicated; choose another antibiotic
	Methotrexate	Elevated serum methotrexate concentrations	Avoid using doxycycline in patients taking high-dose methotrexate
Penicillins (amoxicillin)	Erythromycin, tetracyclines	Decreased effectiveness of penicillin	Do not take at same time; give the penicillin a few hours before the tetracycline.
	Probenecid (Benemid): drug for gout	Inhibits penicillin excretion	Can take together; make sure penicillin levels are not excessive.
	Oral contraceptives	May interfere with contraceptive effects	May not be clinically significant; some say to use alternative birth control methods.
	Methotrexate	Reduced clearance with high doses of penicillins	Only seen in a small group; not enough evidence to avoid. Monitor and consult with physician.
Erythromycins Erythromycin & clarithromycin	Theophylline	Increased theophylline levels	Avoid together; consult with physician; reduce theophylline dosage to avoid toxicity.

(continued)

Table 5.5 (cont'd)

Drug	Interacting drug	Effect	What to do
	Advir Diskus, HFA	Increase levels of salmeterol increasing risk of ventricular arrhythmias and increases levels of fluticasone	Avoid coadministration
	Carbamazepine (Tegretol)	Increased carbamazepine levels seen as ataxia, vertigo, drowsiness	Avoid concurrent use.
	Statins: atorvastatin (Lipitor), simvastatin (Zocor). lovastatin (Mevacor), including combination drugs (amlodipine/atorvastatin)	Increases statin levels (increased myopathy, including muscle pain)	Either switch to azithromycin or to another statin drug like lovastatin (Mevacor) or pravastatin (Pravachol).
	Oral contraceptives	Interfere with contraceptive effects; altered enterohepatic recirculation	Some sources recommend alternative birth control.
	Digoxin	Increased digoxin levels (see increased salivation and visual disturbances) Increased	Switch antibiotic to penicillin. Monitor for signs of digoxin toxicity or switch antibiotic.
	Cyclosporine	Cyclosporine toxicity	Cyclosporine doses may need reduction.
	Ergot alkaloids [e.g., ergotamine (Bellergal-S, Cafergot)] (for migraine headache)	Toxic ergot levels (ergotism; pain, tenderness, and low skin temperature of extremities)	Use azithromycin or another antibiotic.
	Benzodiaepines: including alprazolam (Xanax) midazolam (Versed) triazolam (Halcion)	Increased sedation	Avoid combination; use alternative drugs.
	Citalopram (Celexa)	Dose-dependent prolongation of the QT interval with increased risk of ventricular arrhythmias	Avoid concurrent use.
	Calcium channel blocker: disopyramide (Norpace)	Prolongation of QTc interval	Switch to another antibiotic or monitor for development of arrhythmias.
	Class 1A (disopyramide, quinidine, procainamide) and Class III antiarrhythmia drugs (amiodarone, dofetilide, sotalol)	Causes dose-related prolongation of the QT interval with increased risk of ventricular arrhythmias	Avoid concurrent use.
	Warfarin (Coumadin)	Increases anticoagulant (bleeding) effect	Switch to another antibiotic such as clindamycin or penicillin or monitor for INR values; contact physician.

(continued)

Table 5.5 (cont'd)

Drug	Interacting drug	Effect	What to do
	Haloperidol (Haldol)	Causes dose-related prolongation of the QT interval with increased risk of ventricular arrhythmias	Avoid concurrent use.
	Methadone	Increased risk of QT prolongation with increased risk of ventricular arrhythmias due to an additive effect	Avoid use both drugs together/use alternative.
Azithromycin	Food delays absorption of azithromycin capsules, however tablets may be taken without regard to food.	Decreased absorption resulting in a major reduction in bioavailability	Take on an empty stomach (1 hour before or 2 hours after meals).
	Aluminum and magnesium antacids	Decrease the rate but not the extend of azithromycin absorption	Take antacid 1 hour before or 2 hours after azithromycin.
	Warfarin	Increases bleeding	Contact physician; monitor INR values or switch to another antibiotic that does not interact with warfarin.
	Pimozide (Orap): typical antipsychotic to control repeated movement caused by Tourette's disorder	Increased risk of QT prolongation with increased risk of ventricular arrhythmias due to an additive effect	Contraindicated to use both drugs together.
	Dronedarone (Multaq): for atrial fibrillation	Increased risk of QT prolongation with increased risk of ventricular arrhythmias due to an additive effect	Contraindicated to use both drugs together.
	Phenothiazine antipsychotics (e.g., chlorpromazine, fluphenazine, promethazine, thioridazine)	Increased risk of QT prolongation with increased risk of ventricular arrhythmias due to an additive effect	Contraindicated to use both drugs together.
	Class 1A (disopyramide, quinidine, procainamide) and Class III antiarrhythmia drugs (amiodarone, dofetilide, sotalol)	Causes dose-related prolongation of the QT interval with increased risk of ventricular arrhythmias	Avoid concurrent use/use alternative antibiotic.
	Haloperidol (Haldol)	Causes dose-related prolongation of the QT interval with increased risk of ventricular arrhythmias	Avoid concurrent use.

(continued)

Table 5.5 (*cont'd*)

Drug	Interacting drug	Effect	What to do
	Methadone	Increased risk of QT prolongation with increased risk of ventricular arrhythmias due to an additive effect	Avoid use both drugs together/use alternative.
Fluoroquinolones [ciprofloxacin (Cipro), levofloxacin (Levaquin)	Di-and trivalent cations (e.g., antacids, iron, calcium, zinc)	Decreases fluoroquinolone effect because of decreased absorption	Do not take together; space dose apart either 4 hours before or 2 hours after the fluoroquinolone dose.
	Caffeine	Increases caffeine effects	Do not take together.
	Warfarin	Increases anticoagulant effect	Monitor INR more frequently; consult with patient's physician.
	Steroids (e.g., prednisone)	Increased risk of tendinitis and tendon rupture (Achilles tendon)	Caution is recommend when fluoroquinolones are taken at same time with steroid. Best to avoid.
	Pimozide (Orap)	Increased risk of QT prolongation with increased risk of ventricular arrhythmias due to an additive effect	Contraindicated to use both drugs together.
	Pimozide (Orap): typical antipsychotic to control repeated movement caused by Tourette's disorder	Increased risk of QT prolongation with increased risk of ventricular arrhythmias due to an additive effect	Contraindicated to use both drugs together.
Clindamycin (Cleocin)	Neuromuscular blockers (succinylcholine)	Increased neuromuscular blocking effect	Since most dental patients are not taking these drugs, there are no special precautions.
	Oral contraceptives	Reduced efficacy of oral contraceptive	Caution advised; limited evidence with clindamycin.
Metronidazole (Flagyl)	Alcohol (drinking alcohol, using alcohol mouthrinse, alcohol in foods)	Severe disulfiram-like reaction with headache, flushing and nausea	Avoid alcohol up to at least 3 days after discontinuing metronidazole.
	Warfarin	Inhibits warfarin metabolism; increased anticoagulant effect	High risk: Contact physician; adjustment of warfarin dosage or select different antibiotic.
	Lithium	Lithium excretion inhibited resulting in toxic levels	Contact physician.
	Phenytoin	Increased phenytoin levels	Contact physician.

Note: Most drug–drug or drug–food interactions occur when two or more drugs are taken at the same time. To avoid these interactions most drug dosing is spaced so as not to administer them concurrently. If in doubt, the patient's physician should be contacted. www.drugs.com.

Q. Is there a drug interaction between alcohol and metronidazole?

A. Yes. Ingestion of alcohol when taking metronidazole and for 1 week after metronidazole is stopped can result in a disulfiram-like reaction. Disulfiram (Antabuse) is a medication used to wean individuals off alcohol. Chronic alcoholics are treated with disulfiram. If alcohol is ingested while on disulfiram an acute psychoses (hallucinations) and confusion, abdominal cramps, nausea, facial flushing and a headache can occur. These are similar reactions that also occur with metronidazole.

Q. Can alcohol-containing mouthrinses be used while taking metronidazole?

A. No. Any product containing alcohol is contraindicated. This includes alcohol-containing mouthrinses, foods with alcohol and skin-to-skin contact with perfumes.

Q. How long after finishing the course of metronidazole can alcohol be started?

A. About 3 days after the metronidazole is finished.

Q. Is there a drug interaction if antibiotics are initiated in patients taking warfarin (Coumadin; an anticoagulant)?

A. Yes. There is an increase in both the incidence and degree of over-anticoagulation with certain antibiotic use in patients taking warfarin. In these cases there is an elevation of international normalized ratio (INR) associated with a change in bleeding events. It is suggested that all antibiotics should have warning labels about an increased warfarin effect, the most common antibiotics/antifungal agents causing this drug interaction include: metronidazole, tetracyclines, trimethoprim/sulfamethoxazole (Bactrim), ciprofloxacin (Cipro) azithromycin (Zithromax) and fluconazole (Diflucan). In 2009, the FDA approved label revisions for azithromycin, warning of a potential interaction with warfarin. The exact cause of this interaction is not clear. However, there are a few proposed mechanisms: (1) these antibiotics can decrease the metabolism of warfarin (warfarin is metabolized in the liver by CYP2C9), primarily inhibitors of CYP2C9, resulting in bleeding or (2) antibiotics inhibit gastrointestinal flora which produce vitamin K_2, which is associated with the body's natural clotting factors. With less absorption of vitamin K due to the antibiotic there can be an increase in anticoagulation when warfarin is administered concurrently. Signs of this interaction include increased bruising and bleeding. Even a modest inhibition in warfarin metabolism could lead to a considerable risk of bleeding. Dosage reduction of warfarin may be necessary. Consultation with the patient's physician is necessary (Sims & Sims, 2007; Glasheen *et al.*, 2005; Rice *et al.*, 2003).

Q. Is there a drug interaction between antibiotics and oral contraceptives?

A. Historically, the first case involving an interaction between oral contraceptives and antibiotics was with rifampin, an antituberculosis drug (Skolnick *et al.*, 1976). Oral contraceptives (OCs) available in the United States include estrogen–progestin monophasic, biphasic, or triphasic combination products and progestin-only products. Reports and concerns exist regarding the hypothesis that oral antibiotics can reduce the efficacy of combination OCs. One of many proposed mechanisms is that about 50% of ethinylestradiol, the estrogen component in OC needs to be activated by intestinal bacteria and undergo enterohepatic circulation (Hansten & Horn, 2003). Once activated it is then reabsorbed as active drug. Antibiotics affect intestinal bacteria so that estrogen cannot be activated. The American College of Obstetricians and Gynecologists concluded that tetracycline (Sumycin), doxycycline (Vibramycin, Doryx), metronidazole (Flagyl) and quinolones do not affect OC steroid levels in women taking combination OCs. (American College of Obstetricians and Gynecologists, 2006) However, dental literature has implicated amoxicillin, metronidazole and tetracycline in reducing the effective of oral contraceptives (ADA Council on Scientific Affairs, 2002; Hersh, 1999). The World Health Organization (WHO) (2004) states that there have been suspicions that broad-spectrum antibiotics may lower OC effectiveness based on case reports, but that pregnancy rates are similar among women on OCs and women on both OCs and antibiotics. Essentially, it is a rare interaction but can occur (DeRossi & Hersh, 2002). Today's concentration of estrogen is much lower than years ago. However, a small decrease in efficacy especially in the "low-dose" (<35 μg estrogen) combination OCPs when taken with an oral contraceptive has been documented (Burroughs & Chambliss, 2000).

The ADA Council on Scientific Affairs recommends advising patients of the potential risk of the antibiotic reducing the effectiveness of the oral contraceptive and advising the patient to discuss with her physician the use of an additional nonhormonal type of contraception and to continue compliance with oral contraceptives while on antibiotics (ADA Council on Scientific Affairs, 2002). In any case, it is best to advise the female patient taking OCs to select a nonhormonal back-up birth control for at least 2 weeks after discontinuation of the antibiotic or through the end of the current cycle, whichever is longer, switch the patient to an OC with a higher dose of estrogen and progestin for one cycle or to abstain from sexual activity (Horn & Hansten, 2003; Osborne, 2002).

Q. What is the mechanism of the drug interaction between metronidazole and lithium?

A. It is a pharmacokinetic interaction whereby metronidazole decreases the renal clearance of lithium resulting in elevated lithium plasma levels.

Q. Are clarithromycin and azithromycin both inhibitors of the cytochrome P450 enyzmes?

A. Clarithromycin is a potent inhibitor but azithromycin is much less involved resulting in less drug–drug interactions (Schrader *et al.*, 2004).

III.   Analgesic drug interactions in dentistry

Q. What are common significant analgesic drug–drug interactions that can be seen in the dental practice?

A. Table 5.6 lists common analgesic drug–drug interactions.

Q. If a patient is taking warfarin is it safe to give ibuprofen as an analgesic after a dental procedure?

A. No. This is a synergistic drug–drug interaction where both the warfarin and ibuprofen increase the risk for bleeding. Warfarin is an anticoagulant that inhibits the vitamin K-dependent clotting factors and ibuprofen and aspirin are antiplatelet drugs that inhibit the formation of thromboxane A_2 by inhibiting the cyclo-oxygenase enzyme. The better choice for an analgesic for a patient taking warfarin would be acetaminophen alone or in combination with a narcotic such as acetaminophen with codeine or acetaminophen with hydrocodone. However, there is also a drug–drug interaction between warfarin and acetaminophen. If a patient is taking warfarin and acetaminophen is recommended, the prothrombin time should be measured once or twice a week and should not exceed an INR of 4.0 beyond which there is an increased incidence of bleeding. So, if acetaminophen is recommended in a patient taking warfarin notifying the patient's physician with careful patient monitoring is necessary. Additionally, the lowest dose for the shortest duration is advised (Bell, 1998; Hylek *et al.*, 1998).

Q. What is the mechanism of the interaction between an NSAID such as ibuprofen and warfarin?

A. When an NSAID and warfarin are taken together the NSAID decreases plasma protein binding of warfarin, resulting in an increase in the circulation or plasma levels of warfarin because the NSAID displaces warfarin from the proteins in the plasma.

Q. Is there a drug interaction between ibuprofen and antihypertensive medications such as diuretics, ACE inhibitors and beta-blockers?

A. Yes. NSAIDs such as ibuprofen and naproxen (Aleve) alter the effectiveness of certain antihypertensive medications including diuretics, ACE inhibitors, and beta-blockers, but not calcium channel blockers (e.g., nifedipine, amlodipine, diltiazem, verapamil). NSAIDs inhibit renal prostaglandin synthesis, thus blocking the antihypertensive's mechanism of action. It is recommended that NSAIDs be used only short term (not for more than 5 days) if taking the offending antihypertensive drug but are contraindicated in patients with congestive heart failure or in patients with low

Table 5.6 Analgesic drug–drug interactions.

Drug	Interacting drug	Effect	What to do?
Aspirin and nonsteroidal anti-inflammatory drugs (NSAIDs) (ibuprofen, naproxen)	Warfarin	Synergistic anticoagulant effects with aspirin and NSAIDs (increased bleeding)	Avoid concurrent use/contact patient's physician.
	Angiotensin-converting enzyme (ACE) inhibitors (e.g., enalapril, captopril); beta-blockers, angiotensin II receptor blockers (ARBs)	With NSAIDs: decrease antihypertensive response (lowers blood pressure). Short-term course (5 days) may not significantly increase blood pressure. This drug interaction does not occur with aspirin or low-dose aspirin	Interaction causes lowering of blood pressure. Monitor blood pressure. Use alternative analgesic such as acetaminophen or narcotic after 5 days or more of use of NSAIDs.
	Lithium	NSAIDs inhibits renal clearance of lithium	Decrease lithium dosage. Best to use diflunisal (Dolobid).
	Oral antidiabetic drugs (occurs with aspirin)	Aspirin and NSAIDs increase hypoglycemic effects	Limited importance.
	Furosemide (Lasix)	Decreased diuretic effect	Monitor patient.
	Venlafaxine (Effexor)	Possible serotonin syndrome	Avoid concurrent use.
	Phenytoin (Dilantin)	Decreased hepatic phenytoin metabolism (increased serum levels)	No special precautions.
	Aspirin or NSAID	Synergistic effect (increased bleeding)	Contraindicated.
	Low-dose aspirin + ibuprofen	Ibuprofen may inhibit cardioprotective effect of low-dose aspirin	Avoid concurrent use.
Acetaminophen	Alcohol	Increase incidence of hepatotoxicity (liver disease)	Contraindicated in alcoholics; avoid taking together.
	Carbamazepine (Tegretol)	Increase risk of acetaminophen toxicity	Avoid concurrent use or maximum amount of acetaminophen use <2 g/day.
	Warfarin	Increased anticoagulant effect	Avoid concurrent use. May require adjustment of warfarin dosage. Contact physician.
Narcotics (codeine, hydrocodone, oxycodone, meperidine)	fluoxetine (Prozac), sertraline (Zoloft) and paroxetine (Paxil)	These selective serotonin reuptake inhibitors (SSRIs) are potent inhibitors of CYP2D6 and can delay the metabolism of codeine resulting in less of an analgesic response because codeine and its derivatives require metabolism to be effective	Do not take together; An increase in the codeine dosage or a different analgesic agent may be necessary in patients requiring therapy with CYP450 2D6 inhibitors. Or space doses apart or prescribe the parent compound such as hydromorphone.

(continued)

Table 5.6   *(cont'd)*

Drug	Interacting drug	Effect	What to do?
	Other depressants such as alcohol or drugs (e.g., benzodiazepines, CNS depressants)	Increase sedative properties	Do not take together or limit the amount of alcohol.
	Amiodarone (Cordarone) and quinidine (medicines for cardiac arrhythmias)	These medications are potent inhibitor of CYP2D6. Pain relief would not occur, but there will unpleasant side effects	Do not take together; An increase in the codeine dosage or a different analgesic agent may be necessary in patients requiring therapy with CYP450 2D6 inhibitors. Or space doses apart or prescribe the parent compound such as hydromorphone.
	Haloperidol (Haldol)	This typical antipsychotic is a potent inhibitor of CYP2D6	Do not take together; An increase in the codeine dosage or a different analgesic agent may be necessary in patients requiring therapy with CYP450 2D6 inhibitors. Or space doses apart or prescribe the parent compound such as hydromorphone.
	Indinavir (Crixivan) (an HIV protease inhibitor for HIV/AIDS).	potent inhibitor of CYP2D6	Do not take together; An increase in the codeine dosage or a different analgesic agent may be necessary in patients requiring therapy with CYP450 2D6 inhibitors. Or space doses apart or prescribe the parent compound such as hydromorphone.

concentrations of kidney renin. In these cases, it is best to use acetaminophen (Hass, 1999). On the other hand, aspirin does not alter the effectiveness of antihypertensive medications (Bautista & Vera, 2010).

Q. If a patient is taking ibuprofen but finds it not effective in reducing the pain, can another NSAID be taken such as Aleve or acetaminophen to increase the analgesic effectiveness?

A. No. The addition of another NSAID or acetaminophen if you are already taking an NSAID may increase the chance of developing renal damage in long-term use. Short duration using this combination is less likely to cause kidney damage. It is recommended that acetaminophen or another NSAID not be taken within 3 days of another NSAID (Haas, 1999; Henrich *et al.*, 1996).

IV. Sympathomimetic agents and drug interactions in dentistry

Q. What are common significant vasoconstrictor/drug interactions that can occur in dental practice?

A. Table 5.7 lists common sympathomimetic (in local anesthetics)–drug interactions.

Q. What are the effects of epinephrine on the sympathetic receptors in the body?

A. Theoretically epinephrine binds to all sympathetic receptors (α_1, α_2, β_1, β_2) in the body. Epinephrine in low concentrations (two to three cartridges) achieved systemically after anesthetic injections in dentistry is fairly selective for beta receptors rather than α-receptors. The β_2-receptors, when activated, cause peripheral vasodilation in skeletal muscle blood vessels, thus lowering total peripheral resistance and therefore diastolic blood pressure which is governed by peripheral vascular resistance. At the same time, the β_1- (and β_2)-receptors in the heart are activated to increase cardiac output and therefore systolic blood pressure; this is influenced by peripheral vascular resistance as well, but is also heavily influenced by the cardiac output, which epinephreine increases strongly. With an increase in systolic blood pressure and a decrease in diastolic blood pressure, there is no real change in mean blood pressure; these two influences cancel each other out regarding mean blood pressure. A couple of cartidges (two or three) typically will cause a slight or no rise in systolic BP and a slight fall in diastolic BP.

However, in higher doses (more than three or four cartridges) α_1-receptors are also stimulated. Since there are more of them, the net effect is vasoconstriction throughout the body, and an increase in peripheral resistance. This results in an increase in both systolic and diastolic blood pressure, and a possible reflex slowing of the heart mediated by the vagus nerve releasing acetylcholine onto the sinoatrial node (Hersh & Giannakopoulos, 2010; Yagiela, 1999).

Q. Is there an interaction between epinephrine and noncardioselective beta-blockers such as propranolol and timolol?

A. Yes. Although rare it can happen. The interaction is due to the nonselective blocking of both β_1- and β_2-adrenoceptors (named after the adrenergic nerves that innervate them) allowing the binding of epinephrine to α_1-receptors, which results in vasoconstriction and possible increase in blood pressure (hypertension). It is important to avoid intravascular injection of the local anesthetic (Hersh & Giannakopoulos, 2010).

Q. What is the mechanism of the interaction between epinephrine in a local anesthetic and a tricyclic antidepressant?

A. The hypothesis of depression is that there is a decrease in the amount of norepinephrine and serotonin in the brain. Tricyclic antidepressants, such as amitriptyline (Elavil) and clomipramine (Anafranil), work by inhibiting the reuptake of norepinephrine from the synapse by blocking the noradrenergic reuptake pump allowing more of norepinephrine to stay in the neuronal synapse. Injected epinephrine can be terminated by two ways: metabolized by catechol-*O*-methltransferase (COMT) and neuronal reuptake by the noradrenergic reuptake pump, the same pump that takes up norepinephrine. Thus, if the pump is not removing epinephrine from the synapse it will accumlate. Accumulation of epinephrine from the local anesthetic could essentially cause cardiac arrhythmias and hypertension in a patient taking a tricyclic antidepressant. The amount of epinephrine should be limited to two cartridges of 1:100 000 (Goulet *et al.*, 1992).

Q. Is there an interaction between epinephrine and other antidepressants such as selective serotonin reuptake inhibitors (SSRIs) such as Zoloft or Lexapro?

A. No. The same is not true for SSRIs such as fluoxetine (Prozac), fluvoxamine (Luvox), citalopram (Celexa), escitalopram (Lexapro), paroxetine (Paxil), and sertraline (Zoloft), because SSRIs stop the movement of serotonin back into neurons by inhibiting the serotonin reuptake pump and not the noradrenergic reuptake pump so that SSRIs have no affect on epinephrine.

Q. Is epinephrine contraindicated in patients taking monoamine oxidase (MAO) inhibitors?

A. No. Theoretically, there are no restrictions for using epinephrine in patients taking MAO inhibitors such as isocarboxazid (Marplan), phenelzine (Nardil), tranylcypromine (Parnate), and selegiline (Eldepryl). MAO inhibitors do not affect the noradrenergic reuptake pump.

Table 5.7 Sympathomimetic drug–drug interactions.

Drug	Interacting drug	Effect	What to do?
Epinephrine (contained in local anesthetics)	Nonselective ($\beta_1\beta_2$) beta-blockers such as propranolol (Inderal), nadolol (Corgard), timolol (Blocadren) and sotalol (Betapace)	Elevated blood pressure and heart rate because these drugs block both β-receptors allowing epinephrine to bind to alpha-receptors which causes vasoconstriction of skin and mucous membranes. Care must be taken when injecting to avoid intravascular administration. The patient's vital signs should be recorded before the injection and five minutes afterward. If there are no cardiac changes additional local anesthetic can be administered.	Epinephrine should be used cautiously. Limit the amount used to 0.04 mg (two cartridges of a local anesthetic with 1:100 000 epinephrine).
	Selective beta-blockers (β_1) such as atenolol(Tenormin), metoprolol(Lopressor), acebutolol(Sectral) and betaxolol(Kerlone)	No elevation in blood pressure because these drugs bind only to the β_1-receptors.	No concerns especially in the controlled hypertensive.
	Tricyclic antidepressants [e.g., amitriptyline (Elavil)]	Hypertension (enhances sympathomimetic effects)	Treat similar to the cardiac patient; maximum amount is two cartridges of a local anesthetic containing epinephrine 1:100 000.
	Typical phenothiazidine antipsychotics (α-receptor blockers) such as haloperidol and chlorpromazine (Thorazine). The "newer" atypical antipsychotics [e.g., risperidone (Risperdal), olanzapine (Zyprexa), quetiapine (Seroquel), aripiprazole (Abilify) and ziprasidone (Geodon)]	"Older" typical antipsychotic blocks α_1-receptors resulting in orthostatic hypotension. Epinephrine in low doses causes β_2 stimulation which may worsen the hypotension. This interaction is rare but if accidental intravascular injection there is a possibility for a hypotension episode. The "newer" atypical antipsychotics have much less α-receptor blocking action and thus less incidence of orthostatic hypotension. These atypical antipsychotics are more prescribed today because of less adverse effects from binding to the different receptors.	Use epinephrine cautiously; use as low a dose as possible especially with the typical antipsychotics because of its actions on alpha receptors.
	Cocaine	Increased heart contraction leading to death	Do not use epinephrine if the patient used cocaine within 24 hours.
	Marijuana (cannabis)	Seriously prolongs tachycardia in an intoxicated patient. Peak blood levels occur within 10 minutes	Best to use a local anesthetic without vasoconstrictor if you suspect the patient has just used marijuana.
	Methamphetamine	Methamphetamine is an amphetamine which is an adrenergic receptor agonist which increases norepinephrine release. Duration of action can be from 8 to 12 hours.	Avoid using epinephrine which can result in a severe myocardial infarction. Use a local anesthetic without a vasoconstrictor.

*Note: these are the more commonly severe drug interactions. www.drugs.com.

Q. Are there any interactions with lidocaine?

A. Yes. Lidocaine is contraindicated in patient with known hypersensitivity to amide local anesthetics, a severe degree of SA, AV or intraventricular heart block (if not with pacemaker), or Adams-Stokes syndrome. There is controversial regarding Wolff-Parkinson-White syndrome.

Q. Can epinephrine be used safely in patients taking antipsychotics?

A. First, there are two types of antipsychotics indicated for the treatment of schizophrenia: "older" typical antipsychotics and the "newer" atypical antipsychotics. The typical antipsychotics include phenothiazines such as chlorpromazine (Thorazine), and other neuroleptic drugs such as haloperidol (Haldol), trifluoperazine (Stelazine) and control the acute symptoms but not the emotional response.

The typical "older" antipsychotics such as haloperidol have high affinity to α_1-receptors, which causes the adverse effect of orthostatic hypotension. Theoretically, epinephrine stimulates β_2-receptors causing vasodilation and hypotension. It is a rare event. The "newer" atypical antipsychotics include:

- Risperidone (Risperdal)
- Olanzapine (Zyprexa)
- Quetiapine (Seroquel)
- Aripiprazole (Abilify)
- Ziprasidone (Geodon)
- Lurasidone (Latuda).

Introduced since 1990, some atypicals have much less α_1- and α_2-receptor blocking action and thus fewer incidences of orthostatic hypotension and work primarily by blocking serotonin 5-HT receptors and dopamine receptors. No two atypical antipsychotics have the same binding affinities to the receptors. For instance, risperidone binds much less to alpha receptors than olanzapine and quetiapine (Goulet *et al.*, 1992; Yagiela, 1999).

There are numerous annoying adverse effects because typical and atypical antipsychotics bind to many different receptors. Some adverse effects include (Table 5.8).

Epinephrine has a paradoxical hypotensive effect in persons taking typical antipsychotics. The typical antipsychotics may inhibit or reverse the vasopressor (vasocontrictor) effect of epinephrine. Many of these agents, including the atypical antipsychotics, exhibit α_1-adrenergic blocking activity and produce hypotension as an adverse effect. Use of epinephrine in patients receiving neuroleptic therapy may cause a paradoxical further lowering of blood pressure, since beta stimulation (due to epinephrine in low doses) may worsen hypotension in the setting of alpha blockade. There may be less of an interaction between the atypical antipsychotics because some cause less alpha-receptor blockage because of less binding affinity (e.g., risperidone and less affinity than clozapine, quetiapine and olanzapine). However, it is best to avoid or use a low dose of epinephrine in these patients (http://www.drugs.com/drug-interactions/epinephrine-with-phenergan-989-0-1949-1259.html).

Q. Is there an interaction between epinephrine and drugs for attention deficit hyperactivity disorder (ADHD)?

A. Even though some drugs such as atomoxetine (Strattera) inhibit the noradrenergic reuptake pump similar to tricyclic antidepressants there have not been any adverse reports with the use of injected epinephrine. Other drugs used for

Table 5.8 Adverse effects.

- α-Adrenergic receptor blockade: orthostatic hypotension, reflex tachycardia (body's response to a decrease in blood pressure by increasing heart rate in an attempt to raise blood pressure) and sexual dysfunction
- Muscarinic receptor blockade: xerostomia, confusion
- Histamine receptor blockade: sedation/drowsiness, weight gain
- Serotonin receptor blockade: weight gain
- Dopamine blockade: extrapyramidal side effects

Table 5.9   Anti-anxiety (benzodiazepines) drug–drug interactions.

Drug	Interacting drug	Effect	What to do?
Benzodiazepines Diazepam(Valium) Alprazolam (Xanax) Midazolam (Versed) Triazolam (Halcion)	Grapefruit juice	Inhibits CYP3A4 enzyme, decreasing metabolism of these drugs thus increasing blood levels	The duration of effect of grapefruit juice – do not take juice while on these drugs.
	Cimetidine (Tagamet)	Inhibits diazepam elimination Increases CNS depression	Little clinical importance.
	Opioids (codeine, hydrocodone)	Increases CNS depression	Avoid taking together.
	Clarithromycin	Increase benzodiazepine levels; increased sedation	contraindicated; use alternative drugs.
	HIV protease inhibitors	Increase benzodiazepine levels	Contraindicated.
	HIV efavirenz/ emtricitabine/tenofovir	Increase benzodiazepine levels	Contraindicated.
	Isoniazid (INH)	Increase benzodiazepine levels	Contraindicated.

www.drugs.com.

ADHD include amphetamine or amphetamine-like stimulants which could increase the risk of cardiovascular events in children and adults with preexisting cardiovascular disease. It is recommended to monitor blood pressure and heart rate in these patients and limit the use of epinephrine to 0.4 to 0.54 mg (Hersh & Moore, 2008).

Q. Is epinephrine contraindicated in patients with a true sulfite allergy?

A. Yes. If a patient has a true sulfite allergic another local anesthetic without epinephrine should be used.

V.   Anti-anxiety drug interactions in dentistry

Q. What are common significant anti-anxiety (benzodiazepine) drug–drug/food interactions can be seen in the dental practice?

A. Table 5.9 lists common anti-anxiety drug–drug/food interactions.

Q. Does grapefruit juice alter the metabolism of drugs?

A. Yes. Furanocoumarin compounds found in grapefruit interfere with liver and intestinal cytochrome P450 isoenzymes by inhibiting CYP3A4. Any drug that is metabolized by CYP3A4 will have a decreased breakdown if taken with grapefruit juice which can result in increased plasma levels of the drug (toxicity). Grapefruit juice is also a P-glucoprotein inhibitor. The management of these drug interactions is basically to avoid having grapefruit when taking any medication. The only dental drugs that can be affected by grapefruit juice include: hydrocodone, oxycodone, carbamazepine (Tegretol), and benzodiazepines (diazepam, triazolam, midazolam, alprazolam) (Stump *et al.*, 2006).

References

American Dental Association Council on Scientific Affairs (2002) Antibiotic interference with oral contraceptives. *Journal of the American Dental Association*, 133:880.

American College of Obstetricians and Gynecologists (2006) Use of hormonal contraception in women with coexisting medical conditions. *American College of Obstetricians and Gynecologists Practice Bulletin*, 107:1453–1472.

Bautista, L.E. & Vera, L.M. (2010) Antihypertensive effects of aspirin: what is the evidence? *Current Hypertension Reports*, 12:282–289.

Bell, W.R. (1998) Acetaminophen and warfarin. Undesirable synergy. *Journal of the American Medical Association*, 279:702–703.

Burroughs, K,E, & Chambliss, M.E. (2000)Antibiotics and oral contraceptive failure. *Archives of Family Medicine*, 9:81–82.

Cupp, M.J. & Tracy, T. (1998) Cytochrome P450: new nomenclature and clinical implications. *American Family Physcian*, 57:107–116.

DeRossi, S.S. & Hersh, E.V. (2002) Antibiotics and oral contraceptives. *Dental Clinics of North America*, 46:653–654.

Glasheen, J.J., Fugit, R.V. & Prochazka, A.V. (2005) The risk of overanticoagulation with antibiotic use in outpatients on stable warfarin regimens. *Journal of General Internal Medicine*, 20:653–656.

Goulet, J.P., Pérusse, R. & Turcotte, J.Y. (1992) Contraindications to vasoconstrictors in dentistry. *Part III. Oral Surgery Oral Medicine Oral Pathology*, 74:692–297.

Haas, D.A. (1999) Adverse drug interactions in dental practice: interactions associated with analgesics. Part III in a series. *Journal of the American Dental Association*, 130:397–407.

Hansten, P. & Horn, J. (2003) Drug–drug interaction mechanisms.Available from www.hanstenandhorn.com/article-d-i.html (accessed 13 December 2011).

Henrich, W.L., Agodoa, L.E., Barrett, B., *et al.* (1996) Analgesics and the kidney: summary and recommendations to the Scientific Advisory Board of the National Kidney Foundation from an Ad Hoc Committee of the National Kidney Foundation. *American Journal of Kidney Disease*, 27:162–165.

Hersh, E.V. (1999) Adverse drug reactions in dental practice: interactions involving antibiotics. *The Journal of the American Dental Association*, 130:236–251.

Hersh, E.V. & Giannakopoulos, H. (2010) Beta-adrenergic blocking agents and dental vasococntrictors. *Dental Clinics of North America*, 2054:687–696.

Hersh, E.V. & Moore, P.A. (2004) Drug interactions in dentistry: The importance of knowing your CYPs. *The Journal of the American Dental Association*, 135:298–311.

Hersh, E.V. & Moore, P.V. (2008) Adverse drug interactions in dentistry. *Periodontology* 2000, 46:109–142.

Hylek, E.M., Heiman, H., Skates, S.J., *et al.* Acetaminophen and other risk factors for excessive warfarin anticoagulation. *The Journal of the American Medical Association*, 279:657–662.

Meredith, P.A. & Elliott, H.L. (1992) An additive or synergistic drug interaction: application of concentration-effect modeling. *Clinical Pharmacology & Therapeutics*, 51:708–714.

Osborne, N.G. (2002) Antibiotics and oral contraceptives: potential interactions. *Journal Gynecologic Surgery*, 18:171–172.

Rice, P.J., Perry, R.J., Afzal, Z., *et al.* (2003) Antibacterial prescribing and warfarin: a review. *British Dental Journal*, 194:411–415.

Schrader, S.P., Fermo, J.D. & Dzikowski, A.L. (2004) Azithromycin and warfarin interaction. *Pharmacotherapy*, 24:945–949.

Sims, P.J. & Sims, K.M. (2007) Drug interactions important for periodontal therapy. *Periodontology* 2000, 44:15–28.

Skolnick, J.L., Stoler, B.S., Katz, D.B. *et al.* (1976) Rifampin, oral contraceptives, and pregnancy. *Journal of the American Medical Association*, 236:1382.

Stump, A.L., Mayo, T., Blum, A. (2006) Management of grapefruit-drug interactions. *American Family Physician*, 15(74):605–608.

Weinberg, M,A. (2002) Drug interactions in dentistry. In: *Oral Pharmacology* (eds. Weinberg, M..A., Westphal, C. & Fine, B.F.) pp. 68–96. Pearson, Upper Saddle River NJ.

World Health Organization (WHO) (2004) *Medical Eligibility Criteria for Contraceptive Use*, 3rd edn. Reproductive Health and Research, WHO, Geneva.

Yagiela, J.A. (1999) Adverse drug interactions in dental practice: interactions associated with vasoconstrictors. Part V of a series. *Journal of the American Dental Association*, 130:701–709.

Chapter 6

Evidence-based theory for drug prescribing

I. General considerations

Q. Is it appropriate to prescribe antibiotics against postsurgical infections in implant/periodontal surgery and oral/maxillofacial surgery?

A. Yes and No. It has been reported that presurgical antibiotics and good surgical technique reduced postoperative infection to 1%. The longer the surgical procedure, the higher the incidence of postoperative infection. A single prophylactic antibiotic dose is sufficient and using antibiotics after the surgery is not indicated unless extensive surgery is performed with soft tissue manipulation in which antibiotics is recommended to continue for 3 days following the surgery. The decision to use postsurgical antibiotics depends on the patient (e.g., diabetic patient). So, the clinical situation should be evaluated before any antibiotics are prescribed. Use of an antimicrobial rinse such as chlorhexidine gluconate can also be prescribed pre-and postsurgery (Resnik & Misch, 2008).

Q. For antibiotic prophylaxis how many hours or days before the dental procedure should the systemic antibiotic be administered?

A. To have the maximum effect, the antibiotic should be in the tissues when the bacterial contamination occurs, not after. In order for this to happen, the antibiotic needs to be administered only about 1 to 2 hours before surgery to attain plasma levels 3 to 4 times the minimum inhibitory concentration (MIC) needed to kill bacteria (Peterson, 1990). The antibiotic does not need and should not be given the day before or several days before the surgery (Classen *et al.*, 1992).

Q. What is the usual prophylactic dose of antibiotic that should be prescribed preoperatively?

A. According to Peterson (1990), In order to attain high levels in the plasma for the maximal therapeutic response, the dose is usually twice that of the regular dose; it is equivalent to administering the loading dose. For example, if the usual dose of penicillin VK is 500, prescribe 1 g. or some dentists give the same dose that the American Heart Association recommends for prophylaxis against bacteremia which is 2 g one hours before the dental procedure.

Q. Should there be a concern with development of bacterial resistance when prescribing short-term prophylactic antibiotics before a surgical procedure?

A. No. Selective growth of resistant bacteria begins only once the host's susceptible organisms are killed, which occurs in about 3 days of antibiotic use. Thus, one day/time of antibiotic use does not affect the development of resistant bacteria (Peterson, 1990).

The Dentist's Drug and Prescription Guide, First Edition. Mea A. Weinberg and Stuart J. Froum.
© 2013 John Wiley & Sons, Inc. Published 2013 by John Wiley & Sons, Inc.

Q. Does the selected antibiotic need to be effective against primarily anaerobic or aerobic bacteria?

A. Since the oral environment is usually 2:1 anaerobic to aerobic bacteria it is best to choose an antibiotic effect against both periodontal pathogens (Resnik & Misch, 2008). The rest of the chapter will give recommendations for using specific antibiotics with a specific bacterial infection.

The following reviews the classification of bacteria:

- Gram-positive facultative cocci: *Streptococcus sanguis, mitis, salvarius, Staphylococcus aureus*
- Gram-positive facultative rods: *Actinomyces* (including *A. viscosus, A. naeslundii*)
- Gram-negative facultative rods: *Eikenella corrodens, Capnocytophaga* spp. *Aggregatibacter actinomycetemcomitans* (formerly *Actinobacillus actinomycetemcomitans*).
- Gram-positive obligate anaerobic coccus: *Peptostreptococcus* spp.
- Gram-positive obligate anaerobic rods: *Eubacterium* spp.
- Gram-negative obligate anaerobic rods: *Porphyromonus gingivalis, Prevotella intermedia, Tannerlla forsynthesis* (formerly *Bacteroides forsythus*), *Fusobacterium nucleatum*.
- Gram-negative anaerobic spirochete: *Treponema* spp.
- Obligate aerobic: *Mycobacterium tuberculosis, Pseudomonas aeruginosa.*

Q. What can happen if antibiotics are used indiscriminately?

A. The indiscriminate use of systemic antibiotics could influence the emergence of resistant bacterial strains which would be resistant to eradication by antibiotics. However, as stated in a previous question, development of resistant strains after 1 day of antibiotic use will most likely not happen. Allergies to drugs may also develop.

Q. Is it best to use a single antibiotic or combinations?

A. Depending upon the results of antimicrobial testing and susceptibility combination antibiotic therapy may be necessary in mixed infections. It could be more advantageous to use combination drugs because the simultaneous use of two drugs of the same category (e.g., two bactericidal antibiotics) can achieve bactericidal synergism, allowing a reduction in dose or a shorter duration of therapy. For example, amoxicillin and metronidazole are effect against *Aggregatibacter actinomycetemcomitans*, where either antibiotic alone is ineffective (Jorgensen & Slots, 2000). Combination drugs can also help to reduce the emergence of resistant bacterial strains. A disadvantage of using multiple antibiotics is the increased incidence of adverse effects and potential drug-drug interactions. For example, prescribing a bacteriostatic antibiotic such as tetracycline with a bacteriostatic drug such as amoxicillin is not advised because the bactericidal antibiotic requires active multiplying bacteria in order to destroy the bacteria.

Q. Is it appropriate to start therapy with a broad-spectrum antibiotic?

A. When prescribing antibiotics the risk vs. benefits must be considered. Broad-spectrum antibiotics increase the incidence of superinfections with *Candida* sp., enteric rods, pseudomonads, and staphylococci and increase the emergence of resistant bacterial strains.

Q. Should the prophylactic antibiotic be bactericidal or bacteriostatic?

A. Bactericidal. The antibiotic should kill the bacteria rather than inhibiting multiplication and reproduction.

Q. What is the inoculum effect?

A. The maximum concentration to have a therapeutic effect may be insufficient even with the recommended prescribed dose because of the large number of bacteria present in untreated periodontal pockets. Thus, the minimum inhibitory concentration (MIC) of a certain antibiotic may actually be higher than the standard MIC for that drug.

II.   Prescribing for inflammatory periodontal diseases and periodontal surgical procedures

Q. Do antibiotics have a role in the management of periodontal disease and periodontal therapy?

A. Yes. In some cases antibiotics have been shown to be helpful in the co-management of periodontal diseases and the selective use of antibiotics will help to avoid inappropriate prescribing.

Q. If systemic antibiotics are indicated in the adjunctive management of certain periodontal diseases, when should antibiotics be started during therapy?

A. Antibiotics should never be used alone without accompanied by mechanical debridement (scaling and root planing) and/or periodontal surgery. Sometimes antibiotics can be prescribed following initial therapy (scaling and root planing) and microbiological testing.

Q. Why is it necessary to use antibiotics in conjunction with scaling and root planing?

A. Mechanical debridement is necessary to disrupt the bacterial biofilm (colonies). This makes it easier for the antibiotic to penetrate the bacterial cell.

a.   Gingivitis

Q. What bacteria are primarily found in chronic gingivitis?

A. Predominant bacteria in chronic gingivitis includes *Actinomyces* spp., *Capnocytophaga* spp., *Fusocbacterium* spp. and *Streptococcus* spp. (*S. mitis, S. oralis, S. sanguis, S. gordonii, S. intermedius*) (Teles *et al.*, 2007).

Q. Is antibiotic therapy used for chronic gingivitis?

A. Although chronic gingivitis is a bacterial infection, there is no current literature to support the use of systemic antibiotics because the infection is localized to the gingival unit with shallow probable depths which is easily treatable and reversible with mechanical debridement (scaling) and optimal oral hygiene.

Q. Is there any rationale for using antimicrobial agents for the treatment of chronic gingivitis?

A. There is no rationale for using systemic antibiotics in the treatment of chronic gingivitis. Topical antimicrobials including chlorhexidine gluconate may be used as an *adjunct* to scaling and root planing to help control the gingival inflammation but should never be used without mechanical debridement.

Q. Are there any cons for using systemic antibiotics in chronic gingivitis?

A. Yes. No literature supports the use of antibiotics. Indiscriminate use of antibiotics leads to adverse effects including bacterial resistance and unnecessary adverse effects.

b.   Chronic periodontitis

Q. What are the bacteria found in inflammatory chronic periodontitis?

A. Predominant bacteria in chronic periodontitis (CP), previously referred to as adult periodontitis, include all of the bacteria in gingivitis in addition to obligate anaerobes: *Porphyromonas gingivalis* and *Prevotella intermedii* and facultative anaerobes: *Fusobacterium* spp., *Eikinella corrodens, Tannerella forsythensis* (formerly *Bacteroides forsythus*), *Aggregatibacter actinomycetemcomitans* (*Aa*) (formerly known as *Actinobacillus actinomycetemcomitans*), *Actinomyces naseslundii, Peptostreptococcus* spp., *A. viscosus, Veillonella* spp. and *Treponema denticola*.

Q. Do some bacteria actually invade the gingival tissues (junctional epithelium and gingival connective tissue)?

A. Some bacteria actually invade the inflamed gingival tissues rather than merely staying in the periodontal pocket. The prevalence of *P. gingivalis* and *T. forsythensis* was found not to be significantly different in chronic and aggressive periodontitis patients in either the plaque or the tissues. Prevalence of *Aa* in gingival tissue was higher in the localized aggressive periodontitis (63%) group than in either the chronic periodontitis (16%) or the generalized aggressive periodontitis (38%) group. *A. actinomycetemcomitans* serotype c was detected in 50% of localized aggressive periodontitis tissue samples (Thiha *et al.*, 2007).

Q. Is systemic antibiotic therapy used in the treatment of inflammatory chronic periodontitis?

A. The use of systemic antibiotics in "garden variety" chronic periodontitis is very controversial. Some studies show that the addition of antibiotics to mechanical debridement may reduce the need for further treatment including surgery. In the 1980s Loesche showed a benefit of using antibiotics as an adjunct (or after subgingival debridement) to conventional periodontal treatment in "reducing the need for periodontal surgery" in patients with chronic periodontitis. Actually these patients although defined as having chronic periodontitis could have had refractory periodontitis. In Loesche's studies the need for surgery or extractions was determined 4 to 6 weeks after initial treatment which consisted of scaling and root planing and metronidazole 250 mg, three times a day for 7 days. Results showed a decrease in teeth requiring surgery, pocket probing depths and subgingival bacteria (Bacteriodes and spirochetes) and an apparent gain in periodontal attachment (Loesche *et al.*, 1984, 1991, 1992, 1996). Metronidzole is only effective against obligate anaerobes and not *Aa*, *Eikenella corrodens*, and *Capnocytopha*.

Other studies using amoxicillin plus metrondizole as an adjunct to mechanical debridement have resulted in improved clinical parameters and high percentage of eliminate of *Aa* and *P.gingivalis* in *advanced* chronic and refractory chronic periodontitis (van Winkelhoff *et al.*, 1992).

Sefton *et al.*, (1996), reported that azithromycin (500 mg once daily) consistently reduced spirochetes in chronic periodontitis patients throughout the 22 weeks of the study, but only reduced pigmented anaerobes at 3 and 6 weeks. Additional long-term studies using larger number of subjects need to be performed.

On the other hand, there are some clinical studies that have documented that there are no additional treatment outcome benefits when antibiotics are used as an adjunct to scaling and root planing and periodontal pocket elimination surgery (Slots & Rams, 1990). The first clinical periodontal studies using tetracycline was in chronic periodontitis patients, found no statistically significant differences in probing depth reduction but a slight improvement in attachment levels (Listgarten *et al.*, 1978). Currently, systemic antibiotics are not indication for chronic periodontitis.

Q. Are there any cons for prescribing systemic antibiotics for chronic periodontitis?

A. Yes. Failing to recognize the patient has chronic periodontitis may cause the indiscriminate use of antibiotics which may increase the incidence of bacterial resistance and increased incidence of adverse effects. It must be determined that the chronic periodontitis patient is actually a refractory periodontitis patient and then antibiotics are indicated. For plain "garden variety" chronic periodontitis patients systemic antibiotics offer little or no advantage when used as an adjunct to conventional periodontal therapy.

Q. What is doxycycline 20 mg?

A. Doxycycline 20 mg is considered to be a subantimicrobial dose and is indicated for the management of generalized chronic periodontitis. The trade name was Periostat but it is now available generically as doxycycline hyclate 20 mg. Usual antibiotic doses are 100–200 mg but at 20 mg doxycycline exerts anticollagenase activity rather than antibacterial activity. Doxycycline 20 mg inhibits the synthesis and secretion of collagenase which is an enzyme that breaks down collagen which makes up the periodontium (bone, connective tissue). This anticollagenase property does not depend on the drug's antibacterial actions. Doxycycline 20 mg is indicated for generalized chronic periodontitis especially in cases where scaling and root planing are ineffective in halting the progression of attachment loss.

Q. Clinically, what are the outcomes of prescribing doxycycline hyclate 20 mg?

A. Gain of clinical or periodontal attachment and decreased probing depth.

Q. What does gain of clinical attachment mean?

A. After periodontal therapy (e.g., scaling and root planing) reduction of probing depths as a result of gingival recession and/or removal of inflammatory infiltrate in the gingival connective tissue with reformation of collagen fibers. Healing after conventional periodontal therapy is usually via a long junctional epithelium.

Q. Do the same contraindications/precautions with doxycycline follow with doxycycline 20 mg?

A. Yes. Doxycycline 20 mg should not be used in pregnant women or breast feeding. Inform female patients on oral contraceptives. There is possible development of resistant bacterial strains.

Q. What is the recommended dosage for doxycycline hyclate 20 mg?

A. Taken twice a day (every 12 hours) as an adjunct to scaling and root planing for up to 9 months.

Q. What are specific instructions on how to take the drug?

A. Take on an empty stomach at least 1 hour before or 2 hours after meals. Do not take concurrently with antacids, iron, zinc or multivitamins (wait two hours before or two hours after). Swallow with a full glass of water to prevent esophageal irritation. Dairy products are alright to have with doxycycline.

Q. What should be done if a dose is missed?

A. If the missed dose is close to the next dose, skip the missed dose and proceed with regular dosing regimen. Do not take two doses at once to make up the missed dose.

c.   Ulcerative periodontal diseases

Q. What are ulcerative periodontal diseases?

A. Ulcerative periodontal diseases (UPDs) including necrotizing ulcerative gingivitis (NUG) and necrotizing ulcerative periodontitis (NUP) are bacterial infections caused specifically by *Treponema* spp., *Fusobacterium nucleatum*, and *Prevotella intermedia*.

Q. Does necrotizing ulcerative gingivitis clinical look different from gingivitis?

A. Necrotizing ulcerative gingivitis (NUG) differs from the other periodontal diseases. Three criteria must be present for a diagnosis of NUG: interdental gingival necrosis or "punched out" ulcerative papillae, gingival bleeding and pain (Rowland, 1999). There is usually spontaneous bleeding which occurs when touched or during eating.

Q. Clinically what does NUG look like?

A. NUG is clinically characterized by small, gray, ulcerative lesions that begin at the tips of the interdental papillae and spread to the gingival margin to form punched-out or cratered lesions. There may be a grayish-white pseudomembrane covers the affected area.

Q. Is fever and a bad odor present in NUG?

A. Fever and fetid oral odor are variable findings are not always present.

Q. Why did the disease name change from acute ulcerative necrotizing gingivitis (ANUG) to NUG?

A. Armitage (1999) documented that the word "acute" is a clinical descriptive term and should not be used as a diagnostic classification (Rowland, 1999).

Q. What are some features of NUP?

A. Necrotizing ulcerative periodontitis has the same features as NUG except there is loss of clinical attachment and alveolar bone.

Q. Are necrotizing periodontal diseases seen in immunocompromised patients?

A. Yes. NUG/NUP may be the first sign of HIV infection. Although, not limited to HIV infection, NUPs is often seen in patients who have severe malnutrition and are immunosuppressed. In HIV patients with gingivitis the free gingiva often appears as a distinct red band about 2 to 3 mm in width and is known as linear gingival erythema.

Q. What is the treatment for NUPs?

A. It is the consensus that antibiotics are required to treat UPDs. However, many different antibiotic regimens have been suggested including metronidazole, tetracycline and penicillin (Rowland, 1999).

d.   Refractory and recurrent periodontitis

Q. What is refractory periodontitis?

A. Refractory periodontitis was eliminated as a separate diagnostic term from the latest 1999 periodontal classification (American Academy of Periodontology, 2000). So, refractory periodontitis is not a single diagnostic term and can occur in all periodontal disease categories. It refers to destructive periodontal diseases (e.g., chronic periodontitis) in any patient who has additional attachment loss at one or more sites, despite all efforts and careful monitoring to stop the progression of the disease. Refractory patients generally do not respond to initial therapy (American Academy of Periodontology, 2000).

Q. Are systemic antibiotics indicated in refractory patients?

A. Yes. Antibiotic therapy is usually reserved for periodontal patients having continued periodontal destruction even after mechanical debridement and effective oral hygiene to help reduce the bacterial load and promote periodontal health in patient that do not respond to conventional therapy (American Academy of Periodontology, 2004). Antibiotic susceptibility testing is necessary to determine efficacy of antibiotics against the periodontal pathogens in the patient. (However, this is controversial due to varying lab results.)

Q. Where are oral microbiology testing labs located in the United States?

A. The Oral Microbiology Testing Service (OMTS) Laboratory at Temple University Maurice H. Kornberg School of Dentistry (Dr. Rams) in Philadelphia, Oral Microbiology Testing Laboratory at University of Southern California (Dr. Slots) and Oral Microbiology Laboratory (OML) at the University of North Carolina-Chapel Hill in North Carolina.

Q. What is a DNA probe?

A. DNA probes will detect specific species and determine the antibiotic susceptibility. Molecular DNA testing uses saliva to identify and measure specific types of bacteria in periodontal diseases. Oral DNA Labs (a Quest Diagnostics Company) (www.OralDNAtraining.com) is a company that does oral salivary DNA testing.

Q. What is the difference between recurrent periodontitis and refractory periodontitis?

A. Patients with recurrent periodontitis continue to have signs of periodontitis due poor compliance with oral hygiene and do not come to the office for regular periodontal maintenance. Patients with refractory periodontitis have regular periodontal care and perform adequate oral hygiene but continue to have periodontal tissue breakdown. The etiology of refractory periodontitis is most likely due to periodontal pathogens and the immune response of the host to the pathogens.

Table 6.1   Antibiotics that can be prescribed for refractory periodontitis.

- Clindamycin (Gram-negative) 150 mg q6h for 10 days (Walker *et al.*, 1993; Gordon *et al.*, 1990). Post-antibiotic therapy with clindamycin results in gain of attachment and pocket depth reduction (clindamycin comes in 150 mg cap).
- Metronidazole + amoxicillin/ (Gram-negative obligate/facultative): 500 mg amoxicillin + 250 mg metronidazole: initially take 2 tabs of each, then 1 tab each q8h for 7 days (van Winkelhoff *et al.*, 1992).
- Amoxicillin clavulanate (Gram-positive): 250 mg tid for 10 days.
- Metronidazole (Gram-negative obligate): 250–500 mg tid for 10 days (Loesche *et al.*, 1996; Saxén & Asikainen, 1993; Winkel *et al.*, 2001).

Q. Are systemic antibiotics indicated in recurrent periodontitis?

A. No. Managing the recurrent periodontitis patient involves working with the noncompliant patient on oral hygiene and motivation. Also, it is important to monitor the frequency of periodontal maintenance visits. Using a chlorhexidine rinse as an adjunct to tooth brushing and flossing can help to reduce oral biofilm on the tongue, tonsillar pillars, and gingiva and in saliva where the bacteria reside. After initial therapy is completed and the patient continues to have localized areas with ≥5 mm with bleeding on probing, localized controlled-delivery of Arestin, Atridox or PerioChip can be done (Low, 2006).

Q. What are some recommended antibiotics used in refractory periodontitis?

A. The decision of choice of antibiotic depends on the pathogens present which are determined from DNA testing. Antibiotic therapy is used to help reduce the bacterial load when used in conjunction with scaling and root planing.

Some antibiotics that can be prescribed for refractory periodontitis as an adjunct to scaling/root planing/periodontal surgery include (Table 6.1).

e.   *Aggressive periodontitis*

Q. What is aggressive periodontitis?

A. The older term for aggressive periodontitis was juvenile periodontitis. There is a genetic predisposition to aggressive periodontitis and modified with certain risk factors such as smoking and diabetes. In localized aggressive periodontitis <30% of sites are involved and if >30% of periodontal sites are affected then it is generalized aggressive periodontitis.

Q. Should systemic antibiotics be prescribed in patients with aggressive periodontitis?

A. It is clearer substantiating the use of systemic antibiotics in aggressive periodontitis which has high levels of *Aggregatibacter actinomycetemcomitans*. The use of systemic antibiotics in periodontal infections is based solely on the fact that certain bacteria actually invade into the epithelial cells of the gingiva rather than just staying in the "pocket area" (Revert *et al.*, 1990; Saglie *et al.*, 1982). These bacteria including *Porphyromonas gingivalis* (Pg), *Aggregatibacter actinomycetemcomitans*, and spirochetes invade the gingival and avoid removal by scaling and root planing; hence, systemic antibiotics should be used. *Porphyromonas gingivalis* also has the ability to invade human gingival fibroblasts. Numerous papers supports the adjunctive use of systemic antibiotics in the treatment of localized and generalized aggressive periodontitis because of the invasion of these bacteria into the periodontal tissues, which cannot be eradicated by scaling and root planing or surgery alone.

Q. What systemic antibiotics are recommended in the management of aggressive periodontitis?

A. Since there are many different combinations of periodontal pathogens in periodontitis, at least 10 different antibiotic regimens may be required to specifically target the various pathogen complexes (Beikler *et al.*, 2004). Antibiotics

Table 6.2   Suggested antibiotic dosages used in aggressive periodontics.

• Penicillin VK (250–500 mg qid) + metronidazole (250–500 mg tid) for 8–10 days. (Yek *et al.*, 2010; Walker & Karpinia, 2002).
• Doxycycline hyclate alone: 100 mg bid on day 1, then 100 mg qd for 10–14 days (Saxén *et al.*, 1990).
• Azithromycin (can penetrate into both normal and diseased periodontal tissues and into PMNs and has a post-antibiotic effect): 500 mg qd for 4 to 7 days (Sefton *et al.*, 1996).
• Clindamycin: 150–300 mg q6h for 8–10 days (clindamycin comes in 150 mg cap).
• Metronidazole: 250–500 mg q8h for 8–10 days (metronidazole comes in 250 mg tab (for obligate anaerobic infections).

immediately after scaling and root planing can provide more probing depth reduction and gain of attachment with healing improved up to 6 months (Doğan *et al.*, 2007; Söder *et al.*, 1989). There is no controversy regarding the use of systemic antibiotics in the adjunctive treatment of aggressive periodontitis. However, there may be some questions regarding the selection of the antibiotic. Haffajee *et al.* (2003) reported a significant improvement in periodontal attachment levels with tetracycline, metronidazole and a borderline statistical significance for the combination of amoxicillin and metronidazole.

Q. Can Arestin or Atridox be applied into the periodontal pocket in aggressive periodontitis patients?

A. No. Locally-applied antibiotics have little or no effect on *Aggregatibacter actinomycetemcomitans* and do not penetrate deep into the gingival tissues.

Q. What are some suggested antibiotic dosages used in aggressive periodontics?

A. Some suggested systemic antibiotics in conjunction with scaling/root planing/surgery in aggressive periodontitis patients are given in Table 6.2 (recommendations are from Walker & Karpinia, 2002).

Q. Can metronidazole be prescribed alone?

A. Metronidazole is only effective against obligate or strict or obligate anaerobes so it should be prescribed with penicillin to have better antimicrobial coverage.

f. Periodontal therapy

Periodontal flap surgery: pocket reduction

Q. Are systemic antibiotics necessary after pocket reduction periodontal surgery?

A. The primary rationale for using systemic antibiotics during surgical therapy is based on the fact that there may be an increased risk of complications including infection, pain and delayed wound healing (Arab *et al.*, 2006; Powell *et al.*, 2005). Additionally, the bacterial burden of the host may be lessened with the use of systemic antibiotics (van Winkelhoff, 2005). However, the prevention of infections after periodontal surgery through the routine use of antibiotics seems to be primarily based on empiricism and is very controversial and generally not recommended.

The majority of the literature does not support the use of prophylactic antibiotics in preventing post-operative infection in patients undergoing periodontal osseous surgery including full thickness flaps, degranulation, osteoplasty or ostectomy and sutures (Arab *et al.*, 2006; Checchi *et al.*, 1992). Powell *et al.* (2005), reported that there was no statistical difference in the incidence of postoperative infections in patients undergoing periodontal surgery that did not take an antibiotic (1.81%) and those who received antibiotics pre- and/or postoperatively (2.85%). Very few studies support the use of antibiotics after periodontal osseous surgery to reduce pain swelling and improve wound healing (Peterson, 1990).

Q. Why do dentists prescribe antibiotics after periodontal surgery?

A. Many dentists may base their decision to use antibiotics pre- and/or postoperatively empirically. Do antibiotics reduce the incidence of infections post osseous surgery? According to Powell *et al.* (1990), the overall incidence of infections following different periodontal surgeries was 2.09%. Patients who received antibiotics had a 2.85% incidence of infections compared to 1.81% where antibiotics were not used. Thus, it is the consensus and the opinion of the authors that there is no benefit in using antibiotics for the sole purpose of only purpose of prevention of postosseous surgery infections.

Bone/bone substitutes grafting procedures

Q. Should antibiotics be prescribed for bone grafting procedures?

A. The difference between periodontal osseous resective surgery and periodontal surgery using bone grafts or bone substitute materials is that in osseous resective surgery native bone is being either removed (ostectomy) or reshaped (osteoplasty) and the remaining bone retains its blood and lymph supply. The concern is that in periodontal surgery which involves the placement of bone grafts (autogenous, bovine, freeze-dried bone) or bone substitutes (hydroxyapatite, anorganic bovine bone, bioactive glass) without an established blood supply into an infrabony defect that already has an intact blood supply. An infrabony defect is type of intrabony vertical defect with 3 bony walls bordering the tooth (Weinberg & Eskow, 2000). Thus, until this grafted bone material can establish a blood supply rich in inflammatory and immune cells antibiotics may be required to aid in preventing postsurgical infections. Additionally, optimal repair and regeneration of the periodontium has been shown to be enhanced when there is suppression of the microbiota during healing (Giannopoulou *et al.*, 2006).

During the healing phase, by 18 hours there is an accumulation of polymorphonuclear leukocytes (PMNs) which are the first inflammatory cells to move into the wound area (Zipfel *et al.*, 2003). After blood clot formation and inflammation, there is a 2-day period of fibroblast-like mesenchymal cell chemotaxis which is driven by growth factors (Zipfel *et al.*, 2003). By 5 to 9 days, blood vessel components are observed. By day 10 the first osteoblasts with new bone formation observed (Zipfel *et al.*, 2003). Thus, until inflammatory and immune cells are established with blood vessel formation, it may be prudent to give antibiotics 1 hour before the surgery and for 9 days after surgery to likely prevent postoperative infection. The reason for starting the antibiotic only 1 to 2 hours before is because most antibiotics are absorbed into the blood and show peak blood levels 1 to 2 hours after the first dose. This dose will also provide blood levels that will infiltrate the graft site. It is not necessary to start the antibiotic many days before. The duration of antibiotic therapy is for 10 days when new bone has formed.

Most of the research done on the preoperative and postoperative use of antibiotics with bone grafts/bone substitutes evaluated the clinical outcomes of the surgery, namely looking at probing depths reduction and clinical attachment gain. Some studies showed increased graft success with antibiotics while others did not support the routine administration of antibiotics (Sculean *et al.*, 2001).

Q. What would be the rationale for using preoperative/postoperative systemic antibiotics for bone grafting procedures?

A. To reduce postoperative infection. However, using aseptic techniques and good surgical techniques are two important factors in reducing the incidence of postoperative infections (Resnik & Misch, 2008). Until blood vessel formation can be established with inflammatory and immune cells, antibiotic coverage is recommended to reduce the incidence of postoperative infection.

Some clinical trials reported that the use of systemic antibiotics in conjunction with bone material or enamel matrix proteins did not produce statistically significant pocket depth reduction and gain of clinical attachment (Sculean *et al.*, 2001).

Q. Does research recommend the use of prophylactic antibiotics when performing surgery with enamel matrix proteins (Emdogain®)?

A. There is no standard protocol for the adjunctive use of antibiotics, pre- or postsurgery, with Emdogain®. A 2001 clinical article found that there was no advantage in prescribing systemic antibiotics as an adjunct to Emdogain® infrabony surgery (Sculean *et al.*, 2001).

Q. Should an antibiotic be mixed in the bone graft/bone substitute material for periodontal osseous defects?

A. There is no standardized protocol for mixing an antibiotic (e.g., opening a tetracycline or doxycycline capsule) with a bone graft or bone substitute material. Additionally, some clinicians compound a 5 or 10% solution of tetracycline powder with normal saline, sterile water or local anesthetic without actually knowing the exact dilution to demineralize the root surface, burnish onto the root surface to remove the smear layer and fibrin and exposing the collagen matrix (Delazari *et al.*, 1999). This indication for topical use of tetracycline is controversial when used for periodontal regeneration. Some cases have caused root resorption and may induce an inflammatory response (Ben-Yehouda, 1997; Haddad-Houri *et al.*, 2004). The pharmacist can make up a 5% solution which is 50 mg/mL (pH 1.6) or a 10% solution, which is 100 mg/mL. Tetracycline and doxycycline are basic compounds but after reconstituted with water the pH of doxycycline becomes 1.6–3.3. It is noted that bone forms best with an alkaline pH.

Periodontal regenerative surgery: Guided tissue regeneration (GTR)

Q. Is it recommended to prescribe systemic antibiotics for guided tissue regenerative surgery?

A. It depends. Powell *et al.* (1990) reported a 2.99% postoperative infection rate after guided tissue regeneration (GTR). In 1993 Mombelli *et al.* reported that not only was bacterial colonization of the treated sites common but there were high total bacterial counts at the time of membrane removal (using nonbioabsorbable membranes) and on exposed membranes. The numbers of *Porphyromonas gingivalis*, *Prevotella intermedia*, *Tannerella forsythensis*, and *Aggregatibacter actinomycetemcomitans* on retrieved expanded polytetrafluoroethylene (e-PTFE) membranes (Gore-Tex®, Gore®) were high (Ling *et al.*, 2003). Upon membrane retrieval bacteria were found in the collar part of the membrane, which was partly exposed supragingivally during the healing time (DeSanctis *et al.*, 1996). Additionally, even in cases where the barrier material had remained unexposed during the entire healing time, bacteria were found in the collar part of the membrane. DeSanctis *et al.* (1996) concluded that it is actually bacterial colonization rather than bacterial contamination from the surgical procedure which may alter healing following membrane exposure (Hung *et al.*, 2002). The type of barrier material used is critical to the incidence of bacterial contamination. Bioabsorbable polylactic acid (Guidor®) shows less bacterial colonization than ePTFE (Zucchelli *et al.*, 1999). Sela *et al.* (2009), found that cross-linked collagen membranes (e.g., Biomend Extend™, Ossix™) are primarily broken down by proteolytic enzymes of *Porphyromonas gingivalis*, but they are more resistant to proteolysis than collagen membranes that were not cross-linked (e.g., Bio-Gide®). Early destruction of membranes greatly influences the success of the GTR surgery. Additionally, chlorhexidine, doxycycline and minocycline were found to inhibit the breakdown from the proteolytic enzymes and metronidazole had no effect. It was concluded that the use of antibacterial agents with cross-linked collagen membranes may significantly inhibit the breakdown of the membranes.

Q. Is chlorhexidine oral rinse recommended for patients after guided tissue regeneration (GTR) surgery?

A. Yes. Chlorhexidine has been found to reduce and delay, but not prevent, the early bacterial accumulation on membrane materials especially when it becomes exposed to the oral environment which may result in surgical failure or incomplete regeneration. Additionally, chlorhexidine is likely not the primary factor in reducing bacterial accumulation but rather the type of membrane material used (Chen, 2003; Zucchelli *et al.*, 2000).

Q. What are recommended antibiotics for guided tissue regenerative surgery?

A. Different antibiotic regimens have been suggested. Since it was been found that *P. gingivalis* and *Aa* are the primary bacteria that colonize membranes, an antibiotic that is specific to these bacteria is recommended. Metronidazole is very effective against Gram-negative obligates (*P. gingivalis*) but not facultative anaerobes (*Aa*). Amoxicillin plus clavulanate potassium (Augmentin®) was been documented to be 98.8% to 100% effective against obligate anaerobes as well as facultative anaerobes. These bacteria have a high resistance against clindamycin (Ardila *et al.*, 2010). It has been suggested that coverage should be for 8 days. In penicillin allergic patients, azithromycin can be used.

Q. When should the antibiotic be started?

A. According to Nowzari *et al.* (1995) 500 mg amoxicillin/clavulanic acid (Augmentin) was started 1 hour before GTR surgery, followed by 500 mg tid for 8 days afterward (Nowzari *et al.*, 1995).

Q. Can locally-applied antibiotics such as Atridox® or Arestin® be used with GTR?

A. No. There is lack of penetration of the locally-applied (into the periodontal pocket) antibiotic in the deeper parts of the tissues.

III. Prescribing for dental implant surgery

Q. Is there a standard protocol for the use of prophylactic antibiotics for dental implant placement?

A. No. The use of prophylactic antibiotics for dental implant placement remains controversial, as does the coverage of antibiotics after implant surgery (Pye *et al.*, 2009). One of the earlier articles advocating the use of preoperative antibiotic prophylaxis for routine implant placement found a significantly higher survival rate at each stage (stage 1 healing; stage 2 surgical uncovering; stage 3 before loading of the prosthesis; and stage 4 loading of prosthesis) of implant treatment in patients who had received preoperative antibiotics (Laskin *et al.*, 2000). In 2003, a Cochrane Review failed to find evidence to recommend or discourage the use of prophylactic antibiotics to prevent complications of implant placement and implant failure (Esposito *et al.*, 2003). However, a 2008 Cochrane review determined that there was some evidence that 2 g of amoxicillin administered 1 hour before implant placement significantly reduced early implant failure. Further research is still needed (Esposito *et al.*, 2008). In 2008, Resnik & Misch recommended prophylactic use of systemic antibiotics with good surgical technique in dental implant placement and bone grafting procedures to help reduce postoperative infections. On the contrary, some researchers claim that there is little or no advantage to using antibiotics presurgically (Mazzocchi *et al.*, 2007).

Resnik & Misch (2008) concluded that in healthy patients a single dose of antibiotic presurgically is sufficient and that it is not necessary to continue antibiotic coverage after surgery except in extensive cases such as placement of multiple implants including immediate implants and bone grafting with membranes. In these cases, Resnik & Misch (2008) recommend after the loading presurgical dose antibiotics should be continued as 3 postsurgical doses per day for 3 consecutive days.

Wagenberg & Froum (2006) found a better success rate in implant survival in patients that were prescribed amoxicillin than were not. Additionally, a 2009 systematic review concluded that 2 g of amoxicillin administered orally one hour before implant placement surgery significantly reduced the rate of implant failure (Geisler, 2009).

Q. Is there concern that the use of small doses before implant surgery can increase the incidence of bacterial resistance?

A. No. Selective growth of resistant bacteria begins only once the host's susceptible organisms are killed, which occurs in about 3 days (48 hours) of antibiotic use. Thus, one day/time of antibiotic use does not affect the development of resistant bacteria (Peterson, 1990).

Q. It seems to be an evidence-based consensus that presurgical antibiotic prophylaxis for routine implant placement is a common procedure in reducing/preventing infections following surgery. What is the protocol for continuing the antibiotic after the surgery is completed?

A. Postoperative use of systemic antibiotics for implant placement is unclear and controversial; however, Wagenberg and Froum (2006) in a retrospective study of 1925 consecutively placed immediate implants from 1998 to 2004 showed three times more implant failure if no antibiotics were given postsurgery. In particular, they found that penicillin was a more effective antibiotic for implant survival than alternative antibiotics (e.g., if the patient were allergic to penicillin another antibiotic was prescribed).

Q. What is the definition of peri-implantitis?

A. Peri-implantitis is an inflammatory process that affects the peri-implant bone around a dental implant that is in function (Albrektsson & Isidor, 1994).

Q. What are the definitions of the ailing, failing, and failed implant?

A. An ailing implant is referred to as peri-implant mucositis where only the gingiva is inflamed around the implant. There is no mobility or bone lost. A failing implant is referred to as peri-implantitis where there is bone loss (two to three threads exposed) around the implant. A failed implant is mobile. The first sign of a failing implant is pain and discomfort which indicated mobility (el Askary *et al.* 1999).

Q. What is the pharmacologic management of the ailing, failing, and failed implant?

A. Presently, there is not enough evidence to support which is the most effective therapy to treat peri-implantitis. However, it was noted that even though there is little evidence suggesting the most effect therapy for treating peri-implantitis, currently used treatments may still be effective (Esposito *et al.*, 2006, 2010; Pye *et al.*, 2009; Norowski & Bumgardner, 2009; Lindhe & Meyle, 2008). According to the Sixth European Workshop on Periodontology, there is limited evidence that the adjunctive use of systemic antibiotics could resolve many peri-implantitis lesions. Also, regenerative procedures had no additional beneficial effects on treatment outcomes (Lindhe & Meyle, 2008). Klinge *et al.* (2005) relates peri-implantitis as a site-specific infection comparable to chronic periodontitis and the incidence of peri-implantitis varies according to implant design and surface characteristics with the different implant systems. Suggested treatments for peri-implantitis include:

1. Peri-implant mucositis (ailing implant) is treated with mechanical debridement, oral hygiene instruction, chlorhexidine gluconate rinse/irrigation (for about 3–4 weeks or until the inflammation has resolved) and maintenance.
2. Failing implant: Presently, there is no consistent treatment regimen for treating a failing implant. There are many references and proposed treatments including: mechanical debridement, chlorhexidine rinse/irrigation, controlled-locally delivered antibiotics (Arestin®, Atridox®), systemic antibiotics (metronidazole 250 mg tid for 10 days; amoxicillin 250 mg tid for 7 days) and surgery to detoxify or deplaque the implant surface. Even though in past literature there has been much clinical improvement with regenerative procedures a most recent study on regenerative surgical procedures using a bone graft or enamel matrix derivative (Emdogain®) covered with a collagen membrane found promising results (Froum *et al.*, 2012).
3. Failed implant: removal of implant (Pye *et al.*, 2009).

a.   Prescribing for sinus floor elevation surgery

Q. Is the maxillary sinus sterile?

A. There is conflicting information regarding the presence of bacteria in healthy maxillary sinus cavities. It was once thought that the maxillary sinus was sterile (Hamad *et al.*, 2009). However, now it is confirmed that the normal flora of the maxillary sinus includes *Staphylococcus aureus*, α and γ hemolytic streptococci, *Bacteroides* spp., *Fusobacterium* spp., and *Propinonibacterium acnes*.

Q. What is the etiology of early infection following sinus floor elevation surgery?

A. Early infection following sinus floor elevation surgery and subsequent graft and/or implant failure can occur due to many factors including:

1. Contamination of the sinus by sinus or oral cavity pathogens
2. Existing chronic sinusitis
3. Patient smokes resulting in delayed incision healing
4. Perforation of the membrane

5. Graft becomes contaminated with saliva
6. Lack of aseptic technique.

Q. Are prophylactic antibiotics recommended for sinus elevation surgery?

A. Yes. Complications during and following sinus lift surgery include bacterial contamination at the time of implant placement, perforating the Schneiderian membrane followed by sinus infection, oroantral fistula, and infection of the graft. As mentioned earlier in the book, it is important for the antibiotic to be present before the infection develops. As the sinus fills with fluid, bacteria trapped in this moist, warm environment find it an excellent place to grow. The bacteria begin to multiply and cause infection. Since it is unknown whether complications will arise, antibiotic prophylaxis is given to patients.

Q. What is the rationale for using preoperative antibiotics for sinus floor elevation surgery?

A. To have the antibiotic present at the time of bacterial contamination for the prevention of postoperative infection of the sinus and graft or soft tissue perforation. Using a loading dose at least one hour before surgery will impart blood levels that will infiltrate the grafted site.

Q. What antibiotic should be prescribed before sinus elevation surgery?

A. The selection of the antibiotic is based on the fact if the membrane is perforated the maxillary sinus will be exposed and the patient will most likely develop an acute sinusitis. The antibiotic of choice should be based on the current guidelines for management of acute sinusitis. The cultivable bacteria should be known. Review of sinus aspiration studies performed in adults with acute sinusitis suggests that *Streptococci pneumoniae* is isolated in approximately 20% to 43%, *Haemophilus influenzae* in 22% to 35%, and *Moraxella catarrhalis* in 2% to 10% of aspirates. Other bacterial isolates found in patients with acute sinusitis include *Staphylococcus aureus* and anaerobes. Local resistance patterns vary widely, but about 15% of *S. pneumoniae* has intermediate penicillin resistance and 25% is highly resistant (Rosenfeld *et al.*, 2007; Sinus and Allergy Health Partnership (SAHP), 2004). Therefore, broad-spectrum amoxicillin (1 g taken 1 hour before surgery) would be most appropriate. If the patient has a past history of chronic or periodontic sinus infections amoxicillin/clavulanate potassium is recommended. (Tasoulis *et al.*, 2011) The azalides (azithromycin, clarithromycin) or clindamycin (300 mg 1 hour before surgery) may also be used for patients with penicillin allergy (Rosenfeld *et al.*, 2007; Tasoulis *et al.*, 2011). The spectrum of activity of penicillin VK is narrow and does not cover *H. influenza* or *Moraxella catarrhalis*. This is why amoxicillin is useful for sinus infections (Rosenfeld *et al.*, 2007).

Q. What are the dosages of the antibiotics and what is the duration of therapy?

A.
Dosages: amoxicillin: 1 or 2 g 1 hour before surgery on day 1, then 500 mg every 8 hours for 10 days. (amoxicillin is supplied as 500 mg capsules)
   If allergic to penicillin: azithromycin or clarithromycin: 500 mg 1 hour before surgery on day 1, then 250 mg once a day for 3 to 10 days. (generic available; supplied as 250 mg and 500 mg tablet) (Farhat *et al.*, 2008); clindamycin 300 mg 1 hour before surgery on day 1, then 150 mg every 6 hours for 3 to 10 days..
   Duration of therapy: The antibiotic should be continued after the sinus surgery. Most trials of acute bacterial rhinosinusitis (ABRS) administer antibiotic for 10 days (e.g., amoxicillin 500 mg tid) (Rosenfeld *et al.*, 2007). No significant differences have been noted, however, in resolution rates for ABRS with a 6–10-day course of antibiotics compared with a 3–5-day course (azithromycin) up to 3 weeks after treatment.

Q. What happens if the patient was previously taking an antibiotic in the past 4 to 6 weeks?

A. This increases the chance for bacterial resistance. Guidelines from the Sinus and Allergy Partnership recommend to use high-dose amoxicillin/clavulanate (Augmentin; can write the prescription for the generic) (Rosenfeld *et al.*, 2007) (Sinus and Allergy Health Partnership (SAHP), 2004).

Table 6.3 How a prescription for methylprednisolone is written.

> Rx Methylprednisolone Dosepak
> Disp: 1 package
> Sig: Use as directed in the instructions on the package.

Q. What should be done if the infection does not respond to the given antibiotics?

A. Once the graft is infected and there is pus the graft area must be irrigated and the patient placed on an antibiotic for up to 3 weeks. If the infection has not resolved the graft may have to be removed. Once the infection is eliminated the area can be regrafted (Misch, 1992; Smiler, 1997).

Q. What other medications should be given preoperatively to sinus surgery?

A. Some symptoms/signs of sinusitis include infection (purulent exudates), nasal congestion and headache (Katranji *et al.*, 2008). Patients with existing chronic sinusitis have a higher incidence of sinusitis after sinus surgery.

Prescribing nasal decongestants can help to reduce the incidence of developing obstruction of the ostium after surgery.

- Nasal decongestants:
  - Afrin (oxymetazoline) nasal spray (starting a few days before surgery and continues for 10 to 14 days after surgery). Starts working within 10 minutes and lasts for about 12 hours. It works by causing vasoconstriction of the nasal mucosa.
- Anti-inflammatory (to minimize postoperative swelling) medications:
  - ibuprofen 800 mg q8h for 5 days (if there are no contraindications for ibuprofen such as peptic ulcer disease, asthma (aspirin insensitivity), or patient taking warfarin.
  - methylprednisolone dose pack (follow tapering dosage instructions on pack) *or* dexamethasone 8 mg (Decadron) starting 1 hour before surgery, then 4 mg for 2 days.

Q. How is a prescription for methylprednisolone written (Table 6.3)?

A. The brand name is Medrol but it can be substituted for the generic. If a patient is a poor candidate for corticosteroids (e.g., uncontrolled diabetes, peptic ulcer disease, osteoporosis, Cushing's syndrome, preexisting wide angle glaucoma, systemic viral disease, and psychiatric disorders) it is highly recommended that the patient's physician should be contacted.

- Antimicrobial rinse:
  - Chlorhexidine gluconate 0.12% rinse (Farhat *et al.*, 2008)

Q. What is the ostium?

A. The ostium is the opening from the sinus above the first molar into the nose through the middle meatus (turbinate) of the nose. The maxillary sinus drains through the ostium.

Q. What can happen if the bone graft material was overpacked in the sinus?

A. The lower part of the sinus is where the bone is placed. Normal sinus drainage is not normally interfered with because the ostium is located about 28.5 mm from the sinus floor (Greenstein & Cavallaro, 2011; Uchida *et al.*, 1998). Overpacking or graft migration can cause blockage of the ostium resulting in a sinusitis.

Q. What other conditions can cause obstruction or blockage of the ostium?

A. Inflammation of the sinus tissues.

Q. What happens if the sinusitis is not resolved?

A. If the sinusitis is not cured after 2 weeks then referral to an ENT specialist is recommended (Katranji *et al.*, 2008).

IV.   Prescribing for oral surgery

Q. What are the most likely bacteria causing an infection after oral and maxillofacial surgery?

A. *Streptococci*, anaerobic Gram-positive cocci and anaerobic Gram-negative rods.

Q. Do antibiotics routinely need to be prescribed with extractions?

A. No. A review of controlled studies for mandibular third molar surgery found little or no evidence of benefit from antibiotic prophylaxis to prevent local infection for most dentoalveolar surgery in medical healthy patients (Lawler *et al.*, 2005). Every patient must be assessed individually. It is normal to have some inflammation with pain, swelling, redness and trismus (limitation of jaw opening) following an extraction. This is not diagnostic of an infection (Sancho-Puchades *et al.*, 2009).

Q. When should antibiotic prophylaxis be needed for third molar extractions?

A. There are few adequate reviews of clinical studies on antibiotic prophylaxis in oral surgery. In 2007, a Task Force of the American Association of Oral and Maxillofacial that reviewed different aspects of third molar extractions did not even mention anything about antibiotics prophylaxis or antibiotics after extractions. Surgeons recommend that in routine nonimpacted third molar extractions antibiotic prophylaxis is probably not necessary. Antibiotic prophylaxis using a narrow-spectrum, single, high dose of antibiotic (e.g., penicillin VK) may be indicated for deep bony impactions.

Q. What is the rationale for prescribing after third molar surgical extraction?

A. Ideally, extraction procedures should be of short duration with minimal soft and hard tissue damage. Complications following surgical extraction can include inflammation and infection. The more osteotomy, tissue manipulation and longer procedures may benefit from a pre-operative antibiotic prophylaxis (single dose). However, there is no literature showing this (Schwartz & Larsen, 2007).

Q. What constitutes an infection following tooth extraction?

A. Hot intense swelling, presence of fluctuation, purulent discharge from the extraction site for more than 72 hours after surgery. Pain and swelling that gets worse or does not improve 48 hours after surgery (Lawler *et al.*, 2005; Pogrel, 1993).

Q. Is dry socket an infection of the socket?

A. No. Dry socket or alveolar osteitis is not considered to be an infection but rather a consequence of early wound healing with increased fibrinolytic activity. This condition does not require antibiotics.

V.   Prescribing for odontogenic infections

Q. Are odontogenic infections composed of many bacteria?

A. Yes. Odontogenic infections are polymicrobial. Studies have documented that there is an average of 4 to 6 different bacterial pathogens. The bacteria found in the early stages of an odontogenic infection are primarily aerobic and in the later, chronic stages (days later) it is converted from aerobic to anaerobic colonies.

Q. What is an abscess?

A. An abscess is a collection of pus or dead neutrophils (PMNs) formed by the tissue and is caused by an infection involving bacteria which are usually slow growing. The body walls-off (to prevent the spread of the infection) an abscess with host cells such as PMNs, which can reduce the ability of the antibiotic to penetrate the bacteria. Thus, it is important, when possible to perform an incision and drainage (I & D) before the antibiotic is administered; it is most important to remove the reservoir of infection and reduce the bacterial load.

Q. What is the antibiotic regimen for prescribing antibiotics for periodontal or endodontic abscesses?

A. There are two schools of thought concerning the optimal duration of antibiotic therapy: either the duration of therapy should be for 3 days (high dose; short term) or for 7 to 10 days. Of course it depends on the severity of the infection and if there is systemic involvement.

Using antibiotics at high dose for short periods of time (e.g., 3 or 5 days versus 10 days) has been suggested because it increases patient adherence as well as targets both sensitive and most resistant bacteria (due to the high dose) reducing both the development of resistance and the amount of antibiotic delivered to the environment. If antibiotics are prescribed over a long time period (e.g., >7 to 10 days) there is increased incidence of bacterial resistance (Pallasch, 1996) because any bacteria that survive low doses of antibiotics most likely are resistant. Medical literature favoring 3-day therapy claims that prolonged exposure to antibiotics increases the risk of adverse effects, and the development of antibiotic resistant bacteria (El Moussaoui *et al.*, 2006; Paul, 2006).

Following the short-term therapy recommendations for odontogenic infections: the loading dose (LD) for penicillin should be 1.0 g on the first day, followed by a maintenance dose of 500 mg qid after the LD. The loading dose for clindamycin should be 600 mg on the 1st day, following by 300 mg after the LD (American Academy of Periodontology, 2004).

Some medical literature recommends that longer durations, 10 days, of treatment may be required if the initial therapy was not active against the offending bacteria. It should be noted that this article reviewed antibiotic duration in adults hospitalized with community-acquired pneumonia (Cunningham *et al.*, 2009). These authors found that there was no difference in the risk of treatment failure between the short-term versus long-term antibiotic therapy and maybe it depends on the antibiotic chosen. It should be noted that these patients were hospitalized with mild to moderate community-acquired pneumonia, a potentially life-threatening condition. One of the cons for using short-term therapy is that after 3 or 5 days the patient may relapse.

Another clinical study comparing 4–5 days versus 10 day antibiotic therapy in patients with group a streptococcal tonsillopharyngitis found shorter courses of penicillin were inferior to 10 days of penicillin (Casey & Pichichero, 2005).

There is no published dental literature on clinical trials concerning antibiotic duration of therapy for dental infections. Since only medical literature is available information must be extrapolated for dental purposes.

Q. What does the term "selective pressure" of antibiotics mean?

A. Selective or selection pressure of antibiotics has led to the emergence of resistant bacteria while the susceptible bacteria die. Antibiotics can affect normal flora (bacteria not associated with the disease) which leads to the emergence of resistant bacteria inhabiting the same environment. So, antibiotics are actually selected for resistant strains (Albrich *et al.*, 2004).

a.   Prescribing for endodontic abscess

Q. How do bacteria gain access to the pulp?

A. Normally, bacteria enter the pulp through decay.

Q. Are the same bacteria in both an endodontic and periodontal abscess?

A. It is a mixed anaerobic (facultative and obligate) bacterial infection. The bacteria are similar but every endodontic infection has a different combination of bacteria; no two infections are the same. Some bacteria types include:

- Facultative Gram-positive cocci (*Streptococcus* spp.)
- Anaerobic Gram-positive cocci (*Peptostreptococcus* spp.)
- Gram-negative anaerobic rods (e.g., *Prevotella* spp., *Fusobacterium necrophorum*, *Bacteroides vulgaris*).
- (Khemaleelakul *et al.*, 2002).

Q. What is the capacity of the pulp to heal?

A. The pulp has limited capacity to heal because it has a limited blood supply; it represents terminal circulation. When bacteria enter the pulp an inflammatory reaction occurs, which does not heal. After the inflammatory process is initiated it eventually leads to necrosis of the pulp.

Q. Why does a patient still feel pain after in an irreversible pulpitis?

A. In an irreversible pulpitis (which is an acute inflammatory response) the pressure from the inflammation causes a lot of pain because there is no place for the inflammation to expand in a hard structure to relieve the pain (http://www.endomail.com/articles/jv05pulp.html).

Q. In irreversible pulpitis which thermal response increases pain?

A. The first or initial phase of irreversible pulpitis, cold increases the pain and heat decreases it. On the second phase, cold relieves the pain and heat increases the pain.

Q. What are the different endodontic diagnoses and specific treatments?

A. Table 6.4 lists different endodontic diagnosis terminology according to the American Board of Endodontics (ABE). A complete endodontic diagnosis is made up of two parts: pulpal diagnosis and periapical diagnosis (www.aae.org/certboard).

Q. Is there a difference between a sinus tract and a fistula?

A. Yes, there is a difference between a sinus tract and a fistula and it depends on the lining of each tract. These two terms are often confusing to the dentist. A fistula is an internal connection between two epithelial surfaces such a tract between the epithelial lining of the intestines and the skin epithelium. On the other hand, a sinus tract is a connection between bone (e.g., periapical lesion) and an epithelial surface (e.g., alveolar mucosa), which discharges purulent exudates (Harrison & Larson, 1976). Draining sinus tracts are commonly lined with granulation tissue, not epithelium, which is chronic inflammatory tissue produced from chronic inflammation from bacterial contaminated root canals. Days after root canal therapy, microscopic analysis shows that the tract is completely gone because it is lined with chronic inflammatory granulation tissue rather than epithelium (Harrison & Larson, 1976). When the source of the inflammation, the granulation tissue, is removed via endodontic procedures, the lesion will heal. On the other hand, since a fistula is lined with epithelial tissue the lesion would probably not heal because the epithelial tissue it not a product of inflammation. Thus, in dental diagnosis the term "fistula" is discouraged in favor of the more correct term "sinus tract" (Harrison & Larson, 1976). By definition, a chronic apical abscess is a sinus tract. Because the pus is draining, sinus tracts are usually not accompanied by pain or swelling (Slutzky-Goldberg *et al.*, 2009). On the other hand, asymptomatic apical periodontitis has an apical radiolucent area not associated with a sinus tract.

Q. How does a sinus tract develop?

A. A sinus tract develops as a result of a periapical lesion when the inflammatory process expands concentrically and it is closer to the buccal than lingual plate. Development of a sinus tract usually does not cause pain because it is actually drainage of the infection (http://www.endomail.com/articles/jv05pulp.html). If the infection is not allowed to drain through a pulpal opening (through the tooth), sinus tract or an incision, extraoral swelling and lymph node involvement will likely develop as the abscess spreads beyond the local confines of the periapical area and into the facial planes. Sinus tracts are usually associated with chronic apical abscesses (Baumgartner, 2004). Radiographically, radiolucency is usually seen apical to the abscessed tooth.

Q. Why is the tooth sensitive to touch and pressure?

A. The tooth may still feel sensitive to pressure, since the periodontal ligament (PDL) fibers may still be inflamed due to the presence of the adjacent irritating necrotic debris of the pulp.

Table 6.4   Classification of endodontic lesions.

Diagnosis	Signs and symptoms	Treatment	Antibiotics required
Pulpal diagnosis			
Normal pulp	None + cold + heat + electric pulp testing	None	None
Reversible pulpitis	++ cold (but does not linger) ++ heat (but does not linger)	Inflammation will resolve and its own and pulpal tissues returns to normal	None
Irreversible pulpitis (symptomatic and asymptomatic)	Symptomatic: vital inflamed pulp. Lingering thermal (cold and heat) pain; spontaneous pain; + electric pulp testing Asymptomatic: no clinical symptoms but inflammation due to caries or trauma	Pulpectomy or extraction	No antibiotic is required because the infection is contained within the pulpal tissue or just around the tissue. There are no signs of an infection such as fever, facial swelling or purulence.
Pulp necrosis	Nonvital pulp; asymptomatic Electric pulp testing	Root canal treatment if the tooth is restorable	None
Previously initiated therapy	Could be symptomatic	Finish endodontic therapy	None
Previously treated	Could be symptomatic or asymptomatic	Retreat if necessary	None
Periapical diagnosis			
Normal apical tissues	No symptoms	No treatment	None
Symptomatic apical periodontitis	Pain on percussion and biting; may or may not be associated with an apical radiolucent area	Endodontic therapy	None
Asymptomatic apical periodontitis	Apical radiolucent area; no clinical symptoms (tenderness, thermal reaction, percussion)	Endodontic therapy	None
Acute apical abscess	Spontaneous, rapid onset of pain, tenderness of tooth to pressure, pus formation and swelling	Endodontic therapy	Antibiotics are needed to prevent the spread of the infection before treatment of the tooth. Medical attention may be necessary.
Chronic apical abscess	Little or no discomfort to percussion with some discharge of pus through sinus tract	Endodontic therapy	None. Pus is being drained through the sinus tract.

Adapted from www.aae.org/certboard.

Q. What does the radiolucency around the apex indicate?

A. Periradicular bone destruction. The infected necrotic pulp is contained in the canal by either an epithelial plug or a layer of neutrophils (white blood cells) at the apical foramen which attempts to prevent the bacteria from invading the periradicular area. The invasion of bacteria past the apical foramen into the periradicular area causes the production of an abscess or cellulitis (Baumgartner, 2004).

Q. How does the periapical radiolucency develop?

A. First, the radiographic PDL widening is due to edema, resulting in accumulation of inflammatory exudates in the collagen (connective tissue) of the PDL. The PDL widening is referred to as apical periodontitis. This PDL widening can be caused by occlusal trauma (e.g., primary occlusal trauma is caused by a "high" restoration on a tooth with adequate periodontal support), orthodontic movement or tooth extrusion. Additionally, inflammatory cells present in the exudates include PMNs, which are the first inflammatory cells to arrive at the site of injury which is the pulp (e.g., due to bacterial caries involvement). The function of PMNs is to rid the microbial invasion but unfortunately it is a "double-edged sword" because while attempting to kill the bacteria they also cause host tissue damage during the acute phases of apical periodontitis. It is the dead PMNs within the root canal that release enzymes such as phospholipase A that induces prostaglandin E_2-mediated bone resorption. Also, proinflammatory cytokines including interleukin-1 (IL-1) and tumor necrosis factor (TNF-α) secreted by PMNs and macrophages play an additional role in periapical bone resorption and increase in collagenase production.

Q. How does an endodontic infection occur?

A. The dental pulp is sterile. The most common way bacteria enter the pulp is via dental caries. Other ways of bacterial entry into the pulp include mechanical or traumatic exposure, lateral and furcal canals or exposed noncarious dentinal tubules, cracks in the enamel–dentine junction and periodontal exposure of dentinal tubules (Baumgartner, 2004). The necrosis starts from the pulp chamber and then goes through the pulpal canal to the apex.

Q. Why do some periapical lesions show radio-opacity?

A. If the bone surrounding a lesion shows osteosclerosis most likely this is caused by resistance to the pathologic process resulting from osteoblastic activity.

Q. What is the difference between an acute versus a chronic apical abscess?

A. An acute lesion produces pain on biting and percussion while a chronic lesion produces little to no discomfort.

Q. When are antibiotics indicated in an endodontic infection?

A. There must be systemic signs and symptoms of infection or spread of infection: increased swelling, cellulitis, malaise, fever >37.8° C (100° F), lymphadenopathy, persistent infection or osteomyelitis (American Association of Endodontists, 2006). According to the American Association of Endodontists, swellings increasing in size should be incised for drainage and adjunctive antibiotics used (American Association of Endodontists, 2006). Antibiotics are indicated when the diagnosis is acute apical abscess. Also, antibiotics are recommended in immunocompromised patients.

Q. When are antibiotics not indicated?

A. Antibiotics are not indicated in endodontic therapy in the following cases (American Association of Endodontists, 2006; Crumpton & McClanahan, 2003):

- There is pain without signs and symptoms (e.g., swelling) of infection.
- Irreversible pulpitis with or without symptomatic apical periodontitis (older term was acute periradicular periodontitis).
- Necrotic pulp with a draining sinus tract (this acts as a pathway of drainage) (e.g., chronic apical abscess – older term was chronic periradicular abscess.
- Necrotic pulp with chronic periradicular periodontitis without swelling.

Q. Are systemic antibiotics indicated in irreversible pulpitis?

A. No. In irreversible pulpitis, antibiotics do not significantly reduce the pain, percussion perception or the quantity of pain medication needed. The best way to relieve the pain is to perform a pulpotomy which will remove the inflamed pulp (Fedorowicz *et al.*, 2005).

Q. Are antibiotics necessary in treating a combined perio/endo lesion?

A. No. Management of a combined lesion is based on basic endodontic and periodontal therapy. Remember that antibiotics are not a substitute for mechanical debridement of the root canal and root surface (Longman *et al.*, 2000).

Q. Why are endodontic infections difficult to treat with antibiotics?

A. Infections in areas of poor blood supply (avascular), such as abscesses, necrotic areas and sinus infections are difficult to treat because of poor distribution and concentration of the antibiotic into these regions. Additionally, the diversity of pathogens in the canal and their different sensitivities makes the ideal antibiotic choice difficult.

Q. What is the antibiotic of choice for an acute apical abscess?

A. Although there are no specific guidelines suggesting an ideal antibiotic there are some recommendations based on current evidence and microbiology. Penicillin VK is the antibiotic of choice for an acute apical abscess because most bacteria are susceptible to it and it a narrow-spectrum antibiotic which is all that is required for the bacterial profile in an endodontic abscess. (It has been recommended to prescribe a high dose for a short period of time to be effective and help reduce the development of resistance (Roberson & Smith, 2009; Baumgartner & Xia, 2002; Karlowsky *et al.*, 1993).

- The dose of penicillin VK is: a loading dose: 1000 mg stat on day 1, followed by 500 mg every 6 hours after the LD up to day 5, 7 or 10 as needed.
- If the patient is allergic to penicillin,
  clindamycin: LD: 600 mg followed by 300 mg every 6 hours for 5 to 7 days.
  or
  azithromycin: LD: 500 mg on day 1, then 250 mg once a day for 2 to 5 days
  or
  clarithromycin: LD: 500 mg followed by 250 mg every 12 hours for 5 to 7 days.

Q. Why is clindamycin recommended in patients allergic to penicillin?

A. Clindamycin is highly effective against anaerobic bacteria and penetrates bone well (Levine, 2003).

Q. What is a recommended antibiotic if the infection is not confined and is spreading?

A. Augmentin (amoxicillin/clavulanic acid) 875 mg bid. If allergic to penicillin then prescribe: Z-pack 250 mg (2 tabs day 2 and one tab days 2 to 5).

Q. Are any bacteria resistant to penicillin?

A. Yes. Some anaerobic bacteria from endodontic lesions are resistant to penicillin. The only way to determine this if a culture and sensitivity test was not performed is that the patient will not be getting clinically better in a few days. In these cases it is necessary to switch to another antibiotic such as amoxicillin/clavulanic acid or clindamycin, which penetrates bone very well.

Q. How long should antibiotics be prescribed?

A. 5 to 7 days, even though clinical signs and symptoms will start to decrease within 2 to 4 days. Not longer than 7 days because of potential destruction of normal oral flora.

Q. Does the severity of the abscess influence the dose of an antibiotic?

A. Yes. The larger the extent of infection, the greater the dose and concentration of the antibiotic will be.

Q. Why is penicillin VK the best antibiotic, in nonallergic, nonimmunocompromised patients, for the management of an endodontic abscess?

A. It is ideal to choose a narrow-spectrum antibiotic. Penicillin VK is well distributed into most soft tissues sites, saliva and abscesses. Penicillin VK is effective against facultative bacteria including streptococci and anaerobic bacteria. Even though there are many more strains present in an infection that cannot be identified in susceptibility tests, penicillin VK is effective against many of the strains of bacteria in a polymicrobial infection. Also, by choosing a narrow-spectrum antibiotic like penicillin it allows the patient's immune response to cope with the remaining strains. This is why incision and drainage (I & D) and debriding the root canal to remove the reservoir of infection is important and reduces the bacterial load. However, if the patient is immunocompromised, then a broad-spectrum antibiotic like amoxicillin is indicated. However, a broad-spectrum antibiotic may select for resistant organisms elsewhere in the body including the gastrointestinal (GI) and genitourinary (GU) tract. These resistant organisms may be detrimental to the patient in the future. This is why the narrower spectrum of penicillin VK is recommended unless it is a life threatening infection or the patient is immunocompromised (Baumgartner, 2011).

Q. What patient instructions are important for penicillin VK?

A. Take penicillin with a full glass of water 1 hour before or 2 hours after meals. Take with yogurt or acidophilus tabs.

Q. Why is amoxicillin not the drug of choice for an odontogenic infection?

A. Amoxicillin is not needed in the treatment of routine odontogenic infections because it shows slightly less activity against Gram-positive cocci but increased efficacy against aerobic Gram-negative cocci and bacilli, bacteria not commonly involved in odontogenic infections (Karlowsky *et al.*, 1993).

Q. Are cephalosporins effective in treating periapical infections?

A. No. Cephalosporins are broad-spectrum antibiotics with limited activity in periapical infections because most periapical infections are mixed bacterial infections predominated by obligate anaerobic bacteria. Cephalosporins are not highly effective against these bacteria with less activity against many anaerobics than penicillin (Levine, 2003).

b. Prescribing for periodontal abscess

Q. What is the treatment for a periodontal abscess?

A. The initial treatment of a periodontal abscess consists of establishing drainage, which is usually through the gingival pocket. Following effective drainage of pus, removal of the cause, which is usually subgingival calculus, is performed through scaling and root planing. The area can be irrigated with chlorhexidine or saline. Antibiotics are indicated if there is systemic involvement (e.g., fever, lymphadenopathy) or the infection has spread (e.g., cellulitis). Have the patient return to the office in about 3 days to evaluate. Further treatment (e.g., periodontal surgery or extraction) may be necessary.

Q. Can an antibiotic be prescribed for a periodontal abscess without scaling and root planing?

A. No. An antibiotic should never be prescribed without physical removal of the bacterial load. An antibiotic cannot penetrate the bacterial cell wall if the biofilm is not disrupted. Additionally, scaling and root planing before the start of antibiotics may minimize the microbial regrowth because microorganisms could spread and grow onto other oral surfaces.

References

Albrich, W.C., Monnet, D.L., Harbarth, S. (2004) Antibiotic selection pressure and resistance in *Streptococcus pneumoniae* and *Streptococcus pyogenes*. *Emerging Infectious Diseases*, 10:514–517.

American Academy of Periodontology (2004) Position Paper. Systemic Antibiotics in Periodontics. *Journal of Periodontology*, 75:1553–1565.

American Academy of Periodontology (2000) Parameter on "refractory" periodontitis. American Academy of Periodontology *Journal of Periodontology*, 71:859–860.

American Association of Endodontists (2006) Antibiotic and the treatment of endodontic infections. *Endodontics Colleagues for Excellence*, Summer:1–6.

Arab, H.R., Sargolzaie, N., Moeintaghavi, A., *et al.* (2006) Antibiotics to prevent complications following periodontal surgery. *International Journal of Pharmaceutics*, 2:205–208.

Ardila, C.M., López, M.A. & Guzmán, I.C. (2010) High resistance against clindamycin, metronidazole and amoxicillin in *Porphyromonas gingivalis* and *Aggregatibacter actinomycetemcomitans* isolates of periodontal disease. *Medicina Oral Patologia Oral y Cirugia Bucal*, 1:e947–951. www.eapd.gr/Guidelines?Guidelines_Antibiotics.htm

Armitage, G.C. (1999) Development of a classification system for periodontal diseases and conditions. *Annual of Periodontology*, 4:1–6.

Baumgartner, J.C. (2004) Microbial aspects of endodontic infections. *Journal of the California Dental Association*, 32:459–468.

Baumgartner, J.C., & Xia, T. (2002) Antibiotic susceptibility of bacteria associated with endodontic abscesses. *Journal of Endodontics*, 29:44–77.

Beikler, T., Prior, K., Ehmke, B., *et al.* (2004) Specific antibiotics in the treatment of periodontitis – A proposed strategy. *Journal of Periodontology*, 75:169–175.

Ben-Yehouda, A. (1997) Progressive cervical root resorption related to tetracycline root conditioning. *Journal of Periodontology*, 68:432–435.

Casey, R.R., & Pichichero, M.E. (2005) Metaanlysis of short course antibiotic treatment for group a streptoccal tonsillopharyngitis. *The Pediatric Infectious Disease Journal*, 24:909–917.

Checchi, L., Trombelli, L. & Nonato, M. (1992) Postoperative infections and tetracycline prophylaxis in periodontal surgery: a retrospective study. *Quintessence International*, 23:191–195.

Chen, T.Y. (2003) Attachment of periodontal ligament cells to chlorhexidine-loaded guided tissue regeneration membranes. *Journal of Periodontology*, 74:1652–1659.

Classen, D.C., Evans, R.S., Pestotnik, S.L., *et al.* (1992) The timing of prophylactic administration of antibiotics and the risk of surgical-wound infection. *New England Journal of Medicine*, 326:337–339.

Crumpton B.J. & McClanahan S. (2003) Antibiotic resistance and antibiotics in endodontics. Clinical Update. Naval Postgraduate Dental School. 25(12) December.

Cunningham, K.E., Ellis, S., Kripalani, S. (2009) What is the proper duration of antibiotic treatment in adults hospitalized with community-acquired pneumonia? *The Hospitalist* (online: www.the-hospitalist.org).

DeSanctis, M., Xucchelli, G. & Clauser, C. (1996) Bacterial contamination of barrier material and periodontal regeneration. *Journal of Clinical Periodontology*, 23:1039–1046.

Doğan, D., Cristan, C., Dietrich, T., *et al.* (2007) Timing affects the clinical outcome of adjunctive systemic antibiotic therapy for generalized aggressive periodontitis. *Journal of Periodontology*, 79:1201–1208.

el Askary, A.S., Meffert, R.M., Griffin, T. (1999) Why do dental implants fail? Part I. *Implant Dentistry*, 8:173–185.

el Moussaoui, R., de Borgie, C.A.J.M., van den Broek, P., *et al.* (2006) Effectiveness of discontinuing antibiotic treatment after three days versus eight days in mild to moderate-severe community acquired pneumonia: randomized, double blind study. *British Medical Journal*, 332:1355–1358.

Esposito, M., Grusovin, M.G., Oliver, R., *et al.* (2003) Antibiotics to prevent complications following dental implant treatment. *Cochrane Database of Systematic Reviews*, 3:CD0004152.

Esposito, M., Grusovin, M.G., Coulthard, P., *et al.* (2006) Interventions for replacing missing teeth: treatment of peri-implantitis. *Cochrane Database of Systematic Reviews*, (3)CD004970.

Esposito, M., Grusovin, M.G., Talati, M., *et al.* (2008) Interventions for replacing missing teeth: antibiotics at dental implant placement to prevent complications. *Cochrane Database of Systematic Reviews*, (3):CD004152.

Esposito, M., Grusovin, M.G. Tzanetea, E., *et al.* (2010) Interventions for replacing missing teeth: treatment of perimplantitis. *Cochrane Database of Systematic Reviews*, Issue 6. Art. No.: CD004970. DOI: 10.1002/14651858.CD004970.pub4.

Farhat, F.F., Kinaia, B. & Gross, H.B. (2008) Sinus bone augmentation: A review of the common techniques. *Compendium of Continuing Education in Dentistry*, 29(7):388–392.

Fedorowicz, Z., Keenan, J.V., Farman, A.G., *et al.* (2005) Antibiotic use for irreversible pulpitis. *Cochrane Database of Systematic Reviews*, Issue 2. Art. No.: CD004969. DOI: 10/100214651858.CD004969.pub2.

Geisler, S. (2009) Orally administered amoxicillin decreases the risk of implant failures. *Journal of the American Dental Association*, 140:1294–1296.

Giannopoulou, C. Andersen, E. Brochut, P., *et al.* (2006) Enamel matrix derivative and systemic antibiotics as adjuncts to non-surgical periodontal treatment: biologic response. *Journal of Periodontology*, 77:707–713.

Gordon, J.M., Walker, C., Hovlaris, C., *et al.* (1990) Efficacy of clindamycin hydrochloride in refractory periodontitis: 24-month results. *Journal of Periodontology*, 61:686–691.

Greenstein, G, & Cavallaro, J. (2011) Transcrestal sinus floor elevation with osteotomes: simplified technique and management of various scenarios. *Compendium*, 32:14–20.

Haddad-Houri, Y., Karaka, L., Stabholz, A., *et al.* (2004) Tetracycline conditioning augments the in vivo inflammatory response induced by cementum extracts. *Journal of Periodontology*, 75:388–392.

Haffajee, A.D., Socransky, S.S. & Gunsolley, J.C.(2003) Systemic anti-infective periodontal therapy. A systematic review. *Annuals of Periodontology*, 8:115–181.

Harrison, J.W. & Larson, W.J. (1976) The epithelized oral sinus tract. *Oral Surgery Oral Medicine Oral Pathology*, 42:511–517.

Hamad, W.A., Mata,r N., Elias, M., *et al.* (2009) Bacterial flora in normal adult maxillary sinuses. *American Journal of Rhinology & Allergy*, 23:261–263.

Hung, S.H., Lin, Y.W., Want, Y.H., *et al.* (2002) Permeability of *Streptococcus mutans* and *Actinobacillus actinomycetemcomitans* through guided tissue regeneration membranes and their effects on attachment of periodontal ligament cells. *Journal of Periodontology*, 73:843–851.

Jorgensen, M.G. & Slots, J. (2000) Responsible use of antimicrobials in periodontics. *Journal of the California Dental Association*, 28:185–193.

Karlowsky, J. Ferguson, J. & Zhanel, G. (1993) A review of commonly prescribed oral antibiotics in general dentistry. *Journal of the Canadian Dental Association*, 59:292–300.

Katranji, A., Fotek, P. & Wang, H.L. (2008) Sinus augmentation complications: Etiology and treatment. *Implant Dentistry*, 17:339–349.

Khemaleelakul, S., Baumgartner, J.C. & Pruksakorn, S. (2002) Identification of bacteria in acute endodontic infections and their anti-microbial susceptibility. *Oral Surgery Oral Medicine Oral Pathology Oral Radiology Endodontology*, 94:746–755.

Klinge, B., Hultin, M. & Berglundh, T. (2005) Peri-implantitis. *Dental Clinics of North America*, 49:661–676.

Laskin, D.M., Dent, C.D., Morris, H.F., *et al.* (2000) The influence of preoperative antibiotics on success of endosseous implants at 36 months. *Annuals of Periodontology*, 5:166–174.

Lawler, B. Sambrook, P.J., Goss, A.N. (2005) Antibiotic prophylaxis for dentoalveolar surgery: is it indicated? *Australian Dental Journal*, 50 (Suppl 2):S54–S59.

Levine, S.P. (2003) Endodontics. In: Dental Secrets, 3rd edn (ed. *Sonis, S.T.*), pp. 117–137. Hanley & Belfus, Philadelphia.

Lindhe, J. & Meyle, J. (2008) Peri-implant diseases: Consensus Report of the Sixth European Workshop on Periodontology. *Journal of Clinical Periodontology*, 35(Suppl. 8):282–285.

Ling, L.J., Hung, S.L., Lee, C.F. *et al.* (2003) The influence of membrane exposure on the outcomes of guided tissue regeneration: clinical and microbiological aspects. *Journal of Periodontal Research*, 38:57–63.

Listgarten, M.A., Lindhe, J. & Helldén, L. (1978) Effect of tetracycline and/or scaling on human periodontal disease. Clinical, micro-biological, and histopathological observations. *Journal Clinical Periodontology*, 5:246–271.

Loesche, W.J., Giordano, J., Soehren, S., *et al.* (1996) Nonsurgical treatment of patients with periodontal disease. *Oral Surgery Oral Medicine Oral Pathology Oral Radiology Endodontology*, 81:533–543.

Loesche, W.J., Syed, S.A., Morrison, E.C., *et al.* (1984) Metronidazole in periodontitis. I. Clinical and bacteriological results after 15 to 30 weeks. *Journal of Periodontology*, 55:325–335.

Loesche, W.J., Schmidt, E., Smith, B.A., *et al.* (1991) Effects of metronidazole on periodontal treatment needs. *Journal of Periodontology*, 62:247–257.

Loesche, W.J., Giordano, J.R., Hujoel, P., *et al.* (1992) Metronidazole in periodontitis: reduced need for surgery. *Journal of Clinical Periodontology*, 19:103–112.

Longman, L.P., Preston, A.J., Martin, M.V., *et al.* (2000) Endodontics in the adult patient: the role of antibiotics. *Journal of Dentisty*, 28:539–548.

Low, S.B. (2006) Managing the difficult periodontal patient. *Inside Dentistry*, 2:62–65.

Mazzocchi, A., Passl, L. & Moretti, R. (2007) Retrospective analysis of 736 implants inserted without antibiotic therapy. *Journal of Oral and Maxillofacial Surgery*, 65:2321–2323.

Misch, C.M. (1992) The pharmacologic management of maxillary sinus elevation surgery. *The Journal of Oral Implantology*, 18:15–23.

Mombelli, A., Lang, N.P. & Nyman, S. (1993) Isolation of periodontal species after guided tissue regeneration. *Journal of Periodontology*, 64:1171–1175.

Norowski, P.A. & Bumgardner, J.D. (2009) Biomaterial and antibiotic strategies for peri-implantitis. *Journal of Biomedical Materials Research Part B, Applied Biomaterials*, 88:530–543.

Nowzari, H., Matian, F. & Slots, J. (1995) Periodontal pathogens on polytetrafluoroethylene membrane for guided tissue regeneration inhibits healing. *Journal of Clinical Periodontology*, 22:469–474.

Pallasch, T.J. (1996) Pharmacokinetic principles of antimicrobial therapy. *Periodontology 2000*, 10:5–11.

Paul, J. (2006) What is the optimal duration of antibiotic therapy? *British Medical Journal*, 332:1358.

Peterson, L.J. (1990) Antibiotic prophylaxis against wound infections in oral and maxillofacial surgery. *Journal of Oral and Maxillofacial Surgery*, 58:617–620.

Pogrel, M.A. (1993) Infection management. *Oral and Maxillofacial Surgery Clinics of North America*, 5:127–135.

Powell, C.A., Mealey, B.L., Deas, D.E., *et al.* (2005) Post-surgical infections: prevalence associated with various periodontal surgical procedures. *Journal of Periodontology*, 76:329–333.

Pye, A,D,, Lockhart, D.E.A., Dawson, M.P., *et al.* (2009) A review of dental implants and infection. *Journal of Hospital Infection*, 72:104–110.

Resnik, R. & Misch, C. (2008) Prophylactic antibiotic regimens in oral implantology – rationale and protocol. *Dental Implant Summaries*, 17:142–150.

Revert, S.M., Wilström, G., Dahlèn, G., *et al.* (1990) Effect of subgingival debridement on the elimination of *Actinobacillus actinomycetemcomtans* and *Bacteriodes gingivalis* from periodontal pockets. *Journal of Clinical Periodontology*, 17:345–350.

Roberson, D. & Smith, A.J. (2005) The microbiology of the acute dental abscess. *Journal of Medical Microbiology*, 58:155–162.

Rosenfeld, R.M., Andes, D., Bhattacharyya, N., *et al.* (2007) Clinical practice guideline: adult sinusitis. *Otolaryngology – Head and Neck Surgery*, 137:S1–S31.

Rowland, R.W. (1999) Necrotizing ulcerative gingivitis. *Annals of Periodontology*, 4:65–73.

Saglie, R., Newman, M.G., Carranza, F.A. Jr., *et al.* (1982) Bacterial invasion of gingival in advanced periodontitis in humans. *Journal of Periodontology*,53:217–222.

Sancho-Puchades, M., Herrázez-Vilas, J.M., Berini-Aytés, L., *et al.* (2009) Antibiotic prophylaxis to prevent local infection in oral surgery: use or abuse? *Medicina Oral Patologia Oral Cirugia Bucal* , 14:E28–33.

Saxén, L. & Asikainen, S. (1993) Metronidazole in the treatment of localized juvenile periodontitis. *Journal of Clinical Periodontology*, 20:166–171.

Saxén, L., Asikainen, S., Kanervo, A., *et al.* (1990) The long-term efficacy of systemic doxycycline medication in the treatment of *Actinobacillus actinomycetemcomitans* associated periodontitis. *Archives of Oral Biology*, 35:227S–229S.

Sculean, A., Blaes, A., Arweiler, N., *et al.* (2001) The effect of post-surgical antibiotics on the healing of intrabony defects following treatment with enamel matrix proteins. *Journal of Periodontology*, 72:190–195.

Schwartz, A.B. & Larsen, E.L. (2007) Antibiotic prophylaxis and postoperative complications after tooth extraction and implant placement: a review of the literature. *Journal of Dentistry*, 35:881–888.

Sefton, A.M., Maskell, J.P., Beighton, D., *et al.* (1996) Azithromycin in the treatment of periodontal disease. *Effect on microbial flora. Journal of Clinical Periodontology*, 23:998–1003.

Sela, M.N., Babirtski, E., Steinberg, D., *et al.* (2009) Degradation of collagen-guided tissue regeneration membranes by proteolytic enzymes of *Porphyromonas gingivalis* and its inhibition by antibacterial agents. *Clinical Oral Implants Research*, 20:496–502.

Sinus and Allergy Health Partnership (SAHP) (2004) Antimicrobial treatment guidelines for acute bacterial rhinosinusitis. *Otolaryngology-- Head and Neck Surgery*, 30(Suppl):1– 45.

Slots, J. & Rams, T.E. (1990) Antibiotics in periodontal therapy: Advantages and disadvantages. *Journal of Clinical Periodontology*, 17:479–493.

Slutzky-Goldberg, I. Tsesis, I., Slutzky, H., *et al.* (2009) Odontogenic sinus tracts: a cohort study. *Quintessence International*, 40:13–18.

Smiler, D.G. (1997) The sinus lift graft: Basic technique and variations. *Practical Periodontics & Aesthetic Dentistry*, 9:885–893.

Söder, P.O., Frithiof, L., Wikner, S., *et al.* (1989) The effects of metronidazole in treatment of young adults with severe periodontitis. *Journal of Dental Research*, 68:710, abstr 86.

Tasoulis, G., Yao, S.G., Fine, J.B. (2011) The maxillary sinus: challenges and treatment for implant placement. *Compendium*, 32:10–20.

Teles, R.P., Bogren, A., Patel, M., *et al.* (2007) A three-year prospective study of adult subjects with gingivitis II: microbiological parameters. *Journal of Clinical Periodontology*, 34: 7–17.

Thiha, K., Takeuchi, Y., Umeda, M., *et al.* (2007) Identification of periodontopathic bacteria in gingival tissue of Japanese periodontitis patients. *Oral Microbiology and Immunology*, 22:201–207.

Uchida, Y., Goto, M., Katsuki, T., *et al.* (1998) A cadaveric study of maxillary sinus size as an aid in bone grafting of the maxillary sinus floor. *Journal of Oral and Maxillofacial Surgery*, 56:1158–1163.

van Winkelhoff, A.J. (2005) Antibiotics in periodontics: are we getting somewhere? *Journal of Clinical Periodontology*, 32:1094–1095.

van Winkelhoff, A.J., Tijhof, C.J. & de Graaff, J. (1992) Microbiological and clinical results of metronidazole plus amoxicillin therapy in *Actinobacillus actinomycetemcomitans*-associated periodontitis. *Journal of Periodontology*, 63:52–57.

Wagenberg, B. & Froum, S.J. (2006) A retrospective study of 1,925 consecutively placed immediate implants from 1988 to 2004. *The International Journal of Oral & Maxillofacial Implants*, 21:71–80.

Walker, C. & Karpinia, K. (2002) Rationale for use of antibiotics in periodontics. *Journal of Periodontology*, 73:1188–1196.

Walker, C.B., Gordon, J.M., Magnusson, I., *et al.* (1993) A role for antibiotics in the treatment of refractory periodontitis. *Journal of Periodontology*, 64(8 Suppl):772–781.

Weinberg, M.A. & Eskow, R.N. (2000) Osseous defects: proper terminology revisited. *Journal of Periodontology*, 71:1928.

Winkel, E.G., van Winkelhoff, A.J., Timmerman, M.F., *et al.* (2001) Amoxicillin plus metronidazole in the treatment of adult periodontitis patients. A double-blind, placebo-controlled study. *Journal of Clinical Periodontology*, 28:2956–305.

Yek, E.C., Cintan, S., Topcuoglu, N., *et al.* (2010) Efficacy of amoxicillin and metronidazole combination for the management of generalized aggressive periodontitis. *Journal of Periodontology*, 81:964–974.

Zipfel, G.J., Guiot, B.H. & Fessler, R.G. (2003) Bone grafting. *Neurosurgical Focus*, 14:1–8.

Zucchelli, G., Sforza, N.M., Clauser, C. *et al.* (1999) Topical and systemic antimicrobial therapy in guided tissue regeneration. *Journal of Periodontology*, 70:239–247.

Chapter 7

Management of the medically compromised dental patient

I. American Heart Association (AHA) guidelines for antibiotic prophylaxis

a. Prevention of infective endocarditis: Antibiotic prophylaxis for the dental patient

Q. What year are the most current guidelines for prevention of infective endocarditis in dental patients?

A. 2007. Published in *Circulation* (*The Journal of the American Heart Association*). The title of the article is: Prevention of infective endocarditis. Guidelines from the American Heart Asssociation. A guideline from the American Heart Association Rheumatic Fever, Endocarditis, and Kawasaki Disease Committee, Council on cardiovascular Disease in the Young, and the Council on Clinical Cardiology, Council on Cardiovascular Surgery and Anesthesia, and the Quality of Care and Outcomes Research Interdisciplinary Working Group. Online version: http://circ.ahajournals.org.

Q. What are the major changes in the updated recommendations?

A. The Committee concluded that only a very small number of cases of infective endocarditis (IE) might be prevented by antibiotic prophylaxis for dental procedures even if prophylactic therapy were 100% effective.

Q. Why were new recommendations needed?

A. The committee concluded that infective endocarditis was more likely to develop from frequent exposure to random bacteremias associated with daily activities (e.g., intraoral trauma, flossing and brushing) than from bacteremia caused by a dental, GI tract, or genitourinary (GU) tract procedure. Additionally, the committee recommended that maintenance of meticulous oral hygiene may reduce the incidence of bacteremia from daily activities and is more important than prophylactic antibiotics for a dental procedure to reduce the risk of IE.

Q. What are the current medical conditions cited in the 2007 Guidelines that require antibiotic prophylaxis?

A. See Table 7.1.

Q. Does a patient with a cardiovascular implantable electronic device (e.g., pacemaker) require antibiotic prophylaxis according to the American Heart Association (AHA)?

A. There does not seem to be any scientific studies to support the use of antibiotic prophylaxis in these patients for invasive dental procedures (Baddour *et al.*, 2011).

The Dentist's Drug and Prescription Guide, First Edition. Mea A. Weinberg and Stuart J. Froum.
© 2013 John Wiley & Sons, Inc. Published 2013 by John Wiley & Sons, Inc.

Table 7.1   Conditions recommended for prophylactic antibiotics.

---

1) Artificial heart valves
2) A history of infective endocarditis
3) Certain specific, serious congenital (present from birth) heart conditions, including
    Unrepaired or incompletely repaired cyanotic congenital heart disease, including those with palliative shunts and conduits
    A completely repaired congenital heart defect with prosthetic material or device, whether placed by surgery or by catheter intervention, during the first six months after the procedure
    Any repaired congenital heart defect with residual defect at the site or adjacent to the site of a prosthetic patch or a prosthetic device
4) A cardiac transplant that develops a problem in a heart valve
    According to the new guidelines, patients who have taken prophylactic antibiotics in the past but no longer need them include patients with:

Mitral valve prolapse
Rheumatic heart disease
Bicuspid valve disease
Calcified aortic stenosis
Congenital heart conditions such as ventricular septal defect, atrial septal defect and hypertrophic cardiomyopathy.

Q. Are there other medical conditions that may also require antibiotic prophylaxis?

A. Yes. When in doubt get a medical consultation from the patient's physician. Other conditions possibly requiring premedication prior to invasive dental treatment include (Lockart *et al.*, 2007):

- Renal transplants/dialysis
- Hemophilia
- Shunts
- Immunosuppression secondary to cancer and cancer chemotherapy
- Immunosuppression secondary to HIV/AIDS
- Systemic lupus erythematosus
- Poorly controlled insulin-dependent diabetes mellitus.

Q. Is antibiotic prophylaxis required for patients that have been treated for heart disease (e.g., blocked arteries)?

A. No. For patients with blocked arteries angioplasty can be performed to open blocked heart arteries. Stent placement is another option that can be done during angioplasty. A cardiac stent is a small mesh tube used to treat narrow or weak arteries. Balloon angioplasty involves a specially designed catheter with a small balloon tip is guided to the point of narrowing in the artery. Once in place, the balloon is inflated to compress the fatty matter into the artery wall and stretch the artery open to increase blood flow to the heart.

Q. According to the most current 2007 guidelines what dental procedures are required for patients to have antibiotic prophylaxis?

A. See Table 7.2.

Q. Is antibiotic prophylaxis required for patients taking low-dose aspirin?

A. No. Antibiotic prophylaxis is not indicated for patients taking low-dose aspirin.

Q. According to the 2007 guidelines which is the antibiotic of choice for prophylaxis against IE?

A. The bacterium most commonly associated with endocarditis following dental and oral procedures is *Streptococcus viridans* (α-hemolytic streptococci). Amoxicillin remains the most recommended antibiotic for endocarditis prophylaxis.

Table 7.2   Antibiotic prophylaxis recommendations for dental procedures.

Higher incidence	Lower incidence
Dental extractions	Restorative dentistry (operative and prosthodontic)
Periodontal procedures: surgery, scaling and root planing, probing and recall maintenance	Local anesthetic injections (all except intraligamentary)
Implant placement and reimplantation of avulsed teeth	Placement of rubber dams
Root canal instrumentation when beyond apex (endodontics)	Postoperative suture removal
Subgingival placement of antibiotic fibers or strips	Placement of removable prosthodontic/orthodontic appliances
Placement of orthodontic bands (not brackets)	Taking oral impressions or radiographs
Intraligamentary local anesthesia injection	Fluoride treatment
Prophylactic cleaning of teeth and implants	

Walter *et al.* (2007) Prevention of infective endocarditis. Guidelines from the American Heart Asssociation. A guideline from the American Heart Association Rheumatic Fever, Endocarditis, and Kawasaki Disease Committee, Council on cardiovascular Disease in the Young, and the Council on Clinical Cardiology, Council on Cardiovascular Surgery and Anesthesia, and the Quality of Care and Outcomes Research Interdisciplinary Working Group. Circulation, 116(15): 1736–54 with permission from Wolters Kluwer Health. Online version: http://circ.ahajournals.org.

Table 7.3   Prophylactic antibiotic regimens for oral and dental procedures.

Situation	Drug	Regimen (to be taken 30 min to 60 min before dental procedure)
Oral	amoxicillin	adults: 2.0 g / children: 50 mg/kg
Unable to take oral medications	ampicillin or cefazolin, or ceftriaxone*	adults: 2.0 g IM or IV/ children: 50 mg/kg IM or IV adults: 1 g IM or IV/children: 50 mg/kg
Allergic to penicillins or ampicillin-oral	cephalexin* or clindamycin or azithromycin or clarithromycin	adults: 2 g / children: 50 mg/kg adults: 600 mg / children: 20 mg/kg adults: 500 mg / children: 15 mg/kg
Allergic to penicillins or ampicillin and unable to take oral medications	cefazolin or ceftriaxone* or clindamycin	adults: 1 g IM or IV/children: 50 mg/kg IM or IV. adults: 600 mg IM or IV/ children: 20 mg/kg IM or IV

*Cephalosporins should not be given to an individual with a history of anaphylaxis, angioedema, or urticaria with penicillins or ampicillin.
Walter *et. al.* (2007) Prevention of infective endocarditis. Guidelines from the American Heart Association. A guideline from the American Heart Association Rheumatic Fever, Endocarditis, and Kawasaki Disease Committee, Council on cardiovascular Disease in the Young, and the Council on Clinical Cardiology, Council on Cardiovascular Surgery and Anesthesia, and the Quality of Care and Outcomes Research Interdisciplinary Working Group. Circulation, 116(15): 1736–54 with permission from Wolters Kluwer Health. Online version: http://circ.ahajournals.org.

Agents such as ampicillin and penicillin VK have an equal antimicrobial effect against α-hemolytic streptococci, but amoxicillin is better absorbed in the gastrointestinal tract and provides higher, more sustained serum levels than the other penicillins (Lockart *et al.*, 2007).

Q. What are the most current AHA guidelines for antibiotic dosing for prophylaxis against IE?

A. See Table 7.3.

Q. What happens if the patient forgot to take the antibiotic 30 to 60 minutes before the dental procedure?

A. If the dosage of antibiotic was not taken before the procedure, the full amount may be taken up to 2 hours after the dental procedure (Wilson *et al.*, 2007; Dajani *et al.*, 1997).

Q. What happens if a patient is already taking an antibiotic for either a medical or dental reason?

A. Patients receiving antibiotics for other reasons at the time of a routine dental visit who are considered at risk for endocarditis have specific recommendations. The antibiotic that the patient is already taking is not adequate to prevent a dentally induced bacteria. Rather than increasing the dose of the drug currently being used, it is advisable to select an agent from a different class of antibiotic. Remember, if you have to choose another antibiotic, it must have the same bactericidal or bacteriostatic activity as the antibiotic taken for prophylaxis. For instance, if the patient is taking tetracycline (a bacteriostatic drug), he or she cannot take amoxicillin (a bactericidal antibiotic), but can take clindamycin, azithromycin, or clarithromycin, which are all bacteriostatic. If possible, the dental procedure is best postponed until at least 9 to 14 days after completion of the antibiotic. This will allow the normal oral flora to re-establish and help to reduce the incidence of bacterial resistance (Wilson *et al.*, 2007; Dajani *et al.*, 1997).

Q. Can I prescribe erythromycin to a patient who is allergic to penicllin?

A. Erythromycin, which was originally approved as an effective prophylactic agent for endocarditis in cases of penicillin allergy, is no longer among the recommended drugs. Erythromycin can cause severe gastrointestinal upset, and certain formulations (e.g., erythromcyin ethylsuccinate) have complicated pharmacokinetics. Instead, second-generation erythromycins, azithromycin, or clarithromycin can be prescribed because they have better absorption and produces less adverse effects.

Q. Is it advisable to see a patient taking antibiotic prophylaxis more than once a week or even once a week?

A. No. Since repeated use of antibiotics can lead to the emergence of antibiotic-resistant microorganisms in the oral cavity, it is recommended that there be an interval of at least 7 days between dental treatment appointments. There needs to be adequate time for the patient's normal oral flora to be re-established and prevent the development of resistant strains.

Q. How are prescriptions written for the different antibiotics for IE prophylaxis (Wilson *et al.* 2007)?

A. See Table 7.4. If allergic to penicillins then prescribe as shown in Table 7.5.

II.   Antibiotic prophylaxis for total joint replacement

Q. What is the concern about antibiotic prophylaxis for dental patients with total joint replacement?

A. A problem arises in patients with total joint replacements because if an infection develops the bacteria cannot be easily eliminated from a joint replacement implant. Bacteremias can cause hematogenous seeding of a joint implant soon after the surgery and for years afterward. This is why antibiotic prophylaxis is very important in dental patients with total joint replacements.

Q. What are the current guidelines for antibiotic prophylaxis for dental patients with total joint replacements?

A. In 2009, the American Academy of Orthopedic Surgery (AAOS) safety committee recommended that dentists consider antibiotic prophylaxis for all patients with total joint (e.g., knee, hip) replacement before any dental procedure whether or not that person was even at a high risk for developing an infection forever. The AAOS stated that "given the potential adverse outcomes and cost of treating an infected joint, replacement, the AAOS recommends that clinicians consider antibiotic prophylaxis of all total joint replacement patients prior to any invasive procedure that may cause bacteremia" (American Dental Association: American Academy of Orthopaedic Surgeons, 2003). This recommendation followed an earlier guideline by the AAOS and the American Dental Association, who

Table 7.4   How the prescription is written for oral prophylactic antibiotic regimens.

Rx amoxicillin 500 mg
Disp: # 4 (four) caps
Sig: Take four caps po 30 minutes to 1 hour before dental procedure

Table 7.5   How the prescription is written for oral prophylactic antibiotic regimens if allergic to penicillin.

Rx clindamycin 300 mg
Disp: # 2 (two) caps
Sig: Take two caps 30 min to 1 hour before dental procedure

OR

Rx clarithromycin 250 mg
Disp: # 2 (two) tabs
Sig: Take two tabs 30 min to 1 hour before dental procedure

OR

Rx azithromycin
Disp: # 2 (two) caps
Sig: Take two caps 30 min to 1 hour before dental procedure

in 2003 said that antibiotic prophylaxis should only be considered *within 2 years post-implant surgery* in high-risk patients who have high-risk dental procedures such as dental extraction, periodontal procedures, endodontic procedures, initial placement of orthodontic bands, implant placement and oral prophylaxis with anticipated bleeding. Readers are referred to this article to review (American Dental Association: American Academy of Orthopaedic Surgeons, 2003). It is emphasized that dentists must use their own clinical judgment in determining whether a patient requires antibiotic prophylaxis.

Q. Why is there controversy regarding the use of antibiotic prophylaxis in patients with total joint replacement?

A. There is some controversy regarding the 2009 guidelines. A recent article suggests that the 2009 guidelines should not replace the 2003 guidelines until further review (Little *et al.*, 2010). Some sources say that staphylococci, the most common cause of prosthetic joint infection, are relatively uncommon commensals of the oral flora and have been rarely implicated in bacteremia occurring after dental procedures. On the other hand, viridans-group streptococci make up most of the facultative oral flora and are the most common cause of transient bacteremia after dental procedures that result in trauma to the gingival or oral mucosa. However, viridans-group streptococci account for only 2% of all hematogenous prosthetic joint infections. Additionally it is stated that concerns about promoting antimicrobial resistance and about adverse reactions from antimicrobial use may outweigh any hypothetic benefit related to prevention of prosthetic joint infection (Deacon *et al.*, 1996). (http://www.ccjm.org/content/78/1/36.short). Another 2011 article, reported that dental procedure are not associated significantly with a risk for prosthetic joint infections (PJIs) and the use of prophylactic antibiotics in these patients may be questioned (Skaar *et al.*, 2011).

Q. What is the suggested antibiotic prophylaxis 2009 AAOS regimen for dental patients with total joint replacement?

A. See Table 7.6.

Table 7.6   Suggested antibiotic prophylaxis regimen in dental patients with total joint replacement.

Type of patient	Recommended drug	Drug dosage
Oral: Patients not allergic to penicillin	Cephalexin, cephradine or amoxicillin	2 grams orally (po) 1 hour prior to dental procedure
Parenteral: Patients are not allergic to penicillin but cannot take or tolerate oral medications	Cefazolin or ampicillin	Cefazolin 1 gram or ampicillin 2 grams intramuscularly (IM) or intravenously 1 hour prior to the dental procedure
Oral: Patients who are allergic to penicillin	Clindamycin	600 mg orally (po) 1 hours prior to the dental procedure
Parenteral: Patients who are allergic to penicillin but cannot take or tolerate oral medications	Clindamycin	600 mg intravenously (IV) 1 hour prior to the dental procedure

Adapted from: American Dental Association; American Academy of Orthopedic Surgeons (2003) Advisory Statement. Antibiotic prophylaxis for dental patients with total joint replacements. *Journal of the American Dental Association* 134: 895–898. Prevention of infective endocarditis. Guidelines from the American Heart Association. A guideline from the American Heart Association Rheumatic Fever, Endocarditis, and Kawasaki Disease Committee, Council on cardiovascular Disease in the Young, and the Council on Clinical Cardiology, Council on Cardiovascular Surgery and Anesthesia, and the Quality of Care and Outcomes Research Interdisciplinary Working Group. Online version: http://circ.ahajournals.org.

Table 7.7   How the prescriptions are written for oral antibiotic prophylaxis for total joint replacement.

Rx cephalexin 500 mg

Disp: # 4 (four) caps

Sig: Take 4 caps po 30 min to 1 hour before dental procedure.

OR

Rx amoxicillin 500 mg

Disp: # 4 (four) caps

Sig: Take 4 caps po 30 min to 1 hour before dental procedure.

Q. How are prescriptions written for antibiotics used as prophylaxis for dental patients with total joint replacement?

A. Oral antibiotic prophylaxis for total joint replacement
Standard regimen (Table 7.7).
If allergic to penicillin (Table 7.8).

Q. Why is cephalexin suggested as an antibiotic?

A. Cephalexin (Keflex) is a cephalosporin that has excellent bone penetrating properties and is an ideal antibiotic in patient with total joint replacement. However, there is approximately a 10% cross sensitivity between penicillins and cephalosporins, which precludes the prescribing a cephalosporin to patients allergic to penicillins. In these cases an alternative antibiotic is clindamycin (see Table 7.6).

Q. Is a patient with a titanium rod or plate in the neck required to have antibiotic prophylaxis?

A. No. According to the American Dental Association and the American Academy of Orthopedic Surgeons (AAOS) antibiotic prophylaxis is not indicated for dental patients with pins, plates, screws or rods (American Dental Association: American Academy of Orthopaedic Surgeons, 2003; Rubin *et al.*, 1976).

Table 7.8 How the prescriptions are written for oral antibiotic prophylaxis for total joint replacement if allergic to penicillin.

Rx clindamycin 300 mg
Disp: # 2 (two) caps
Sig: Take 2 caps po 30 min to 1 hour before dental procedure.

Table 7.9 Classification of high blood pressure.

Blood pressure classification	Diastolic BP (mmHg)	Systolic BP (mmHg)
Normal	<120 AND	<80
Prehypertension	120–139 OR	80–89
Stage 1 hypertension	140–159 OR	90–99
Stage 2 hypertension	≥160	≥100

Reprinted from Chobanian *et al.* (2003) with permission from Wolters Kluwer Health.

Q. Is antibiotic prophylaxis indicated for patients with pins, plates, or screws?

A. No. Antibiotic prophylaxis is not indicated for dental patients with pins, plates or screws in any part of the body (American Dental Association: American Academy of Orthopaedic Surgeons, 2003).

Q. If the patient is allergic to penicillin can cephalexin be prescribed?

A. No. If the patient is allergic to penicillin, cephalexin, which is a cephalosporin, should not be prescribed as there is a 10% cross-sensitivity in patients allergic to penicillin. Instead, clindamycin can be prescribed (Table 7.8).

III.   Cardiovascular diseases

a. Hypertension

Q. What is the most current classification of blood pressure for adults?

A. The 2003 Joint National Committee on Prevention, Detection, Evaluation, and Treatment of High Blood Pressure (7th Report) classifies blood pressure as shown in Table 7.9.

Q. Should blood pressure be taken on all dental patients?

A. Blood pressure should be taken on all new patients on the initial visit and hypertensive patients at every dental visit (Yagiela & Haymore, 2007).

Q. What are the effects of epinephrine on the sympathetic receptors in the body?

A. Theoretically, epinephrine binds to all sympathetic receptors (α_1, β_1, β_2) in the body. The α_1-receptors are locate predominantly on blood vessels under the skin, mucous membranes and GI tract. The β_2-receptors are located predominantly on blood vessels on certain internal organs like the lungs, liver and brain, and in blood vessels in skeletal muscle. β_1-receptors are primarily located on the heart. The coronary arteries have both α_1-and β_2-receptors.

   Epinephrine in low concentrations (up to two or three cartridges) achieved systemically after anesthetic injections in dentistry is fairly selective for β_2-receptors rather than α-receptors. Epinephrine has some α_1-receptor effects resulting in vasoconstriction. The β_2- receptors, when activated by epinephrine, cause a decrease in peripheral vascular resistance by selectively causing vasodilation in skeletal muscle blood vessels. This opposing vasodilation of epinephrine limits the potential vasopressor effects thus lowering peripheral resistance and therefore diastolic blood pressure which is governed by peripheral vascular resistance. At the same time, the β_1- (and β_2)-receptors in the heart are activated to increase cardiac output and therefore systolic blood pressure; this is influenced by peripheral vascular resistance as well, but is also heavily influenced by the cardiac output, which epinephreine increases strongly. With an increase in systolic blood pressure and a decrease in diastolic blood pressure, there is no real change in mean blood pressure; these two influences cancel each other out regarding mean blood pressure.

Higher doses, as used to treat anaphylaxis, stimulate α_1-receptors. Since there are more of them, the net effect is vasoconstriction throughout the body, and an increase in peripheral resistance. This results in an increase in both systolic and diastolic blood pressure, and a possible reflex slowing of the heart mediated by the vagus nerve releasing acetylcholine onto the SA node (Yagiela, 1999).

Q. If more than three cartridges are needed in these patients is it adequate to space the doses apart rather than injecting all at one time?

A. When epinephrine is injected and absorbed into the blood it is rapidly converted to inactive metabolites. So, injections can be administered over minutes (e.g., 30 minutes) to avoid having too much cumulative doses (Yagiela & Haymore, 2007).

Q. It is a major concern of dentist whether to use epinephrine in hypertensive patients. Does the amount of epinphrine need to be limited in the controlled hypertensive patient?

A. By knowing the mechanism of how epinephrine effects the α and β receptors in the body in low and high doses should help with answering this question. See above question and answer. Remember, epinephrine is an endogenously produced neurotransmitter so that there is no real total contraindication for its use. The question that arises then, is how much epinephrine can be injected? It also depends on the medication used to treat the hypertension.

There is no real need to limit the amount of epinephrine used in dental local anesthesia in hypertensive patients who are controlled so long as there are no drug interactions and no intravascular injections; however, the American Dental Association recommends that the total dosage of epinephrine be limited to 0.04 mg (two or three cartridges) in cardiac risk patients. In uncontrolled hypertensive patients, studies have shown that a few cartridges (up to two or three cartridges) of lidocaine with 1:100 000 epinephrine can be used without changing the blood pressure; however, it is recommended to delay dental treatment in uncontrolled hypertensive patients until the blood pressure is under control. Of course, extra care must be taken aspirate to avoid intravascular injection (Yagiela & Haymore, 2007; Budenz, 2000).

Q. Can levonordefrin be used instead of epinephrine?

A. Levonordefrin (Neo-Cobefrin) is half as potent a vasoconstrictor as epinephrine. However, it primarily stimulates α-adrenergic (sympathetic) receptors, with little to no effect on the α-adrenoceptor. Stimulation of α_1-receptors on tissues/ organs causes vasoconstriction of blood vessels, resulting in hypertension (increased systolic and diastolic blood pressure). Epinephrine produces a greater stimulation of β_2 -receptors than β_1-receptors, causing vasodilatation and decreasing diastolic blood pressure. Higher doses produce more vasoconstriction and increased blood pressure. Since it is less effective/ potent than epinephrine, it is used in higher concentrations (e.g., 2% mepivacaine with 1:20 000 levonordefrin) and has similar adverse effects as 1:100 000 epinephrine. So, levonordefrin can be used in patients taking nonselective beta-blockers.

Q. Is there a local anesthetic that contains less of a concentration than 1:100 000 epinephrine as a vasoconstrictor?

A. Yes. Recommendations in cardiac patients include administering block anesthesia with mepivacaine 3% (Carbocaine, Polocaine plain) and then infiltrating with articaine 4% (Septocaine) that contains 1:200 000 epinephrine, which is half the concentration of 1:100 000 epinephrine.

Q. What is a safe way to administer epinephrine in a hypertensive patient?

A. It is best to inject a small amount of anesthetic solution containing epinephrine and to wait about 5 minutes while monitoring the patient.

Q. Can gingival retraction cord be used safely in hypertensive patients?

A. Gingival retraction cord is made of cotton with a range of options of nonimpregnated and chemically impregnated cords that have astringent (contraction–retraction; shrinkage of gingival tissues and sulcular displacement) or hemostatic (vasoconstriction; coagulation) actions. Examples of astringent/hemostatic agents include aluminum chloride, aluminum sulfate, and aluminum potassium sulfate, racemic epinephrine [equal amounts of dextrorotatory (*d*) and levorotatory (*l*) isomers] and ferric sulfate. 20–25% aluminum chloride and 15.5–20% ferrie sulfate are most commonly used (Strassler & Boksman, 2011). The ADA has been stated that 5 to 10% aluminum chloride is safe and effective (American Dental Association, 2002). Gingival retraction cords are also impregnated with epinephrine. About 92% of the epinephrine is systemically absorbed (Malamed, 1993; Kellam, *et al.* 1992; Pallasch, 1998). In fact, the amount of epinephrine absorbed may be equal to about 3.9 cartridges of a local anesthetic with 1:100000 epinephrine (Kellman *et al.* 1992). This provides a concentration of about 4% (equals 40 mg/ml) of active epinephrine which is about 40 times the concentration given for cardiac arrest or allergic anaphylaxis (Malamed, 1993). Since there is controversy regarding the adverse effects of epinephrine-impregnated gingival retraction cord, it is advised to limit or avoid their use especially in in cardiac patients.

Q. What is the different classification of medications the patient could be taking for hypertension and what are common dental adverse effects and how are they managed in the dental office?

A. See Table 7.10.

Q. If a patient is taking multiple antihypertensive medications, are the adverse effects additive?

A. Yes. If a patient is taking more than one antihypertensive drug that causes xerostomia, the xerostomia effect will be greater (Yagelia & Haymore, 2007).

Q. Are many of these antihypertensive medications also used for other heart conditions?

A. Yes. Some are used as anti-arrhythmic drugs, for angina, and for congestive heart failure.

Q. If a patient is taking a nonselective beta-blocker can epinephrine be administered?

A. There are nonselective and selective cardiac beta-blockers. Non-cardioselective beta blockers block both β_1 and β_2 receptors, which means that both β-receptors will be blocked allowing binding to the α-receptors, which cause vasoconstriction and possible hypertensive effects. Non-cardioselective beta-blockers include: propranolol (Inderal), timolol (Blocadren), and nadolol (Corgard). Epinephrine should be limited to 0.04 mg or two cartridges of 1:100 000 epinephrine.

Cardioselective beta blockers selectively block only β_1-receptors. Thus, there is little concern for using epinephrine in these patients.

Q. Which cardiac drugs can cause gingival enlargement?

A. Calcium channel blockers especially nifedipine (Adalat, Procardia), amlodipine (Norvasc) and less likely, diltiazem (Cardizem) can cause gingival enlargement.

Q. Is the correct term for gingival enlargement gingival hyperplasia or hypertrophy?

A. No. Hyperplasia is a histologic term defined as an abnormal increase in noncellular connective tissue components of the gingiva (Yagiela & Haymore, 2007). Hypertrophy is a term describing the enlargement of an organ or tissue from the increase in size of its cells. Both terms are used incorrectly when describing drug induced gingival enlargement.

Table 7.10 Dental management of patients taking drugs for hypertension.

Antihypertensive drug	Adverse effects	Dental management
Diuretics Thiazide diuretics Chlorothiazide (Diuril) Hydrochlorothiazide (Hydrodiuril) (HCTZ) Loop Diuretics Bumetanide (Bumex) Furosemide (Lasix) Potassium-sparing Diuretics Amiloride (Midamore) Spironolactone (Aldactone) Triamterene (Dyrenium) Combination Diuretics Aldactazide (HCTZ + spironolactone) Dyazide (HCTZ + triamterene) Maxzide (25/50 mg HCTZ + 37.5/75 mg triamterene) Moduretic (HCTZ + amiloride)	Xerostomia (loop diuretics cause the most xerostomia) Orthostatic hypotension Drug interaction with NSAIDs Lichenoid reactions (e.g., lichen planus-like lesions)	*Xerostomia* ✓ Xerostomia: monitor for caries, candidiasis and periodontal disease ✓ If xerostomia is severe, contact patient's physician to change to a different classification of medication ✓ For xerostomia: recommend OTC products • Saliva substitutes: effects only last for a few hours. Most contain either carboxymethylcellulose or hydroxyethylcellulose (e.g., Moi-Stir® spray or oral Swabsticks, Optimoist® spray, Salivart® aerosol;, Xero-Lube® spray OR • mucopolysaccharide solutions (e.g., MouthKote® spray) OR • Saliva stimulants: Natrol Dry Mouth Relief • Saliva lubricants/moisturizers: Biotene Dry Mouth: toothpaste, mouthwash, gum, moisturizing gel ✓ drink plenty of water ✓ chew sugarless gum or candy ✓ use of sodium fluoride gels or rinses ✓ if severe, prescribe salivary stimulants (cholinergic agents) such as pilocarpine (Salgan) or cevimeline HCL (Evoxac) • Pilocarpine is contraindicated in patients with uncontrolled asthma, narrow-angle glaucoma or iritis. Pregnancy category C. Adverse effects include excessive sweating and gastrointestinal distress. Recommended dose: Comes in 5 mg tabs: Initial dose 5 mg tid or qid; up to 3 to 6 tabs per day; not to exceed 2 tabs (10 mg) per dose. Can take up to 6 to 12 weeks to see results. • Cevimeline (Evoxac) contraindicated in patients with uncontrolled asthma, narrow-angle glaucoma or iritis. Pregnancy category C. Adverse effects include sweating and nausea.

(continued)

Table 7.10   (cont'd)

Antihypertensive drug	Adverse effects	Dental management
		Orthostatic hypotension
		✓ Make slow, careful changes in position.
		✓ After being in a supine position for dental care slowly raise the dental chair to an upright position and have the patient sit in the upright position for a few minutes before getting out of the chair.
		✓ Assistance in helping the patient out of the chair is important.
		✓ Monitor vital signs.
		NSAIDs use
		✓ Reduce effectiveness of antihypertensive drug
		✓ Limit use of NSAID to 5 days. Have blood pressure monitored.
		Lichenoid reactions
		✓ Refer to patient's physician for either treatment of the reaction with topical corticosteroids or change in medication
		Use of epinephrine
		✓ No precautions or contraindications with the use of epinephrine with these medications.
		✓ Take vital signs.
		✓ Medical consultation is required if hypertension is not controlled.
		Medical consultation is required if hypertension is not controlled.
Beta-blockers Acebutolol (Sectral) Atenolol (Tenormin) *Carvedilol (Coreg) *Labetalol (Normodyne) Metoprolol (Lopressor) *Nadolol (Corgard) *Pindolol (Visken) *Propranolol (Inderal) *Sotalol (Betapace) *Timolol (Blocadren) ――――――――― *Nonselective cardiac beta-blockers (blocks both β_1 and β_2-adrenergic receptors)	Xerostomia, dizziness, oral lesions, orthostatic hypotension	*Xerostomia*: see above recommendations *Orthostatic hypotension*: see above recommendations *NSAIDs use* ✓ Limit use of NSAID to 5 days. Have blood pressure monitored. *Oral lesions* (Kalmer, 2009) ✓ Lichen planus-like lesions, pemphigus like lesions (especially with propranolol) *Use of epinephrine* ✓ Take vital signs. ✓ Noncardiac selective beta-blockers: limit epinephrine to two cartridges of 1:100 000 because nonselective beta- blockers block both β_1 and β_2 receptors leaving α receptors for binding which causes increased blood pressure. Medical consultation is required if hypertension is not controlled.

(*continued*)

Table 7.10   *(cont'd)*

Antihypertensive drug	Adverse effects	Dental management
α-Adrenergic blockers Doxazosin (Cardura) Prazosin (Minipress) Tamsulosin (Flomax) Terazosin (Hytrin)	Xerostomia, dizziness, vertigo	*Xerostomia*: see above recommendations *Orthostatic hypotension*: see above recommendations *NSAIDs use*: see above recommendations *Use of epinephrine* ✓ No precautions or contraindications with the use of epinephrine with these medications.
ACE inhibitors Benazepril (Lotensin) Captopril (Capoten) Enalapril (Vasotec) Fosinopril (Monopril) Lisinopril (Zestril, Prinivil) Quinapril (Accupril) Ramipril (Altace)	Cough (highest incidence with ramipril), orofacial angioedema (swelling of the oral cavity; tongue, soft palate and uvula) (Yagiela & Haymore, 2007), less xerostomia	Orthostatic hypotension: see above recommendations NSAIDs use: see above recommendations *Orofacial angioedema*: refer to physician or hospital (Rees & Gibson, 1997). Orofacial angioedema is a condition with lip, facial or oral swelling. The danger of this condition is the possibility of airway obstruction (laryngeal edema). (Scully & Porter, 2003). *Use of epinephrine* ✓ No precautions or contraindications with the use of epinephrine with these medications. *Oral vesiculobullous lesions*: *Pemphigoid like lesions*: captopril
Calcium channel blockers Amlodipine (Norvasc) Diltiazem (Cardizem) Felodipine (Plendil) Nisoldipine (Sular) Nifedipine (Adalat, Procardia) Nicardipine (Cardene) Isradipine (DynaCirc) Verapamil (Calan, Isoptin)	Gingival enlargement, dizziness	*Orthostatic hypotension*: see above recommendations *Use of epinephrine* ✓ No precautions or contraindications with the use of epinephrine with these medications. *Gingival enlargement* ✓ More commonly seen with nifedipine and amlodipine ✓ Strict home care (plaque control) ✓ Surgical removal of gingiva, if necessary (as long as the patient is taking the calcium channel blocker the gingiva will return to an overgrowth state).
Angiotensin receptor blockers (ARBs) Candesartan (Atacand) Eprosartan (Teveten) Irbesartan (Avapro) Losartan (Cozaar)	Dizziness, cough	*Orthostatic hypotension*: see above recommendations *NSAIDs use*: see above recommendations *Use of epinephrine* ✓ No precautions or contraindications with the use of epinephrine with these medications.
Central anti-adrenergic Clonidine (Catapres) Methyldopa (Aldomet)	Rebound hypertension, orthostatic hypotension, oral lichenoid lesions, xerostomia	*Xerostomia*: see above recommendations *Orthostatic hypotension*: see above recommendations *NSAIDs use*: see above recommendations *Oral lesions*: Pemphigoid-like oral reaction *Use of epinephrine* ✓ No precautions or contraindications with the use of epinephrine with these medications.

Q. What is the mechanism of calcium channel blocker-induced gingival enlargement?

A. The exact mechanism of action is not clear. However, a proposed hypothesis involves inflammatory factors within the gingival tissue whereby numerous inflammatory cells in the connective tissue are replaced by collagen. An alteration of the intracellular calcium level in gingival cells by nifedipine, local inflammatory factors (plaque or biofilm accumulation), is important in causing gingival enlargement (Ciancio, 2004).

Q. What is the treatment of calcium channel blocker induced gingival enlargement?

A. It is recommended to teach the patient optimum oral home care. If there is no underlying periodontal disease and adequate keratinized gingiva, a gingivectomy can be performed but it must be understood that as long as the patient is taking the drug the gingival enlargement will return. If there is underlying periodontal disease, then periodontal flap surgery is advised. Referral to the periodontist may be necessary.

Q. What are dental implications if the patient is taking antihypertensives?

A. See Table 7.10.
A. Xerostomia or dry mouth is a common adverse effect of heart medication, especially diuretics, but it may not be so severe to interfere with oral function. Orthostatic hypotension is common. There are no drug–drug interactions with epinephrine except for noncardiac selective beta blockers, where the maximum amount of 1:100 000 epinephrine is two cartridges.

Q. Many antihypertensive drugs cause orthostatic hypotension. What precautions should the dentist follow?

A. According to the American Autonomic Society, orthostatic hypotension or postural hypotension is defined as a systolic blood pressure decrease of at least 20 mmHg or a diastolic blood pressure decrease of at least 10 mmHg within 3 minutes of standing (Bradley & Davis, 2003). Many cases of orthostatic hypotension are due to antihypertensive medications. Most antihypertensives, except calcium channel blockers, can potentially cause orthostatic hypotension. Medications that can cause orthostatic hypotension include: Diuretics; beta-blockers, alpha-blockers; angiotensin-converting enzyme (ACE) inhibitors; erectile dysfunction drugs: sildenafil (Viagra), vardenafil (Levitra), and tadalafil (Cialis); antidepressants (tricyclic antidepressants).

Q. How do beta-blockers cause orthostatic hypotension?

A. Beta-blockers block the β-adrenoceptor in the body, preventing the heart from speeding up, preventing the heart from contracting as forcefully, and dilating blood vessels. All three of these effects affect the ability of the body to react to position changes.

Q. When can orthostatic hypotension happen in the dental patient?

A. **1)** When lying down in a supine position and quickly sitting up in an upright position and then standing.
  2) Immediately after intravenous sedation (due to vasodilation).
  3) After nitroglycerin or other medication use.

Q. How can orthostatic hypotension be managed in the dental patient?

A. Make slow, careful changes in position. After being in a supine position for dental care slowly raise the dental chair to an upright position and have the patient sit in the upright position for a few minutes before getting out of the chair. Assistance in helping the patient out of the chair is important. Vital signs must be monitored.

Q. Is angioedema of the oral cavity dose related?

A. No. Angioedema from ACE inhibitors can occur at any time during therapy (Yagiela & Haymore, 2007).

Table 7.11   Dental management of patients taking drugs for angina.

Drug	Mechanism of action	Dental management
Nitrates Nitroglycerin (Nitro-Bid, Nitrostat, Nitro-Dur) Isosorbide dinitrate (Isordil)	Dilates and relaxes coronary blood vessels	Headache, dizziness, and/or flushing, orthostatic hypotension. Monitor blood pressure. Allow patient to sit in an upright position in dental chair for a few minutes before dismissing them.
		Epinephrine can be used but limit to two cartridges of 1:100 000 because of increased risk of developing tachycardia.
Calcium channel blockers Amlodipine (Norvasc) Bepridil (Vascor) Diltiazem (Cardizem) Nifedipine (Procardia, Adalat) Verapamil (Calan, Isoptin)	Slows heart rate and dilates coronary arteries	Orthostatic hypotension: Allow patient to sit in an upright position in dental chair for a few minutes before dismissing them.
		Gingival enlargement (especially with nifedipine and amlodipine).
		No special precautions with epinephrine and no drug interactions.
Cardioselective beta$_1$-blockers Atenolol (Tenormin) Metoprolol (Lopressor) Nadolol (Corgard) Propranolol (Inderal)	Reduces cardiac load and thus oxygen demand	NSAIDs such as naproxen sodium and ibuprofen can decrease the effectiveness of the action of the antihypertensive, resulting in rapid elevation of blood pressure. Limit use of NSAID to 5 days.
		Orthostatic hypotension: Monitor blood pressure. To avoid dizziness/fainting when a patient goes from the supine position have the patient sit in an upright position for a few minutes before dismissing the patient.
		Vesiculobullous oral lesions (propranolol).
		No special concerns with epinephrine and no drug interactions.

b.   *Angina and other ischemic cardiac conditions*

Q. What is angina?

A. Angina pectoris occurs when the metabolic demands of the heart exceed the ability of the coronary arteries to supply adequate blood flow and oxygen to the heart. There are different types of angina: stable angina (angina upon exercise); unstable angina (angina at rest); variant angina (Prinzmetal's angina) due to a hart vasospasm, often occurring during sleep.

Q. What drugs are used to treat angina pectoris?

A. The purpose of medication for angina pectoris is to increase blood flow and oxygen to the heart. Table 7.11 reviews drugs are used in the management of angina:

Q. What adverse effects should be recognized in patients taking these medications?

A. Orthostatic hypotension (except for aspirin). Have the patient sit in an upright position for a few minutes before getting up from the dental chair. It is important to monitor for gingival enlargement in patients taking calcium channel blockers especially nifedipine and amlodipine.

Q. Is epinephrine contraindicated in patients with angina?

A. Management of stable angina patients without a history of a myocardial infarction includes the reduction of stress and anxiety so that epinephrine should be used for stress control but is limited to two cartridges of 1:100 000 epinephrine to avoid increased tachycardia. Profound anesthesia is necessary to prevent stressful situation whereby large amount of endogenous epinephrine are synthesized and released from the adrenal medulla in response to pain. A local anesthetic with 1:200 000 epinephrine can also be used (e.g., articaine 4% or prilocaine 4%). In a 1.7 ml cartridge, 1:200 000 dilution concentration contains 0.0085 mg of epinephrine versus 0.017 mg in 1:100 000 concentration. Short appointments are recommended. Mild or moderate (conscious) sedation may be indicated.

Epinephrine should be avoided and no elective dental treatment in patients with unstable angina or in stable angina with myocardial infarction within 6 months of recent coronary artery bypass graft surgery. Medical consultation with the patient's physician is recommended.

Q. What local anesthetic should be administered if emergency dental treatment is necessary in the unstable angina patient or had a myocardial infarction within the last 6 months?

A. Stress and anxiety reduction is important, as mentioned above, so it is safe to limit the amount of local anesthetic to one or two cartridges.

Q. Why is there 1.7 ml of local anesthetic in one cartridge?

A. Most US manufacturers of local anesthetics made a labeling change in 2005. Each anesthetic cartridge contains a minimum of 1.7 ml and a maximum of 1.8 ml and 1.7 ml is printed on the cartridge. The majority of cartridges are labeled 1.7 ml.

Q. If patients are taking nitroglycerin do they need to have it with them at every dental visit?

A. Yes. It should be out on the table in case it is needed quickly. However, the nitroglycerin in the emergency medical kit in the dental office may have "fresher" nitroglycerin than the pills the patient is taking.

c.   Congestive heart failure

Q. What is heart failure?

A. Heart failure occurs when decreases in contractility prevent the heart from pumping forcefully enough to deliver blood to meet the body's demands. Decreases in cardiac output activate reflex responses in the sympathetic nervous system, which attempt to compensate for the reduced cardiac output.

Q. What is the dental management of patients taking medications for heart failure?

A. See Table 7.12.

Q. Can epinephrine be used safely in a patient with congestive heart failure?

A. It is advised to limit the amount of epinephrine to two cartridges of 1:100 000 epinephrine especially if taking digoxin.

Q. Is lidocaine contraindicated in patients with heart failure?

A. Yes. Lidocaine is contraindicated in patient allergic to lidocaine, heart failure, cardiogenic shock, second-or third -degree heart block (if no artificial pacemaker), Wolff-Parkinson-White syndrome (this may be controversial), and Stokes-Adams syndrome.

d.   Patient on low-dose aspirin and other antiplatelet drugs

Q. Should the term "baby aspirin" be used?

A. No. All products containing 81 mg are called "low-dose aspirin" and not "baby aspirin" because it was ambiguous and many people would give the "baby" aspirin to babies. All labeling is now "low-dose" aspirin. Low-dose aspirin products contain 81 mg of aspirin.

Table 7.12   Dental management of patients taking medications for heart failure.

	Dental management
Diuretics Thiazides Hydrochlorothiazide (Hydrodiuril) Loop diuretics furosemide (Lasix)	NSAIDs such as naproxen sodium (Aleve) and ibuprofen (Advil, Motrin) can decrease the effectiveness of the antihypertensive action of the thiazide diuretic, resulting in rapid elevation of blood pressure. Only use NSAIDs for 5 days. Monitor blood pressure. Orthostatic hypotension: Monitor blood pressure. To avoid dizziness/fainting when a patient goes from the supine position have the patient sit in an upright position for a few minutes before dismissing him or her. Monitor blood pressure. Xerostomia: monitor for dental caries, periodontal disease and candidiasis; monitor salivary consistency No drug interactions with the use of epinephrine.
Cardiac glycosides Digoxin (Lanoxin**)**	No interactions with NSAIDs No xerostomia Limit amount of local anesthetic to two cartridges of 1:100 000 epinephrine because epinephrine may cause arrhythmias in patients taking digoxin Avoid the concurrent use with clarithromycin (Biaxin) and tetracyclines. Use penicillin, clindamycin or azithromycin.
Adrenergic receptor agonist Dobutamine (Dobutrex)	Orthostatic hypotension: Monitor blood pressure. To avoid dizziness/fainting when a patient goes from the supine position have the patient sit in an upright position for a few minutes before dismissing him or her. Monitor blood pressure. Xerostomia: monitor for dental caries, periodontal disease and candidiasis; monitor salivary consistency. No special precautions or interactions with the use of epinephrine.
Vasodilators Hydralazine (Apresoline)	NSAIDs such as naproxen sodium (Aleve) and ibuprofen (Advil, Motrin) can decrease the effectiveness of the antihypertensive action of the ACE inhibitor, resulting in rapid elevation of blood pressure. Only use for 5 days. Monitor blood pressure. Orthostatic hypotension: Monitor blood pressure. To avoid dizziness/fainting when a patient goes from the supine position have the patient sit in an upright position for a few minutes before dismissing him or her. Monitor blood pressure. Xerostomia: monitor for dental caries, periodontal disease and candidiasis; monitor salivary consistency. No special precautions or interactions with the use of epinephrine.
ACE inhibitors Captopril (Capoten) Enalapril (Vasotec) Lisinopril (Prinivil, Zestril) Quinapril (Accupril) Fosinopril (Monopril)	NSAIDs such as naproxen sodium (Aleve) and ibuprofen (Advil, Motrin) can decrease the effectiveness of the antihypertensive action of the ACE inhibitor, resulting in rapid elevation of blood pressure. Limit use to 5 days. Monitor blood pressure. Orthostatic hypotension: Monitor blood pressure. To avoid dizziness/fainting when a patient goes from the supine position have the patient sit in an upright position for a few minutes before dismissing them. Monitor blood pressure. Xerostomia: monitor for dental caries, periodontal disease and candidiasis; monitor salivary consistency. Lichen planus-like oral lesions: captopril – develop oral lesions that mimic or resemble idiopathic lichen planus (Kalmer, 2009). No special precautions or interactions with the use of epinephrine.

(continued)

Table 7.12   (*cont'd*)

	Dental management
Calcium channel blockers Diltiazem (Cardizem) Verapamil (Calan, Isoptin) Amlodipine (Norvasc) Felodipine (Plendil) Isradipine (DynaCirc) Nicardipine (Cardene) Nifedipine (Adalat, Procardia) Nisoldipine (Sular)	OK to recommend or prescribe NSAIDs. Orthostatic hypotension: Monitor blood pressure. To avoid dizziness/fainting when a patient goes from the supine position have the patient sit in an upright position for a few minutes before dismissing him or her. Monitor blood pressure. Monitor for gingival enlargement especially with nifedipine and amlodipine. Xerostomia: monitor for dental caries, periodontal disease and candidiasis; monitor salivary consistency. No special precautions or interactions with the use of epinephrine.

Q. Is aspirin an antiplatelet or anticoagulant drug?

A. Aspirin is an antiplatelet drug with a totally different mechanism of action than warfarin and heparin which are anticoagulant drugs. Aspirin is also used as an antithrombotic agent because of its mechanism of action of inhibiting platelet aggregation.

Q. What are the different antiplatelet drugs?

A. Irreversible platelet inhibitors:

* Aspirin (acetylsalicylic acid or ASA)
* Clopidogrel (Plavix)
* Ticlopidine (Ticlid)
* Prasugrel (Effient)
* Aspirin-dipyridamole (Aggrenox).

Reversible platelet inhibitors
* Dipyridamole (Persantine).

Q. Which is the newest antiplatelet drug?

A. Prasugrel (Effient) is a antiplatelet (aggregation inhibitor) indicated to reduce the rate of thrombotic cardiovascular events such as stent thrombosis in patients with unstable angina, non-ST-segment elevation MI (myocardial infarction), or ST-elevation MI (STEMI) managed with percutaneous coronary intervention. There is a **Black Box Warning** that prasugrel may cause significant or fatal bleeding. Consult with the patient's physician before dental procedures. There is no evidence for discontinuing prasugrel prior to dental surgery. Discontinuing prasugrel as well as any antiplatelet drug may lead to increased risk of cardiovascular events. However, consultation with the patient's physician is important.

Q. What is dipyridamole (Persantine)?

A. Dipyridamole is sometimes used with aspirin to reduce the risk of death after a heart attack and to prevent another heart attack. Dipyridamole is used with other drugs to reduce the risk of blood clots after heart valve replacement. It works by preventing excessive blood clotting.

Q. What is clopidogrel?

A. Clopidogrel (Plavix) is a reversible platelet inhibitor. The combination of aspirin and clopidogrel is usually standard treatment for one month after heart stent placement and long-term use can significanlty reduce the risk of major cardiovascular events after percutaneous coronary intervention (Patrono *et al.*, 2004). Clopidogrel work differently from aspirin by inhibiting the binding of fibrinogen to platelets which is an important step for platelets to clot or aggregate (Awtry & Loscalzo 2000). Clopidogrel is frequently used by patients that cannot tolerate the adverse gastrointestinal effects of aspirin or are allergic or intolerant to aspirin (American Dental Hygiene Association, 2011).

Q. What is the difference between irreversible platelet inhibitors and reversible platelet inhibitors?

A. Irreversible inhibitors of platelet aggregation drugs require new platelets (about 5–10 days) to be produced when the drug is stopped in order to get normal bleeding times. When reversible inhibitors of platelet aggregation drug are stopped the affected platelets regain aggregation function quicker, usually about 2 days (American Dental Association, 2011).

Q. Who should be taking low-dose aspirin?

A. Aspirin is to prevent a heart attack or stroke in individuals who have had a heart attack or stroke, in individuals to prevent a first and second heart attack who currently have coronary heart disease, after coronary bypass surgery, and individuals with stable and unstable angina. No benefit has been shown in men younger than age 45 and women younger than 55 who prophylactically take aspirin. Aspirin interferes with thrombus formation by decreasing platelet formation.

Q. What is the mechanism of action of aspirin's antiplatelet action and does it differ from regular anti-inflammatory/analgesic dose aspirin?

A. Basically, the beneficial antiplatelet effects of aspirin for secondary or primary prevention of cardiovascular disease result from irreversible acetylation of the active site of cyclo-oxygenase (COX) in platelets which prevents the formation of thromboxane A$_2$ (TXA$_2$) resulting in inhibition of platelet aggregation or clotting (http://www.uptodate.com/contents/benefits-and-risks-of-aspirin-in-secondary-and-primary-prevention-of-cardiovascular-disease?source=see_link).   (See "Benefits and risks of aspirin in secondary and primary prevention of cardiovascular disease".)

How does this happen? From a pharmacologic point of view (e.g., arachidonic acid cascade) aspirin inactivates permanently the COX-1 and COX-2 activity in platelets, preventing the formation of TXA$_2$ and in endothelial cells, preventing the formation of prostacyclin (PGI$_2$). COX-1 is considered to be the "protective" enzyme and is normally found in the gastrointestinal tract, kidneys, uterus and platelets. Under the influence of COX-1 prostaglandins maintain and protect the gastric mucosa, maintain normal platelet function and regulate renal blood flow. COX-2 is produced only during inflammation and is found in low amounts in the tissues. The objective of using anti-inflammatory drugs is to reduce the inflammation and pain caused by COX-2. TXA$_2$, found in platelets, strongly induces platelet aggregation and vasoconstriction (prevents bleeding), while prostacyclin, formed in endothelial cells (lining of blood vessels), has the opposite effects of thromboxane and inhibits platelet aggregation and induces coronary artery vasodilation. Thus, prostacyclin has beneficial and desirable effects by protecting cells from platelet deposition and causing coronary artery vasodilation.

The antiplatelet effect occurs when aspirin or acetylsalicylic acid gets hydrolyzed or metabolized to acetic acid and salicylic acid (salicylate). It is the acetic acid that *irreversibly/permanently* binds covalently to the COX enzyme in the platelet. However, in anucleated (without a nucleus) platelets, new COX is formed every about 10 to 14 days, which is how long a platelet lives; the antiplatelet effect will persist about 5 days which is when 50% of platelet function returns to normal. On the other hand, in endothelial cells which have a nucleus, more cyclooxygenase is formed immediately. This allows the endothelial cell to continue to produce prostacyclin (Page, 2005). *Thus, since aspirin is very sensitive at low doses (75 to 325 mg/day) to COX-1 rather than to COX-2 and TXA$_2$ is derived from COX-1 in platelets it can be concluded that aspirin in low-doses and longer dosing intervals has a lasting antiplatelet affect by inhibiting platelet aggregation via inhibition of the formation of TXA$_2$* (Page, 2005).

In contrast, at daily regular analgesic/anti-inflammatory dosages of greater than 1000 mg (this is considered to an be anti-inflammatory dose, not an antithrombotic dose) aspirin inhibits both TXA$_2$ and prostacyclin, which negates the entire antiplatelet effect, while lower doses (antithrombotic) of 75 to 325 mg/day preferentially inhibit TXA$_2$ resulting in the antiplatelet phenomena (Page, 2005). The reason why higher doses and shorter dosing interval is required for an anti-inflammatory/analgesic effect is that COX-2, which is responsible for pain and inflammation, is much less sensitive to the actions of aspirin (Page, 2005). Therefore, regular anti-inflammatory doses most likely will not result in bleeding, while low-dose aspirin could result in bleeding.

Q. How soon after taking aspirin is an antiplatelet effect noticed?

A. Aspirin is absorbed in the upper gastrointestinal tract and within 60 minutes an antiplatelet effect is seen which is associated with a prolonged bleeding time (Awtry & Loscalzo, 2000; Patrono *et al.*, 1998).

Q. Does low-dose aspirin inhibit both COX-1 and COX-2?

A. Yes. Low-dose aspirin inhibits both COX-1 and COX-2 but is a more potent inhibitor of COX-1, thereby suppressing TXA_2 production and irreversibly inhibiting platelet aggregation for the lifetime of the platelet, which is about 10–14 days.

Q. What happens to the antiplatelet effect when nonsteroidal anti-inflammatory drugs (NSAIDs) are given with aspirin?

A. The effect of oral ibuprofen on *in vitro* platelet aggregation was evaluated in a study in which healthy volunteers were treated with aspirin 2 hours before or 2 hours after ibuprofen. When ibuprofen was given before aspirin, TXA_2 production by activated platelets was approximately twofold higher and inhibition of platelet aggregation was negligible at 24 hours. Ibuprofen had no effect on the action of aspirin when given 2 hours after aspirin and neither acetaminophen nor diclofenac affected the activity of aspirin.

Q. Does aspirin cause gastrointestinal tract toxicity (e.g., GI tract bleeding)?

A. Yes. Although aspirin-induced gastrointestinal toxicity is dose-dependent even at lower doses, aspirin can cause serious GI bleeding, especially in preexisting lesions in patients with gastric ulcers (Patrono *et al.*, 2004).

Q. What is the dosage of low-dose aspirin?

A. The accepted dosage of low-dose aspirin is controversial because aspirin is antithrombotic in a wide range of doses (Patrono *et al.*, 2004). Low-dose can be considered to be between 81 mg/day to 325 mg/day or even twice weekly. This dosage is adequate because approximately 10% of the platelets are replenished every day so that once-a-day doing can completely inhibit the formation of TXA_2 (Patrono *et al.*, 2004).

Q. Should I ask every patient if he/she is taking aspirin?

A. Yes. Sometimes patients may take the aspirin on their own without physician supervision. It is important to ask the patient if the aspirin was prescribed by the physician.

Q. Does low-dose aspirin interfere with bleeding time and are patients that take prophylactic low-dose aspirin more prone to bleeding during invasive dental procedures?

A. It has been published that low-dose aspirin may not significantly alter bleeding time (Ardekian *et al.*, 2000; AAP, 1996). Only about 20% to 25% of patients taking aspirin have an abnormal bleeding time (Randall, 2007). The increase in bleeding time lasts for the lifetime of the platelet or until new platelets are formed, which is about 10 to 14 days. About 50% of platelet function returns to normal within 5 days after aspirin is stopped. Consultation with the patient's physician is recommended.

Q. Should aspirin be discontinued before dental surgery (e.g., periodontal/implant/oral surgery) because of the risk of excessive bleeding?

A. It is the consensus that if an antiplatelet drug is used as monotherapy (only one drug) it does not need to be discontinued or alteration in doses. The frequency of oral bleeding complications after invasive dental procedures is low to negligible for patients who were taking antiplatelet drugs. Bleeding will still occur but the risks of altering or discontinuing use of antiplatelet medications outweigh the low risk of postoperative oral bleeding complications resulting from dental procedures and that can be usually controlled with local measures (Napeñas *et al.*, 2009; Brennan *et al.*, 2008; Madan *et al.*, 2005; Ardekian *et al.*, 2000). However, if more than one antiplatelet drug is being taken then the patient's physician or cardiologist must be contacted because in-office procedures may not be possible and the patient may need to be referred to a hospital for treatment.

A clinical study reported that the only significant relationship found between bleeding and all antiplatelet drugs, not just aspirin, was between bleeding and the number of teeth extracted. It was concluded by this research group that no more than three teeth should be extracted at one dental sitting and that the teeth should be adjacent to each other (Cardona-Tortajada *et al.*, 2009).

Q. Does clopidogrel (Plavix) or other antiplatelet agents other than aspirin alter bleeding time?

A. Yes. Antithrombotic/antiplatelet agents may increase the risk of bleeding during invasive dental procedures (Little *et al.*, 2002). In fact, clopidogrel is considered to be a more potent antiplatelet agent and can prolong the bleeding time by 1.5 to 3 times the normal value (Randall, 2007). Also, sensitivity to antiplatelet agents varies in different people (Randall, 2007). Some clinical reports have recommended continuing monotherapy aspirin or clopidogrel or dual therapy with more than one antiplatelet agent for invasive dental procedures (Napeñas *et al.*, 2009). Consultation with the patient's physician is recommended.

Q. Is there an increased risk of bleeding if a patient is taking two antiplatelet agents?

A. Yes. There is an increased bleeding tendency if two antiplatelet agents are used together. This must be taken into consideration before performing invasive dental procedures. Consultation with the patient's physician is recommended.

e. *Anticoagulated patient (patient taking warfarin or heparin)*

Q. What type of patient will be taking anticoagulation drugs?

A. Patients with prosthetic valves, cardiac stents, thromboembolic conditions (pulmonary embolus, deep vein thrombosis), stroke, atrial fibrillation.

Q. What is warfarin?

A. Warfarin, a synthetic derivative of dicoumarol, is an anticoagulant used to decrease the tendency for thrombosis (clot) or as a secondary prophylaxis in individuals who have had a previous thrombosis. Warfarin extends the time for blood to clot. Indications for using warfarin include: stent placement, atrial fibrillation, artificial heart valves, deep venous thrombosis and pulmonary embolism.

Q. What is Coumadin?

A. Coumadin is a brand name for warfarin.

Q. What is the mechanism of action of warfarin?

A. Warfarin inhibits vitamin K epoxide reductase, an enzyme that recycles oxidized vitamin K to its reduced form; it is sometimes referred to as a vitamin K antagonist. Onset of action occurs in a few days until clotting factors in the liver have adequate time to disappear once metabolized. Warfarin inhibits the formation of blood clots within blood vessels by inhibiting the synthesis of liver clotting factors II, VII, IX and X (extrinsic clotting pathway). A single dose of warfarin has a duration of action of about 3 days with a range of 2 to 5 days. The half-life of factor II is about 3 days and that is the longest half-life of all the factors involved (VII, IX and X).

Q. What is INR?

A. INR is referred to as International Normalized Ratio and is a reproducible number that represents the degree of anticoagulation. Prothrombin time (PT) standards vary from different laboratories so INR was developed where a standardized PT could be obtained in different laboratories around the world. It is determined by a simple blood test. The INR must be a certain target number before dental procedures causing bleeding can be performed.

Q. How do patients get their INR values?

A. Usually patients can get their INR values at the cardiologist's office or other medical facility (e.g., lab). Also, there are numerous home testing devices such as INRatio PT Monitoring System (www.hemosense.com) and Philips PT/INR self-testing (Philips Healthcare) that can be used at home or the dentist's office.

Q. When should the INR be taken?

A. It is recommended to measure the INR within 24 hours (the same day) of the dental procedure, but not more than 72 hours (Kassab *et al.*, 2011). This is the time that the earliest changes in INR are seen after warfarin administration (Kuruvilla & Gurk-Turner, 2001). The INR is applicable only for patients who have stable anticoagulant therapy.

Q. What should the INR valve be for dental procedures?

A. It depends on the case but usually it should be 2.0 to 3.0 in patients with pulmonary embolus, deep vein thrombosis, and atrial fibrillation and in a range 2.5 to 3.5 in patients with mechanical heart valves and recurrence of embolism while on warfarin. Individuals not taking warfarin have an INR of 0.8 to 1.2 (Kassab *et al.*, 2011). Anticoagulation drug alteration is required if INR > 4 and invasive surgical procedures are contraindicated until anticoagulant therapy is stable.

Q. Under what conditions can a patient's INR be elevated?

A. An INR can be elevated when a patient is taking warfarin and if the liver is so severely damaged that vitamin K-dependent coagulation factors cannot be synthesized.

Q. For which dental procedures should a patient get an INR?

A. Nonsurgical dental procedures have a significantly lower risk for bleeding than invasive surgical procedures (Kassab *et al.*, 2011).

- Low-risk for bleeding: radiographs, impressions.
- Low-moderate risk for bleeding (INR > 3: do not perform dental procedures): simple restorative procedures, scaling and root planning, endodontic procedures, oral prophylaxis.
- High risk for bleeding (INR > 3.5: do not perform dental procedures): simple extractions for not more than three teeth, periodontal surgery, crown and bridge.

However, Jeske & Suchko (2003) reported that dental procedures can be performed safely on patients with an INR ≤ 4, independent of the type of medical condition and the reason warfarin was prescribed.

Q. Is it necessary to have an INR when performing periodontal probing?

A. It is recommended because of the presence of inflammation, which increases the incidence of gingival bleeding.

Q. Does warfarin have a narrow therapeutic index or window?

A. Yes. A narrow therapeutic index or window is defined as a very close margin between the therapeutic dose in the blood and the lethal/toxic dose of a drug. Drugs that have a narrow therapeutic index include warfarin, lithium, digoxin, phenytoin, clozapine, cyclosporine, metaproterenol, and levothyroxine. The goal of warfarin therapy is to administer the lowest effective dose to maintain the target INR (Kuruvilla & Gurk-Turner, 2001). Initiation of warfarin therapy is difficult and often patients given a loading dose reach a supratherapeutic INR level resulting in prolonged bleeding (Kuruvilla & Gurk-Turner, 2001).

Q. Should warfarin be stopped before a dental procedure?

A. The major risk for thromboembolic events in a patient with atrial fibrillation can occur if warfarin is stopped for 3 days before a dental procedure. Remember that warfarin has a duration of action of about 3 days (range 2 to 5 days) so that if a physician decides to stop warfarin it must be stopped for almost 3 days and not just the day of the procedure because of this prolonged effect; the half-life is 36 hours. The major reason for discontinuing warfarin is prevent bleeding in the patient. Most of the bleeding can be easily treated with local measures. Always get a medical consult from the patient's physician (Jeske & Suchko, 2003).

Q. If warfarin is not stopped is there a higher incidence of postoperative bleeding?

A. Yes. Continuing warfarin during dental surgery will increase the incidence of postoperative bleeding but discontinuing warfarin does not really guarantee that the risk of postoperative bleeding will not happen. (Surgical management of the primary care dental patient on warfarin. UK Medicines Information. http://www.dundee.ac.uk/tuith/Static/info/warfarin.pdf.)

Q. What is hypercoagulation?

A. Stopping warfarin could lead to a "rebound" hypercoagulable state where there is an increase in clotting factors and thrombin activity after discontinuing the warfarin. Warfarin inhibits the synthesis of "new" clotting factors II, VII, IX, and X but does not interfere with already synthesized and circulating factors in the blood. These factors are still able to function until their half-lives are over so that until the remaining coagulation factors disappear there will always be a risk of abnormal coagulation. This results in a transient hypercoagulation. The half-life of factor II is 60 hours; factor VII is 4 to 6 hours; factor IX is 24 hours; and factor X is about 3 days. (http://emedicine.medscape.com/article/821038-overview#a0104).

Q. Besides clotting factors II, VII, IX and X are there any proteins involved in clotting?

A. Yes. Warfarin also inhibits anticoagulant proteins C and S. It takes about 2 days for these proteins to disappear; half-life of protein C is 8 hours and protein S is 30 hours. Thus, a transient hypercoagulation state can also occur due to inhibition of protein C and S soon after treatment with warfarin. Once protein C disappears (shortest half-life) there is a temporary coagulation until warfarin has time to decrease the production of the clotting factors.

Q. Does aspirin and warfarin have the same mechanism of action?

A. No. Both work different and aspirin (an antiplatelet) also causes bleeding and is definitely inferior for anticoagulation.

Q. Why are there so many drug interactions with warfarin?

A. There are several mechanisms of warfarin's drug-drug interactions. Warfarin is metabolized by the liver cytochrome P450 enzymes (CYP1A2) and it is highly protein bound (about 98%) to albumin in the blood which allows other highly protein bound drugs to displace the warfarin.

Q. How do antibiotics interfere with warfarin?

A. Certain antibiotics, especially broad-spectrum antibiotics such as amoxicillin, metronidazole, erythromycin, clarithromycin and azithromycin inhibit bacterial production of vitamin K activity because the antibiotic reduces the normal bacterial flora in the gastrointestinal tract or by decreasing the metabolism of warfarin via cytochrome P450 enzymes in the liver. It is advisable not to prescribe these antibiotics that could result in increased bleeding and consult with the patient's physician if necessary.

Q. What happens if a patient on warfarin needs to have antibiotic prophylaxis?

A. A single 2 g dose of amoxicillin does not cause any interaction. If the patient is allergic to penicillin, a single dose of 600 mg clindamycin will not cause any interaction. Since there is a major interaction between warfarin and clarithromycin and azithromycin, these 2 antibiotics should be avoided due to increased bleeding (www.drugs.com).

Q. What analgesics can be prescribed or recommended to a patient taking warfarin?

A. There is an undesirable synergistic effect when acetaminophen is taken with warfarin resulting dangerously elevated INRs (Bell, 1998). Care must be taken not to prescribe a narcotic-acetaminophen combination drug such as Vicodin. NSAIDs such as ibuprofen or naproxen should be avoided due to increased risk of bleeding.

Q. If a patient is taking warfarin can a NSAID or acetaminophen also be taken?

A. No. when a NSAID or acetaminophen is taken with warfarin the interaction is a synergistic drug interaction with a possibility of increased bleeding. It has been demonstrated that administering acetaminophen to a patient is stable on warfarin may increase the INR within 18 to 48 hours. Thus, careful monitoring of patients taking warfarin and acetaminophen is necessary. Currently there are no specific clinical guidelines to follow when recommending acetaminophen to patients taking warfarin. If a patient requires acetaminophen for mild pain, the dose should be the lowest possible with the shortest duration of acetaminophen therapy (Hylek *et al.*, 1998). It has been recommended that if acetaminophen is necessary at doses >2 g a day for more than 1 day, and an extra INR measurement may be necessary (Hughes *et al.*, 2011).

f.   Low-molecular-weight heparins (LMWHs)

Q. What are low-molecular weight heparins?

A. Low-molecular weight heparins are heparin salts used as an anticoagulant. In patients taking warfarin and are at high risk for developing a thromboembolism they can be given prophylatic LMWHs while the warfarin is stopped. In the past these high-risk patients needed to be hospitalized. Now with the development of LMWHs which are self-administered injections the patient does not need to be hospitalized. Also, since LMWHs have about a 95% bioavailability constant INR testing is not needed. The most common LMWH is enoxaparin (Lovenox). Other LMWHs include tinzaparin (Innohep), dalteparin (Fragmin), and fondaparinux (Arixtra). Patient with prosthetic heart valves needing outpatient oral surgery procedures cannot use LMWHs. The patient's physician must be consulted before any dental procedures because a decision must be made to place the patient on LMWH. Usually dental surgery should be performed 18 to 24 hours after the last dose of LMWH (Ganda, 2008).

Q. What is the best analgesic for a patient taking warfarin?

A. Aspirin and NSAIDs such as ibuprofen or naproxen sodium are contraindicated in patients taking warfarin because of an increased risk for bleeding. Any morphine analogs including hydrocodone (Vicodin) can be used but only for a few days. Extra-strength Tylenol taken with warfarin may cause a substantial increase in INR. So, the recommended analgesic is Regular-strength Tylenol.

g.   Myocardial infarction

Q. How soon after a patient has had a myocardial infarction (MI) can dental treatment be started?

A. As a general rule, treatment should not be started for 6 months post MI and 3 months coronary artery bypass graft surgery (CABG) (Lifshey, 2004).

Q. What medications can a patient that has had a previous MI be taking?

A. In order to reduce the chance of another myocardial infarction, a patient will be taking:

• a low-dose aspirin for its antiplatelet actions.

- a beta-blocker to reduce the workload of the heart by blocking the β_1-receptors on heart muscle cells
  - the beta-blocker binds to the β-receptors on the heart muscle cell and prevents them from being stimulated).
- an ACE inhibitor
  - blocks angiotensin in the blood allowing for vasodilation and lowering blood pressure and having a direct action on the heart which has a protective effect.
- a cholesterol lowering drug such as a "statin"
  - mechanism of action is to reduce the amount of cholesterol made in the liver; does not affect dietary cholesterol.

Q. What should be done if you suspect a patient is having a MI in the dental office?

A. The emergency medical system (EMS) should be activated. Have the patient lie down on the floor and assess the airway, breathing, circulation (ABCs) and monitor vital signs (American Academy of Periodontology, 1996).

h.   Cardiac arrhythmias

Q. What is a cardiac arrhythmia?

A. An arrhythmia occurs when either the impulse rhythm does not start in the sinoatrial node as a normal impulse, or the rate of heartbeats is abnormal (normally the heart beats about 70–80 times per minute), or it is not under automatic control. Classification of arrhythmias is based on the anatomical site of the abnormal rhythm: atrial (atrium), ventricular (ventricle), or supraventricular (atrium or above the ventricles). When the heart is beating too slowly but at a regular rate, it is called sinus bradycardia. If the heart is beating too fast, it is called sinus or ventricular tachycardia. Signs and symptoms of arrhythmia include skipped beats, palpitations, chest pain or shortness of breath.

Q. What drugs are used in the management of cardiac arrhythmias?

A. Many drugs used in the treatment of hypertension and angina are also used in the treatment of arrhythmias. See Table 7.13.

Q. It seems that there are some anti-arrhythmic drugs that can cause vesiculobullous lesions that mimic or resemble the real autoimmune disease?

A. Yes. Clinically, lesions can develop in patients taking certain drugs. This condition is called drug-related lichenoid reactions. See Table A2 (Kalmer, 2009; Scully & Bagan-Sebastian, 2004).

Q. Is epinephrine contraindicated in patients with cardiac arrhythmias?

A. Treatment modification is needed to avoid triggering an arrhythmia. The amount of epinephrine should be limited to two cartridges of 1:100 000 epinephrine to prevent an epinephrine-induced tachycardia.

Q. Is it necessary to get a medical consultation before dental treatment?

A. Yes. If a pacemaker or defibrillator has recently (within 6 months) been implanted, antibiotic prophylaxis may be needed, although there is a low risk for the development of infective endocarditis and the American Heart Association does not recommend antibiotic prophylaxis. With newer pacemakers that are well insulated (shielded) there is most likely no problem with impairing function when an electric dental devices are used, however due to the scarcity of human studies and medico-legal reasons, ultrasonic scaler should be avoided.

i.   Valvular heart disease

Q. What is valvular heart disease?

A. Valvular heart disease includes conditions associated with valvular stenosis and regurgitation. Essentially, it can involve the mitral, aortic, pulmonary or tricuspid heart valves. Valvular heart disease can occur from another pathologic

Table 7.13   Medications used for cardiac arrhythmias.

Common drugs	Common oral adverse effects
Class I: Sodium channel blockers	
Class I-A	
Quinidine (Quinidine)	Lupus erythematosus-like oral lesions
procainamide (Pronestyl)	Lupus erythematosus-like oral lesions
disopyramide (Norpace)	Severe xerostomia
Class I-B	
Lidocaine (Xylocaine)	When given intravenously, nothing related to dentistry
Phenytoin (Dilatin)	Gingival enlargement
mexiletine (Mexitil)	Blood disorders: gingival bleeding
Class I-C	
Flecainide (Tambocor)	Dizziness, fainting (care taken when arising from dental chair)
Propafenone (Rythmol)	Dizziness, metallic taste
Class II β-adrenergic blockers	
Metoprolol (Lopressor)	Nonselective cardiac beta-blocker; limit epinephrine use
	Caution use with antihypertensives (limit to 5 days)
Propranolol (Inderal)	Nonselective cardiac beta-blocker; limit epinephrine use
	Caution use with antihypertensives (limit to 5 days)
	Pemphigus and lichen planus-like oral lesions
Class III Potassium channel blockers	
Amiodarone (Cordarone)	Oral ulcers, neuralgic pain
Dofetilide (Tikosyn)	
Sotalol (Betapace)	Also a beta-blocker
Class IV Calcium channel blockers	
Diltiazem (Cardizem)	Gingival enlargement (less likely than nifedipine)
Nifedipine (Adalat, Procardia)	Gingival enlargement
Verapamil (Calan)	Gingival enlargement (less likely than the other two)

medical condition such as rheumatic fever, congenital heart defects, heart murmur, mitral valve prolapse, Kawasaki's disease, and systemic lupus erythematosus (SLE). With mitral valve prolapse it is important to determine whether there is regurgitation and the degree.

Q. Is antibiotic prophylaxis required for mitral valve prolapse or heart murmur?

A. According to the 2007 Guidelines on Infective Endocarditis from the American Heart Association, mitral valve prolapse and heart murmur do not require antibiotic prophylaxis before invasive dental procedures causing bleeding. If necessary obtain a medical consult from the patient's physician (Wilson *et al.*, 2007).

Q. How is valvular disease treated?

A. Either with medications or valve replacement.

Q. Is antibiotic prophylaxis required for patients with heart valve replacement?

A. Yes. Antibiotic prophylaxis is required for patients with heart valve replacement and palliative shunts, but *not* for cardiac stents. In a baby with congenital heart disease, a shunt diverts blood from one area of the heart to another to allow blood to flow to the lungs to receive oxygen.

Q. What medications are taken by patients with valvular disease?

A. Warfarin, aspirin, clopidogrel (Plavix), Ticlopidine (Ticlid), prasugrel (Effient), aspirin-dipyridamole (Aggrenox). Bleeding is to be monitored. Obtain a consult from the patient's physician. INR is required for warfarin.

Q. What other medical conditions are patients with valvular heart disease are more prone to develop?

A. Heart failure, arrhythmia and infective endocarditis (American Academy of Periodontology, 1996).

IV.   Pregnant and postpartum patient

Q. When is the safest time to treat a pregnant patient?

A. Preventive dental care should be provided to the pregnant patient as early as possible. The first trimester is from week 1 to week 12; second trimester week 13 to week 28 and; third trimester is week 29 to week 40 or delivery.

   Elective dental care is contraindicated in the first 10 weeks of pregnancy because at this time teratogenic risks are greatest. Routine care (e.g., scaling and root planing, restorative procedures) should been performed between 14 and 27 weeks, but it is best early in the second trimester. Emergency care (e.g., active infection or abscess) during the first trimester may outweigh the risks than if treatment was not done. Radiographs can also be taken as needed following all precautions. If there are any reservations concerning treatment of the pregnant patient, consider a consultation with the patient's physician (American Academy of Periodontology, 2004).

Q. Is epinephrine containing local anesthetics safe to administer to the pregnant patient?

A. Yes. As mentioned earlier, epinephrine is a natural hormone produced in the body. Epinephrine acting as a vasoconstrictor actually reduces the toxicity of the local anesthetic. Intravascular injection should be avoided. According to Michalowicz *et al.* (2008), essential dental treatment (e.g., scaling and root planing, temporary or permanent restorations, endodontic therapy or extraction) with the administration of topical anesthetics and local anesthetics containing 1:100 000 epinephrine are safe and did not significantly increase the risk of any adverse events in pregnant women at week 13 to 21 of gestation. In this clinical study, different anesthetics were used including topical 5% lidocaine and 1% dyclonine and injected local anesthetics such as 2% lidocaine with 1:100 000 epinephrine, 4% prilocaine with epinephrine and prilocaine without a vasoconstrictor. The authors conclude that data from larger clinical studies are needed to confirm the safety of dental care in pregnant women.

Q. Is lidocaine the safest local anesthetic to administer to the pregnant patient?

A. Yes. Lidocaine, an amide, is associated with the least medical/dental complications.

Q. Are topical anesthetics safe in pregnant women at 13 to 21 weeks?

A. Caution should be used with ester topical anesthetics since allergic reactions are possible. However, a recent article in the Journal of the American Dental Association reports the use of topical and local anesthetics are safe in pregnant women at 13 to 21 weeks' gestation (Michalowicz *et al.*, 2008).

Q. So, epinephrine is safe to administer during pregnancy?

A. Yes. Lidocaine with 1:100 000 epinephrine (0.017 mg of epinephrine in a 1.7 ml cartridge of lidocaine) is a category B drug in contrast to mepivacaine 3% (without a vasoconstrictor), articaine, and bupivacaine which are a category C. The concern about epinephrine is its effect on uterine muscle but there are no studies to confirm this effect on pregnant women (New York State Department of Health, 2006). Lidocaine can also be administered without epinephrine.

Q. What other precaution should be followed when treating a pregnant patient?

A. During the second and third trimester the patient should be positioned in the dental chair on her left side to avoid or relieve supine hypotensive syndrome. Blood pressure should be monitored in this patient.

Q. Can nitrous oxide be administered safely to a pregnant patient?

A. It is recommended to consult with the patient's prenatal care provider regarding use of nitrous oxide.

V.   Adrenal suppression and thyroid disease

Q. What is cortisol?

A. The adrenal cortex normally produces and secretes cortisol, an endogenous hormone, in the body. When exogenous steroids (e.g., prednisone, methylprednisolone) are taken the adrenal gland shuts off. In the normal, nonstressed person about 20– g of cortisol is produced per day which is equivalent to about 5–7 mg of prednisone. Cortisol is released in a highly irregular manner with peak secretion in the early morning, which then tapers out in the late afternoon and evening. When a person is stressed cortisol production is increased to about 50 to 300 mg a day. Cortisol functions to regulate energy by selecting the right type and amount of substrate (carbohydrate, fat or protein) that is needed by the body to meet the physiological demands that is placed upon it. Cortisol mobilizes energy by moving the body's fat stores (in the form of triglycerides) from one area to another, or delivering it to hungry tissues such as working muscle. During stressful times higher levels of cortisol is released, which has been associated with several medical conditions including suppressed thyroid function and hyperglycemia. However, when taking exogenous steroids there may not be enough endogenous cortisol to handle the body's stressful demands so that patients on long-term systemic steroids have been advised to take supplemental glucocorticoids.

Q. When are systemic glucocorticoid steroids indicated?

A. Chronic persistent asthma, Addison's disease, rheumatoid arthritis, pemphigus, pemphigoid, psoriasis, SLE, and gastrointestinal diseases such as Crohn's disease and ulcerative colitis.

Q. Does a patient taking systemic long-term glucocorticoid steroids such as prednisone or prednisolone need any specific adjustments in dosage during stressful dental procedures?

A. An "older" theory concerning the need for steroid supplementation in patients taking steroids was called the "rule-of-twos" which stated that if the patient was currently on 20 mg of cortisone (equivalent to 5 mg prednisone) daily for 2 weeks or longer within the past 2 years then it was necessary to give supplemental steroids to prevent an adrenal crisis.

Addison's or adrenal crisis is associated with a stressful event that is caused by the failure of cortisol levels to meet the body's increased requirements for cortisol and is primarily a mineralocorticoid steroid deficiency, not a glucocorticoid deficiency. Mineralocorticoids (e.g., aldosterone) maintain the level of sodium and potassium in the body. Adrenal crisis is a medical emergency characterized by abdominal pain, weakness, hypotension, dehydration, nausea and vomiting. Actually, adrenal crisis is primarily due to an insufficiency of mineralocorticoids.

It has been concluded in clinical studies that patients on long-term steroid drugs do not require supplemental "steroid coverage" for routine dentistry, including minor surgical procedures under profound local anesthesia with adequate postoperative pain control. The low incidence of significant adrenal insufficiency precludes the addition of supplemental steroids (Gibson & Ferguson, 2004). For major oral/periodontal surgery under general anesthesia supplemental steroids may be required depending upon the dose of steroid and duration of treatment. It is important to obtain a medical consultation from the patient's physician.

Make sure to schedule the patient in the morning and make sure the patient took the steroid within 2 hours of the dental procedure.

Q. Can epinephrine be used safely in patients taking a systemic steroid such as prednisone?

A. Yes. Epinephrine is synthesized and secreted by the adrenal medulla.

Table 7.14   Dental guidelines for corticosteroid supplementation: preoperative considerations.

Risk category and dental procedure	Supplemental steroids
Minimal risk: e.g., Nonsurgical dental procedures	Not needed – regular steroid dose
Possible risk: e.g. Minor periodontal and oral surgery with local anesthetic	Adrenal insufficiency is prevented when circulating levels of glucocorticoids are about 25 mg of hydrocortisone equivalent/day which is equivalent to a dose of about 5 to 6 mg of prednisone (prednisone is supplied as 1, 2.5, 5, 10, 20, 50 mg tabs). This should be taken 1–2 hours before treatment
Moderate to major risk: e.g., Major dental surgery (multiple extractions, quadrant periodontal surgery, multiple implants under general anesthesia longer than 1 hour (usually in the hospital)	Need glucocorticoid levels of 50 to 100 mg per day of hydrocortisone equivalent on the day of surgery and for at least 1 day after surgery. Intramuscular injection of 100 mg hydrocortisone 1 hour prior to surgery. Prescribe 25 mg hydrocortisone for 24 hours, then return to normal dose.

Data from Little, J.W., Fallace, D.A., Miller, C.S. & Rhodus, N.L. (2008) *Dental Management of the Medically Compromised Patient*, 7th edn. Mosby, St. Louis, pp. 236–247.
National Endocrine and Metabolic Diseases Information Service. Available at: http://endocrine.niddk.nih.gov/pubs/addison/addison.htm (accessed 18 May 2012).

Q. What is the appropriate corticosteroid supplementation for a patient taking steroids and undergoing dental treatment?

A. The final conclusion is that adrenal crisis is a rare event in dentistry, especially for patients with secondary adrenal insufficiency who develop this condition from taking steroids for common medical conditions. Most routine dental procedures, including nonsurgical periodontal therapy (scaling and root planing) and restorative procedures can be performed without glucocorticoid supplementation. See Table 7.14.

Q. Are there any precautions or contraindications for thyroid patients?

A. In most cases, hypothyroid patients receiving thyroid medication and have normal blood levels are treated without any special requirements and no antibiotic prophylaxis is needed. If the hypothyroid patient is untreated it is best to obtain a medical consult and postpone dental treatment until the condition is under control.

In patients who are hyperthyroid and untreated it is advised to avoid any surgical procedures as well as epinephrine because it could cause hyperthyroid crisis (elevated blood pressure and cardiac arrhythmias). Since there is sympathetic overactivity in the hyperthyroid patient, epinephrine's effects will be additive. Epinephrine should *not* be used if the patient is currently being treated for hyperthyroidism with propylthiouracil (PTU), Tapazole or methimazole. Once the patient with hyperthyroidism is treated and is euthyroid (normal thyroid) then precede as normal with no special requirements and epinephrine can be used but limited to two cartridges of 1:100 000.

VI.   Asthma

Q. What medications are taken in the management of asthma?

A. There are two classifications of asthma medications: rescue inhalers for bronchospasm and anti-inflammatory/bronchodilators drugs for long-term control. See Table 7.15.

Q. How is an asthma patient managed in the dental chair?

A. If the patient is using an inhaler for acute bronchospasm it should be on the treatment table in easy reach if an attack occurs. Ask the patient when the last attack was and what triggered it. Be prepared if the patient has an asthmatic attack in the dental chair. Dental care is performed only on well-controlled asthmatics.

Table 7.15 Medications for short-term and long-term control of asthma.

Rescue inhalers (bronchodilators) for bronchospasm (intermittent asthma)
Adrenergic (short-acting)   Albuterol (Proventil, Ventolin)   Pirbuterol (Maxair)   Terbutaline (Brethine, Brethaire)   Metaproterenol (Alupent)   Levalbuterol (Xopenex)
Anticholinergics   Ipratropium bromide HFA (Atrovent)   Ipratropium bromide and albuterol sulfate (Combivent)   Tiotropium bromide (Spiriva)
Long-term control of asthma   *Corticosteroids*   *(anti-inflammatory)*   Beclomethasone dipropionate (Beclovent, Vanceril)   Budesonide (Pulmicort)   Flunisolide (AeroBid)   Fluticasone (Flovent, Advair)   Mometasone (Asmanex)   Triamcinolone (Azmacort)
Selective β_2-agonists (long-acting)   *(bronchodilator)*   Salmeterol (Serevent)   Formoterol (Foradil)
Methylxanthines (bronchodilator)   Theophylline (Slo-Phyllin, Theo-Dur, Theo-24)
Mast cell stabilizers   *(anti-inflammatory)*   Cromolyn sodium (Intal)   Nedocromil (Tilade)
Leukotriene modifiers   *(anti-inflammatory)*   Zafirlukast (Accolate)   Montelukast (Singulair)   Zileuton (Zyflo)   *Immunomodulators*   *(anti-inflammatory)*   Omalizumab (Xolair)

Q. What should be done if the patient is taking corticosteroids for long-term use?

A. See section on adrenal insufficiency. Additionally, an adverse effect of corticosteroids that could affect dental treatment is the development of diabetes. In this case, a medical consultation from the patient's physician is advised to determine if the patient needs cortisone supplementation.

Q. Is epinephrine contraindicated in asthma patients?

A. This is very controversial. 1:100 000 epinephrine is safe to use in a well-controlled asthmatic patient. Actually, there are some OTC products for asthma (e.g., Primatine Mist) contains epinephrine. Epinephrine is also used for the treatment of acute exacerbations refractory to bronchodilator inhalers.

Some articles have reported not to use vasoconstrictors in asthmatic patients because of sodium metabisulfite, a sulfite preservative/antioxidant for the vasoconstrictor to avoid it from being degraded by light; however, epinephrine has been used safely in these patients. Methylparaben is only added to multiple-dose vials (Steinbacher & Glick, 2001).

Q. Can a patient be allergic to epinephrine?

A. No. because epinephrine is an endogenous hormone produced by the adrenal medulla in the body.

Q. Are there any dental materials that can exacerbate an asthmatic attack?

A. Yes. Fissure sealants, methyl methacrylate, dentifrices.

Q. What is Samter's triad?

A. Samter's triad is a medical condition characterized by the presence of asthma + aspirin (and NSAID) sensitivity + nasal polyps. This condition can occur in asthmatic patients who experience worsening of asthma after taking aspirin or NSAIDs. Patients who have Samter's triad also have nasal polyps. Before recommending or prescribing an analgesic to an asthmatic it is important to confirm that the patient does not have nasal polyps and if there has been no problem taking NSAIDs before. Acetaminophen is the preferred analgesic for asthmatic patients.

Q. What antibiotics should not be prescribed to an asthmatic?

A. If the patient is taking theophylline for asthma, erythromycin and clarithromycin (Biaxin) are *contraindicated*. This is a severe drug–drug interaction that can result in death.

VII.   Diabetes mellitus

Q. What is the classification of diabetes mellitus?

A. Type I and type II. The underlying cause of type I diabetes is autoimmune destruction of the beta cells in the pancreas. Since the beta cells do not produce any insulin exogenous insulin must be used to replace the insulin not being produced. Insulin is needed in the body because it helps the blood glucose get into the tissue cells which uses it for energy. When this does not happen glucose stays in the blood resulting in hyperglycemia. After a meal, excess glucose not taken up by the tissue cells, is stored in the liver in the form of glycogen and can be used later on when energy is required. Type I diabetics are prone to diabetic ketoacidosis where fat is broken down to glycerol and fatty acids due to energy needs. The fatty acids are converted to elevated ketone levels which are excreted in the urine. Most type I diabetics need insulin.

Risk factors for type II diabetes include genetics, obesity, and increasing age. Insulin is being produced but there is insulin resistance where insulin is not recognized by the tissue cells, resulting in hyperglycemia, which can cause the pancreas to produce more insulin, resulting in hyperinsulinemia. Type II diabetics do not need exogenous insulin since it is being produced but require oral forms of medications that act differently so that an individual may be on more than one oral medication. See Table 7.16.

Q. What are some important diabetic complications associated with dentistry?

A. Diabetics are at an increased risk for macrovascular (arteries) complications including coronary artery disease and microvascular (the terminal ends of blood vessels of capillaries and arterioles) complications of the eye (retinopathy), gingiva (periodontal disease), kidneys, nerves (neuropathy) and extremities (e.g., foot ulcers). This occurs because of excessive accumulation of glycated proteins (referred to as AGEs or advanced glycation end products) in the walls of

Table 7.16   Oral medications for diabetes mellitus.

Sulfonylureas

First-generation agents: stimulate release of insulin from beta cells

Chlorpropamide (Diabinese)
Tolazamide (Tolinase)
Tolbutamide (Orinase)

Second-generation agents: stimulate release of insulin from beta cells

Glipizide (Glucotrol)
Glyburide (DiaBeta, Micronase)
Glyburide, micronized (Glynase)
Glimepiride (Amaryl)

Biguanides: shuts off the liver's excess glucose production

Metformin (Glucophage)

Combination drugs

Glyburide/metformin (Glucovance)
Metformin/glipizide (Metaglip)
Metformin/rosiglitazone (Avandamet)

Thiazolidinediones: target insulin sensitivity; mechanism unclear

Pioglitazone (Actos)
Rosiglitazone (Avandia)

Alpha-glucosidase inhibitors: slow postprandial (after meals) carbohydrate absorption in the blood. Used when diet alone is not enough

Acarbose (Precose)
Miglitol (Glyset)

Meglitinides: increases insulin secretion from beta cells, which reduces glucose levels

Repaglinide (Prandin)
Nateglinide (Starlix)

---

large blood vessels. This causes impaired collagen turnover due to accumulation of AGE-modified collagen resulting in increased levels of LDL (low density lipoproteins) and narrowing of the blood vessels.

Q. What has to be known about a diabetic patient before rendering dental treatment?

A. How well-controlled is the patient? Results from two different tests must be known before dental treatment is started: fasting glucose and glycosylated hemoglobin (HbA1c). Hemoglobin A1c provides an average of blood glucose control over a 2 to 3 months and is used in conjunction with home blood glucose monitoring. HbA1c (glycated hemoglobin) levels represents blood glucose that combines with hemoglobin and becomes glycated. Therefore, the average amount of glucose in the blood is determined by measuring a hemoglobin A1c level. A consult with the patient's physician is necessary to know the patient's control and HbA1c levels.

The fasting blood glucose is just as important as HbA1c because it has been documented that the risk of infection may be directly related to fasting blood glucose. Fasting glucose levels are done by the patient (from the fingertip) in the morning before eating. When levels are <206 mg/dl there is no risk for developing infection. With blood glucose levels >230 mg/dl there is an increased risk for developing an infection.
HbA1c levels (Mealey & Oates, 2006):

- Normal level: treatment can precede 5.0–6.0%
- Treatment goal: treatment can precede <7.0%
- Alternative diabetic management required >8.0%.
  - (increased risk for complications such as delayed wound healing)

Q. What dental conditions are diabetics prone to develop?

A. Periodontal diseases, xerostomia, fungal infections (e.g., psuedomembraneous candidiasis – dental sore mouth), taste disturbances, burning mouth syndrome, dental caries, glossadynia.

Q. Should diabetic patients have antibiotic coverage to decrease the incidence of infection and increase wound healing?

A. Patients who are poorly controlled should have delayed dental treatment until control is established. If dental treatment cannot wait antibiotic prophylaxis may help prevent impaired and delayed wound healing. If the patient is well-controlled antibiotic coverage is not necessary (http://www,health.am/db/diabetes-mellitus-and-oral health/#1).

Q. What medical condition in diabetics taking insulin is commonly seen in dental offices?

A. Hypoglycemia usually occurs with insulin treatment but can occur with oral hypoglycemics. It happens due either to too much insulin being injected or improper timing of the injections with meals. Symptoms of hypoglycemia may not be apparent until blood glucose levels falls <60 mg/dl but can occur at any blood glucose level. It is characterized by nervousness, anxiety, sweating, headache, hunger, pallor, coldness, palpitations and tachycardia. Treating hypoglycemia is targeted to getting blood glucose to normal by eating 10 to 20 g (3 to 4 ounces) of carbohydrate in the form of sugar such as orange juice or pure sugar. Also, vital signs must be monitored. If the patient becomes unconscious, call 911. Glucagon 1 mg SC or IM or 20 ml of 50% dextrose IV is administered along with oxygen and monitoring vital signs (Lamster *et al.*, 2008; Ship, 2003).

Q. Is epinephrine safe to administer to diabetics?

A. Many factors may increase the body's insulin requirements which could worsen the diabetic state. Epinephrine, which is released during stressful times, causes gluconeogenesis which is the production of glucose. Also, epinephrine inhibits the release of insulin from the pancreas resulting in less glucose uptake into the cells which is used for energy. The risk of metabolic complications after the administration of small doses of epinephrine used in dentistry is much less than when used in larger doses in medicine. Additionally, there is a higher risk of complications in patients taking insulin than being controlled with di*et al*one or hypoglycemic oral drugs (Pérusse *et al.*, 1992).

VIII.   Psychiatric/neurological disorders

Q. Are there any precautions to follow if a patient is taking antianxiety medications, antidepressants and antipsychotics?

A. Yes. See Table 7.13.

Q. Why is there a limit on the amount of epinephrine in patients taking a tricyclic antidepressant?

A. The current theory depression is that there are low amounts of norepinephrine and serotonin. The "older" tricyclic antidepressants work by blocking the reuptake of norepinephrine by inhibiting the noradrenergic reuptake pump. This allows more norepinephrine to accumulate in the synapse increasing the levels of norepinephrine. Epinephrine functions in a similar manner. Epinephrine is partially inactivated by the noradrenergic pump. So if tricyclic antidepressants inhibit the noradrenergic reuptake pump this allows the accumulation of epinephrine in the synapse which can increase epinephrine levels in addition to norepinephrine substantially resulting in a hypertensive crisis. Therefore, the amount of epinephrine should be limited to two cartridges of 1:100 000. Levonordefrin (in 2% mepivacaine) should not be used. (Yagiela, 1999; Pérusse *et al.*, 1992). Since selective serotonin reuptake inhibitors (SSRIs) only affect serotonin and not norepinephrine, there are no precautions to follow regarding the use of epinephrine.

Q. Do psychiatric medications bind to different receptors?

A. Yes. Adverse effects of tricyclic antidepressants and antipsychotics are caused by the different receptors they block (acting like an antagonist): muscarinic (cholinergic) receptors causes xerostomia; α_1-adrenergic receptors resulting in orthostatic hypotension, reflex tachycardia and myocardial depression; histamine receptors resulting in sedation and weight gain (Weinberg, 2002). It should be noted that different drugs have different affinities to the different receptors so that one drug may not have as many adverse effects as another drug. The SSRIs have a low affinity for adrenergic, histaminic and muscarinic receptors resulting in less adverse effects than the "older" tricyclic antidepressants. In fact, "newer" formulations of "older" medications were developed to be more specific to the targeted receptor resulting in less adverse effects.

Q. Do any psychiatric drugs cause dental related problems?

A. Yes, besides xerostomia, lamotrigine (Lamictal), an anticonvulsant mainly used to treat epilepsy and bipolar disorder has been linked to cleft lip and palate in infants if used during pregnancy. The FDA has issued a drug alert concerning this issue.

Q. Are there any precautions to follow for patients with Parkinson's disease?

A. See Table 7.17.

Q. Are there any precautions to follow for patients on antiseizure medications?

A. See Table 7.19.

Q. Are there any precautions to follow for patients with attention deficit hyperactivity disorder (ADHD)?

A. See Table 7.17.

IX. Organ transplant

Q. Is a medical consultation with the patient's physician necessary before dental care is started?

A. Yes. Several factors are involved in preparing for dental treatment in a patient before dental care is given. Antibiotic prophylaxis may be required to prevent systemic infection. If an antibiotic is needed for either prophylaxis against infection or if the patient has an active infection (e.g., abscess) the choice of the antibiotic should be confirmed with the patient's physician (Segelnick & Weinberg, 2009).

Q. Are organ transplant patients more prone to developing bacterial infections?

A. Yes. Bacterial infections occur in 33%–68% of liver transplant recipients, 54% of lung transplant recipients, 47% of kidney transplant recipients, 35% of pancreas transplant recipients, and 21%–30% of heart transplant recipients, usually within 2 months after transplantation. The risk of infection after transplantation is primarily determined by the transplant recipient's epidemiologic exposures and the degree of immunosuppression. Some sources of infection in the transplant recipient include the environment and the recipient's endogenous flora (Soave, 2001; Rubin *et al.*, 1994; Patel & Paya, 1997).

Q. Should the patient going for a major organ transplant be seen by the dentist before the operation?

A. Yes. It is important to remove any forms of inflammation and infection before the transplantation to reduce the incidence of transplant failure or rejection (Segelnick & Weinberg, 2009). Treatment of dental caries, abscesses, necessary extractions, and periodontal diseases is important before transplantation since postoperative immunosuppression reduces a patient's ability to fight off systemic infection.

Q. Is it important to see the patient after transplantation?

A. Yes. It is definitely important to have the patient post-transplantation return to the dental office for regular maintenance appointment. Usually, the patient should not have any dental care for at least 3 months but up to 6 months post-

Table 7.17   Dental management of patients taking neurologic and psychiatric drugs.

Classification	Drug	Dental care
Antipsychotics (for schizophrenia and other psychiatric disorders including bipolar disorder)	Atypical antipsychotics: Clozapine (Clozaril)	• A medical consultation is required if dental surgery (e.g., extractions, periodontal/implant surgery). • Clozapine has a Black Box Warning because of a significant risk of agranulocytosis, which is a condition involving dangerous leukopenia or lowered white blood cell (WBC) count; infection and delayed healing can occur. It is highly recommended to obtain a physician's consult regarding the WBC count. • Patients usually have blood tests taken every week to determine WBC count and absolute neutrophil count. After 1 year on clozapine blood monitoring can be done once a month. • Thrombocytopenia: low blood platelet count; increased bleeding problems. Reported only in a few case reports. • Postpone dental care until WBC have returned to normal • Xerostomia: monitor caries, periodontal diseases and oral candidiasis • Orthostatic hypotension can occur. Raise the dental chair slowly from the supine position and have patient remain in upright position a few minutes before getting up from the chair. • Extrapyramidal side effects can impair the patient's ability to perform oral home care. • Use vasoconstrictors cautiously; Use low dose epinephrine (two cartridges of 1:100 000)
	Other atypical antipsychotics: Risperidone (Risperdal) Quetiapine (Seroquel), Olanzapine (Zyprexa) Ziprasidone (Geodon)	• Do not have the same risk of lowering WBC or platelets as does clozapine • Use low dose epinephrine (two cartridges of 1:100 000) • Xerostomia: monitor caries, periodontal diseases and oral candidiasis • Orthostatic hypotension can occur. Raise the dental chair slowly from the supine position and have patient remain in upright position a few minutes before getting up from the chair. • Extrapyramidal side effects can impair the patient's ability to perform oral home care.
Antidepressants	Tricyclic antidepressants (TCAs): Amitriptyline (Elavil) Imipramine (Tofranil) Nortriptyline (Aventyl) Doxepin (Sinequan)	• TCAs inhibit the reuptake of norepinephrine so limit the amount of epinephrine to two cartridges of 1:100 000 to avoid hypertensive crisis; monitor heart rate and blood pressure; epinephrine uses the same noradrenergic reuptake pump as norepinephrine
	Selective serotonin reuptake inhibitors (SSRIs): Paroxetine (Paxil) Fluoxetine (Prozac) Sertraline (Zoloft) Citalopram (Celexa)	• SSRIs do not involve norepinephrine and epinephrine; selectively inhibits the reuptake of serotonin; Epinephrine can be used

(continued)

Table 7.17 *(cont'd)*

Classification	Drug	Dental care
	Monoamine oxidase inhibitors (MAOIs): Phenelzine (Nardil) Isocarboxazid (Marplan) Tranylcypromine (Parnate)	• MAOIs act by inhibiting the activity of monoamine oxidase (MAO; MAO-A and MAO-B), an enzyme that breaks down monoamine neurotransmitters (epinephrine, norepinephrine, serotonin, melatonin) • Although the risk of an interaction with epinephrine is low, it is best to limit use to two cartridges of 1:100 000 epinephrine to avoid hypertensive crisis; monitor heart rate and blood pressure
Bipolar disorder	Lithium Carbamazepine (Tegretol) Valproic acid (Depakote) Atypical antipsychotics are also used (see above notes)	• Lithium has a narrow therapeutic index which requires frequent blood test to avoid overdosing and adverse effects including fine hand tremors and polydipsia (excessive thirst) • Modest rise in lithium levels • Avoid metronidazole with lithium • Lithium: Limit to two cartridges of 1:100 000 epinephrine • Epinephrine can be used with carbamazepine and valproic acid • Valproic acid: inhibits platelet aggregation which can causes altered bleeding times; monitor platelet counts and it is recommended to obtain a physician consult for invasive dental procedures
Acetylcholinesterase inhibitors (Alzheimer's disease)	Donepezil (Aricept) Galantamine (Reminyl) Rivastigmine (Exelon) Memantine (Namenda) Tacrine (Cognex)	• Alzheimer's drugs act by increasing the levels of acetylcholine in the brain. • Epinephrine can be used safely
Attention deficit hyperactivity disorder (ADHD)	Atomoxetine (Strattera) Amphetamine or amphetamine-like stimulants: amphetamine (Adderall) methylphenidate (Concerta, Ritalin) dexmethylphenidate (Focalin XR)	• Similar actions as tricyclic antidepressants (inhibits the reuptake of norepinephrine and dopamine and increasing their release from the presynaptic neuron into the synaptic space resulting in an increased level of both catecholamines); limit dosage of epinephrine to two cartridges of 1:100 000 epinephrine
Parkinson's disease drugs	*Dopamine precursors*: Levodopa/carbidopa Anticholinergics: Trihexyphenidyl (Artane) Benztropine (Cogentin) *Dopamine antagonists*: Bromocriptine (Parlodel) Pramipexole (Mirapex) Ropinirole (Requip) *Catechol-O-methyl-transferase (COMT) inhibitors*: Entacapone (Comtan) Tolcapone (Tasmar) *Antiviral*: Amantadine	• Epinephrine can be used but use minimum amount (two cartridges) of 1:100 000 epinephrine with COMT inhibitors. • Avoid clarithromycin, tetracycline, doxycycline with dopamine antagonists

(continued)

Table 7.17   *(cont'd)*

Classification	Drug	Dental care
Antiepileptic drugs	Phenytoin (Dilantin) Carbamazepine (Tegretol) Phenobarbital Clonazepam (Klonopin) Oxcarbazepine (Trileptal) Lorazepam (Ativan) Ethosuximide (Zarontin) Valproic acid (Depakene) Divalproex (Depakote) Levetiracetam (Keppra) Tiagabine (Gabitril) Lamotrigine (Lamictal) Gabapentin (Neurontin) Pregabalin (Lyrica) Felbamate (Felbatol) Topiramate (Topamax) Zonisamide (Zonegran)	• Epinephrine can be used • Phenytoin: monitor for gingival enlargement; optimal oral hygiene and if necessary refer to periodontist. As long as the patient is taking phenytoin, even if the gingival is surgically removed, the gingival enlargement will still occur.

transplantation because this is the time period of the highest risk of organ rejection and the high dosage of immunosuppressant agents taken during this time puts the patient at risk for systemic infections. At every appointment a thorough medical history update is done and the patient should bring in a current list of medications.

Q. Should the post-organ transplant patient receive antibiotic prophylaxis?

A. Yes. Preoperative antibacterial prophylaxis aimed at preventing wound infections.

Q. What local anesthetics can be used in patients who are going to have a liver transplant?

A. Patients who are going to have a liver transplant are treated as patients with liver failure. All injectable local anesthetics used in dentistry are amides and are metabolized in the liver. A consultation with the patient's physician will have blood values for the liver enzymes. Any local anesthetic can be used but a maximum of two cartridges at each dental visit.

Q. Can bleeding be a problem in organ transplant candidates?

A. Yes. Also, excessive bleeding can occur in organ transplant patients either due to organ dysfunction or medications the patient is taking. Many patients may be taking an anticoagulant and have decreased platelet counts. For example, patients with end-stage liver disease may have excessive bleeding because the liver is not making enough clotting factors. A medical consultation with the physician is necessary (National Institute of Dental and Craniofacial Research. Dental Management of the Organ Transplant Patient. www.nidcr.nih.gov).

Q. What drugs are patients taking who had an organ transplant?

A. Patients who had a major organ transplant are taking an immunosuppressant drug such as: azathioprine (Imuran), cyclosporine (Sandimmune), tacrolimus, sirolimus, Prograf/FK506, prednisone.

Q. Are there any concerns or potential adverse effects of azathioprine related to dental care?

A. Azathioprine is an antimetabolite indicated as an adjunct for the prevention of rejection in renal transplantation. It has a mechanism of action to reduce inflammation and interfere with the growth of rapidly dividing cells. There is a warning about chronic immunosuppression with an increased risk of malignancy. It functions to prevent organ rejection by inhibiting the production of blood cells in the bone marrow. Serious infections are a constant concern for patients receiving azathioprine and any other immunosuppressive drug. The medical consultation from the patient's physician should address the potential for severe infections occurring while the patient is taking azathioprine. The dentist should have the most recent results of the complete blood count (CBC) before dental treatment is started. Also, there could be bleeding, oral sores or swelling of the face, lips, tongue or throat. There are no drug interactions that would be of concern in dentistry.

Q. Are there any concerns or potential adverse effects of tacrolimus related to dental care?

A. Tacrolimus is an immunosuppressive (decrease the immune system's response to a transplanted organ) drug used to prevent rejection of liver and kidney organ transplant. There is a warning about *increased susceptibility to infection* and the possible development of lymphoma. The medical consultation from the patient's physician should address the potential for severe infections occurring while the patient is taking tacrolimus. Since hypertension is a common adverse effect, patients may be taking a calcium channel blocker which could cause gingival enlargement. There is a drug interaction with clarithromycin and erythromycin. These two antibiotics should not be taken with tacrolimus. Also, do not take with antifungal drugs such as clotrimazole, fluconazole, and ketoconazole.

Q. What are some adverse effects of cyclosporine?

A. Cyclosporine is a potent immunosuppressive agent that prolongs survival of many transplants such as kidney, liver, and heart. Patients taking cyclosporine usually have hypertension and taking a calcium channel blocker such as nifedipine (Adalat, Procardia) which causes gingival enlargement. So, gingival enlargement is due to both cyclosporine and nifedipine. Meticulous oral home care is important with these patients and maintenance/recare appointments every 3 months. Cyclosporine because it is an immunosuppressant may increase the susceptibility to infection. The medical consultation from the patient's physician should address the potential for severe infections occur while the patient is taking cyclosporine.

Cyclosporine can cause nephrotoxicity (including structural kidney damage) and hepatotoxicity. Ciprofloxacin (Cipro) and naproxen (an NSAID) may potentiate renal dysfunction if taken with cyclosporine. Cyclosporine is a substrate and inhibitor of CYP3A4. If cyclosporine is taken with azithromycin (Zithromax), clarithromycin (Biaxin), erythromycin, fluconazole (Diflucan), or ketoconazole (Nizoral) increased concentrations of cyclosporine may occur.

Q. If the patient is taking cyclosporine and requires antibiotic prophylaxis and is allergic to penicillin, what antibiotic can be prescribed?

A. Do not prescribe clarithromycin because there is a drug–drug interaction. If the patient is allergic to penicillin it is recommended to prescribe clindamycin.

Q. What precautions should be followed if the patient is taking a corticosteroid?

A. Usually the post-transplant patient will be taking many drugs so that the corticosteroid (e.g. prednisone) will probably be taken in a lower dose. Corticosteroids mask inflammation, which may occur less since the dose is lower than the usual one.

Q. Are there any concerns or potential adverse effects of sirolimus related to dental care?

A. Sirolimus (Rapamune) is an immunosuppressant only indicated for kidney transplantation. There is an increased susceptibility to infection with the development of lymphoma or other malignancies. The only dental adverse effect is oral ulcerations. Other adverse effects include hypertension, coughing up blood (hemoptysis), high cholesterol, peripheral edema (swelling of extremities), abnormal healing, and bleeding, low white blood count.

Sirolimus is a substrate for cytochrome P450 3A4 (CYP3A4). Inducers of CYP3A4 decrease sirolimus concentrations and inhibitors of CYP3A4 may increase sirolimus levels. Some dental drug inducers are: carbamazepine (Tegretol; for trigeminal neuralgia). Some strong dental drug inhibitors are: ketoconazole, clotrimazole (antifungal agent), erythromycin and clarithromycin (Biaxin); so avoid prescribing them.

X.   Liver disease

Q. Why is it important to get a physician's consultation for a patient with chronic liver disease?

A. Liver disease can increase the risk of bleeding especially in patients taking warfarin and LMWHs. It is important to get the results of the patient's liver function tests, which is an overview of how the liver is functioning. Albumin, bilirubin and prothrombin time (PT) measure the function of the liver and the capacity to make enzymes. These enzymes include alkaline phosphatase (AP), aspartate aminotransferase (AST), and alanine aminotransferase (ALT), which indicate if there has been any damage to the liver cells but not the function of the liver. Elevated levels of enzymes indicate liver damage. A prolonged PT indicates a deficiency in one of the clotting factors.

   A CBC including platelets is important to have because in liver disease there is usually bleeding with a decrease in platelet count (thrombocytopenia). Additionally, many drugs are metabolized by the liver so if the patient has a compromised liver some antibiotics and analgesics may either need to have dosage adjustment or another drug must be prescribed.

Q. What is the mechanism of increased bleeding?

A. The liver produces clotting factors II, V, VII, IX and X. Vitamin K is the cofactor required to synthesis these clotting factors. Severe liver disease results in lower levels of vitamin K resulting in less production of clotting factors. Bleeding will happen with INR > 1.5. However, the prothrombin time (or INR) becomes deviates from normal when about 80% of liver function is lost which is considered to be severe liver disease. Often the patient will have gingival bleeding and bruises. Partial prothrombin time (PTT) is a test that determines how long it takes for the blood to clot and is measured in seconds.

   Levels of albumin, a water-soluble, coagulable protein may decrease, which will lead to a decrease in clotting ability.

Q. What type of liver disease could bleeding be a problem?

A. Cirrhosis, cancer, hepatitis.

Q. When the medical consult is returned to the dental office, how is it read?

A. Frequently, liver function test values [e.g., Alb (albumin), AST, ALT, AP, Tb (total bilirubin) and Db (direct bilirubin)].

Q. What are the required lab values for INR and PTT before dental procedures can be started?

A. INR < 3.5; PTT < 35 s; platelets at least 60 000.

Q. Are there any precautions to follow with a patient with hepatitis or liver cirrhosis?

A. Yes. Many drugs are metabolized by the liver. In patients with liver disease any type of local anesthetic can be used but the maximum amount is limited to two cartridges.

Q. Which antibiotics are safe to give to patients with liver disease?

A. See Table 3.5. Penicillin VK, amoxicillin, clarithromycin (Biaxin), clindamycin (OK in hepatitis but decrease dose by half in cirrhosis).

Q. Which analgesic is safe to give to patients with liver disease?

A. Acetaminophen is considered to be safe and effective overall and is the recommended analgesic for individuals with liver disease. However, avoid chronic use and only use low-dose therapy for the least time. The maximum daily dose is <2 g per day (Hughes *et al.*, 2011). As mentioned earlier in the Guide, the FDA has made a recommendation that all manufactures of combination narcotic/acetaminophen use only 325 mg of acetaminophen per dosage formulation. It can be toxic to the liver when taken in excessive doses or with alcohol. It is an absolute contraindication in alcoholic cirrhosis. It has been reported that acetaminophen is safe in patients with stable chronic alcoholic liver disease for at least a short period of time (maximum of 48–72 hours) up to the maximum recommended dose (Worrlax & Flake, 2007). *Therefore, it is important to not exceed recommended dosages.* It may be prudent to consult with the patient's physician before taking any analgesics. If a narcotic is needed, any combination narcotic with acetaminophen is safe as long as the maximum recommended dose is not exceeded. Also, hydrocodone + ibuprofen (Vicoprofen) can be prescribed if the dentist or patient does not want to use acetaminophen.

Since the liver is the primary site for opioid metabolism, in patients with liver disease there is a risk of opioid accumulation. Codeine should be avoided because it is a prodrug which is transformed in the liver to morphine, its active metabolite. In cases of liver damage codeine cannot be transformed resulting in inadequate pain relief. For moderate to severe pain hydrocodone is recommended but low-dosage and only 2–3 days of use best. Decrease dose by 50% of usual dose; prescribe 1 tab q6h or q8h (Johnson, 2007).

XI. Chronic kidney disease

Q. Is a medical consultation necessary for a patient with chronic kidney disease?

A. Yes. Before any dental treatment a consultation with the patient's nephrologist is needed to determine the severity of disease, how well controlled the patient is and any potential problems such as bleeding.

Q. What are the different types of chronic kidney disease as the disease progresses?

A. Renal insufficiency which is seen in the early phase of disease, renal failure which occurs when the kidneys cannot function in excretion, and end-stage renal disease (ESRD) with the nephrons losing function and uremia, which leads to malnutrition, altered drug metabolism, electrolyte imbalance, bleeding, anemia and death.

Q. What lab values are evaluated for kidney disease?

A. Serum creatinine, creatinine clearance (CrCl), blood urea nitrogen (BUN) and glomerular filtration rate (GFR). Creatinine and BUN are not useful in detecting early renal insufficiency. CrCl is more sensitive in detecting early renal insufficiency.

Q. What does creatinine clearance show?

A. CrCl, which is measured as ml/min, indicates the function of the kidneys with regards to removing creatinine, a waste product, from the blood into the urine. Both blood and urine are required to determine CrCl. CrCl is not recommended for routine evaluation of kidney function. Normal CrCl is 80–120 ml/min.

Q. What does GFR show?

A. GFR tells how efficiently the kidneys are filtering wasters from the blood. GFR is used to determine the severity of kidney disease. Chronic kidney disease is defined as a GFR < 60 ml/min/1.73 m^2 or a GFR ≥ 60 ml/min/1.73 m^2 together with kidney damage for more than 3 months. Serum creatinine levels are used to measure GFR (Hassan *et al.*, 2009).

Q. How is chronic renal disease classified and staged?

A. According to the National Kidney Foundation K/DOQI Staging System for Chronic Kidney Disease (Table 7.18).

Q. What are some comorbidities in patients with renal disease?

A. Patients with renal disease most likely also have hypertension, diabetes mellitus, congestive heart failure and will be taking medications for these conditions as well.

Table 7.18   Classification of kidney failure.

Stage	Severity	GFR (ml/min/1.73 m²)
Stage 1	Kidney damage with normal or increased GFR	≥90
Stage 2	Mild	60–89
Stage 3	Moderate	30–59
Stage 4	Severe	15–29
Stage 5	Kidney failure	<15 (or dialysis)

Q. Why is it important to know about bleeding problems in renal disease patients?

A. There prolonged bleeding time (altered platelet aggregation) due to uremia (syndrome associated with fluid, electrolyte, and hormone imbalances and metabolic abnormalities changes). The platelet count and hematocrit levels should be known especially if bleeding during dental treatment is anticipated. Thus, a medical consultation with the patient's nephrologist is required before any type of dental surgery.

Q. Do patients with CRD also have anemia?

A. Anemia which is caused by a decrease in erythropoietin production can occur in patients with chronic renal disease.

Q. If a patient with chronic kidney disease with a kidney transplant requires antibiotic prophylaxis, which antibiotic is recommended?

A. For antibiotic prophylaxis no dosing adjustments are required for: azithromycin or clindamycin. Additionally, no dosing adjustments are required for doxycycline, erythromycin or penicillin VK. Amoxicillin requires dosage adjustments. If the patient is taking cyclosporine after the kidney transplant, then clarithromycin and erythromycin should not be prescribed due to risk of cyclosporine toxicity.

Q. Should fluoride topical products such as PreviDent be prescribed to a patient with renal disease?

A. No. PreviDent contains 1.1% sodium fluoride, which is indicated for the prevention of tooth decay, reducing dentinal hypersensitivity and remineralization. Topical fluoride should never be swallowed; it is toxic. Topical fluorides should not be prescribed to a patient with kidney disease because fluoride is highly excreted by the kidneys so the risk of toxicity is greater in patients with impaired kidney function.

Q. What are the treatments for renal disease?

A. Treatments for renal disease include monitoring with diet control, hemodialysis or kidney transplant. Most patients undergo hemodialysis rather than peritoneal dialysis.

Q. How often does a patient usually have hemodialysis?

A. Every 2 to 3 days for 3 to 5 hours.

Q. How soon after a patient undergoes hemodialysis should he/she have dental procedures?

A. A consultation with the patient's nephrologist is necessary. Because of increased risk of bleeding it is best to see the patient on days he/she is not undergoing dialysis. Heparin, an anticoagulant, is injected into the patient before dialysis to facilitate blood cycling through the dialyzer. If heparin has a half-life of 4 hours then it takes about 5 half-lives to be completely eliminated from the body; so about 20 hours. It is best to treat the patient one day after hemodialysis.

Q. Is antibiotic prophylaxis required for a patient having hemodialysis?

A. Not according to the American Heart Association Guidelines. However, it is suggested to get a consultation for the physician or nephrologist regarding this because there are many medical conditions that may require antibiotic prophylaxis. During hemodialysis a surgically produced arteriovenous fistula is made, which may be susceptible to infection.

Q. How do I prescribe medications in a patient with kidney disease?

A. Inappropriate dosing in patients with chronic kidney disease can cause toxicity or ineffective therapy. Dosages of drugs cleared renally are based on renal function (calculated as GFR or creatinine clearance). Dosing guidelines are divided into three broad GFR categories:

- $< 10\,ml/min/\,1.73\,m^2$
- $10–50\,ml/min/1.73\,m^2$, and
- $>50\,ml/min/1.73\,m^2$

It is advisable to contact the patient's physician and a pharmacist when prescribing medications to the patient. It must be determined the type and severity of renal impairment. It is most important to obtain a copy of the patient's blood test to determine the GFR, which is the most reliable value for overall kidney function.

Q. Can local anesthetics be administered to patients with chronic kidney disease?

A. All amide local anesthetics including lidocaine and all other injectable anesthetics are metabolized by the liver. No adjustments are needed.

Q. Are most antibiotics safe to prescribe in renal disease?

A. See Table 3.5. Many antibiotics are capable of inducing renal dysfunction. Acute tubular necrosis (ATN) and interstitial nephritis are the most common types of acute renal failure associated with antibiotic use. Acute interstitial nephritis may occur within minutes of drug exposure or may not develop for several months. Pre-existing renal disease, dose, duration and prior exposure to the offending antibiotic may increase the susceptibility of patients to acute interstitial nephritis. Some antibiotics that can cause this adverse effect include penicillin, amoxicillin, and fluoroquinolones. Tetracycline is contraindicated in patients with renal disease and may cause renal failure (Miller & McGarity, 2009). Azithromycin, clindamycin and doxycycline do not require a dosage or interval change and are safe to use.

XII. Recreational and illicit drugs

Q. Can epinephrine be used in a patient who uses cocaine?

A. Cocaine is the most powerful vasoconstrictor. It works in two ways: as a topical anesthetic and as a recreational drug. As a topical anesthetic, cocaine acts by reversibly binding to and inactivating the sodium channels on the nerve resulting in inhibition of a nerve impulse. As a recreational drug cocaine works similar to tricyclic antidepressants by blocking the reuptake of norepinephrine via the norepinephrine reuptake pump back into the nerve. This will result in excessive cocaine remaining in the synapse which could cause tachycardia, hypertension, diaphoresis, mydriasis, and tremors. Also, cocaine binds to dopamine reuptake transporters on the pre-synaptic membranes of dopaminergic neurons. This binding inhibits the removal of dopamine from the synaptic synapse and its subsequent degradation by monoamine oxidase in the nerve terminal. Dopamine remains in the synapse and binds to postsynaptic receptors which then through nerve impulses, activates the dopaminergic reward pathway leading to the feelings of euphoria and the 'high' associated with cocaine use. Deaths have be causes by inducing heart stimulation; increase blood pressure and arrhythmias. If a local anesthetic containing epinephrine is injected in a patient that just used cocaine, the concentration of norepinephrine plus epinephrine can put the patient in cardiac arrest. Epinephrine should not be used within 48 hours after the last dose of cocaine (Weinberg *et al.*, 2002).

Q. Why is it important to know about patients taking cannabis in the dental practice?

A. Cannabis, also known as marijuana, comes from the dried flowers, leaves and stem of the *Cannabis* plant. Cannabis in the forms of hashish and hash oil is more potent than marijuana. Cannabis is known to contain up to 400 chemicals but the primary psychoactive chemical is tetrahydrocannabinol (THC), which changes the person's perception and mood. Cannabis affects almost every system of the body, particularly the cardiovascular, respiratory and immune systems. Cannabis's vasoactive effects include dose-related tachycardia and increased heart rate which can result in a cardiac ischemia in some individuals. Even in acute doses, marijuana causes tachycardia and peripheral vasodilation (Nahas & Latour, 1992; Horowitz & Nersasian, 1978). There is a mild vasodilation that causes the eye to be "red" in marijuana users. There is a high incidence of xerostomia, which needs to be addressed; improve oral health, monitor for caries and periodontal diseases, avoid alcohol containing mouth rinses such as chlorhexidine. Recommend GUM® chlorhexidine gluconate rinse (this is a nonalcoholic chlorhexidine rinse; OTC).

Smoke from cannabis acts as a carcinogen, which is related to dysplastic changes and premalignant lesions in the oral cavity, Because of its immunosuppressive actions, users may be more prone to oral infections (Cho *et al.*, 2005).

Marijuana users may experience an acute anxiety attack in the dental office due to its parasympathetic response. The dentist must be prepared to handle these situations.

Q. Can epinephrine be used in a patient who uses cannabis?

A. Ask the patient at every dental visit update if he/she used marijuana and when it was last used. Marijuana and epinephrine could have a synergistic effects; marijuana's vasoactive effects in acute doses causes tachycardia and a decrease in blood pressure due to peripheral vasodilation (widening of the blood vessels, which causes a decrease in peripheral resistance to blood flow with a lowering of blood pressure) and the possibility of the patient having an acute anxiety response. Thus, epinephrine may cause an increase in these responses which could be life-threatening.

It is very controversial and unclear exactly how long marijuana stays in the body. However, it has been documented that inhaled marijuana is rapidly resorbed from the bloodstream and metabolized in the body. This is the reason blood testing is not used for the detection of marijuana. Although some metabolites have been detected up to 13 days (http://alcoholism.about.com/od/pot/a/marijuana_test.htm).

Horowitz and Nersasian (1978) recommended that patients stay off marijuana for at least 1 week before epinephrine is used in dental treatment. It is probably safest to use a local anesthetic without a vasoconstrictor.

Q. Is marijuana legal to use?

A. As of May 2011, medical marijuana is legal to use in 17 states (Alaska, Arizona, California, Colorado, DC, Delaware, Hawaii, Maine, Michigan, Montana, Nevada, New Jersey, New Mexico, Oregon, Rhode Island, Vermont, and Washington) as an antiemetic in cancer patients, and an analgesic in chronic pain.

Q. Can nitrous oxide be administered safely in marijuana users?

A. Nitrous oxide also is used for illicit/recreational uses. One study reported that marijuana use could enhance some of the subjective effects induced by nitrous oxide inhalation (Yajnik *et al.*, 1994).

Q. Are there any dental considerations for a patient abusing methamphetamine?

A. Methamphetamine an addictive substance that is closely related chemically to its parent compound, amphetamine, but with more central nervous system effects. The chemical name of methamphetamine or as it sometimes called, methylamphetamine is *n*-methyl-1-phenyl-propan-2-amine. Methamphetamine or "meth" is synthesized illegally in laboratories. Inhaled by smoking, methamphetamine releases high levels of dopamine, which stimulates brain cells, enhancing mood and body movement but also is toxic to brain cells containing dopamine and serotonin. It is referred to as "ice" or "crystal" when inhaled by smoking. With long-term use there seems to be a depletion of dopamine resulting in Parkinson-like symptoms. Methamphetamine is also taken orally, inhaled through the nose or injected.

Amphetamine analogues are prescription drugs (e.g., Adderall, Ritalin) indicated for the management of attention deficit hyperactivity disorder (ADHD). (http://chemistry.about.com/od/medicalhealth/a/crystalmeth.htm)

Methamphetamine is a stimulant that binds to α-receptors throughout the body resulting in sympathetic "fight or flight" response, similar to amphetamine. Methamphetamine causes cardiovascular problems including increased heart rate, increased blood pressure and cardiac arrhythmias. Other long-term effects include respiratory conditions, stroke, dilated pupils, excessive sweating, violent behavior, agitation, panic, hallucination, mood swings, confusion, permanent brain damage and death. Oral signs of specifically methamphetamine abuse include teeth attrition due to bruxism/clenching (due to excessive neuromuscular activity), xerostomia (by binding to α_2 receptors in the salivary glands) and dental caries. So called "meth mouth" was coined in the literature to designate rampant, untreated dental caries found specifically on the buccal and smooth surfaces of posterior teeth and interproximal surfaces of anterior teeth. Meth mouth is due to many factors including decreased salivary flow, poor oral hygiene and consumption of carbonated sugar-containing drinks. The etiology of the rampant caries is due to the possible presence of phosphoric, sulfuric or muriatic acid in the methamphetamine (Muzzin *et al.*, 2010). (http://www.dimen sionsofdentalhygiene.com/ddhright.aspx?id=10018). There is also a high incidence of poor oral hygiene in these patients.

Q. Can epinephrine and nitrous oxide be used in a patient who uses methamphetamine?

A. If the patient is a methamphetamine abuser, a medical consultation is recommended. The adrenergic–sympathetic response in the body caused by methamphetamine can stimulate the synthesis and release of epinephrine and norepinephrine from the adrenal medulla which contributes to the increased heart rate and blood pressure. Care should be taken if the patient recently used meth. The use of epinephrine as a vasoconstrictor in local anesthetics synergistically can create a potentially life-threatening cardiac situation. It is recommended to use a local anesthetic that does not contain a vasoconstrictor for at least 24 hours after the patient's last dose of methamphetamine. This is because the duration of action of methamphetamine is anywhere from 8 to 24 hours depending on how much the patient used. It has been documented that the cardiovascular effects are stopped before the drug is entirely eliminated from the body (Newton *et al.*, 2005). The patient's vital signs (heart rate, blood pressure) should be monitored during each visit. Tolerance to the local anesthetic can occur which requires more of the anesthetic solution. A neutral sodium fluoride mouthrinse, toothpaste, or gel, should be included in the patients' daily home care regimen. Fluoride varnish should be applied to areas of decalcification. Regular maintenance/recare appointment every 3 months should be planned (Goodchild & Donaldson, 2007; Donaldson & Goodchild, 2006; Klasser & Epstein, 2006). Consultation with the physician may be necessary if post-operative analgesics are required due to respiratory depression of the opioids (Goodchild & Donaldson, 2007).

Nitrous oxide should be used cautiously with patients taking methamphetamine.

Q. Are there any precautions to take with a patient who uses heroin?

A. Heroin is a semisynthetic opioid synthesized from morphine by acetylation. When injected intravenously, it produces euphoria or a "rush" rapidly within 10 seconds and the effects last for up to 4 hours. Systemic adverse effects of heroin include; constipation, addiction, physical dependence, "pin-point pupils", bacteremia, xerostomia, tongue discoloration, low blood pressure, bluish-colored lips and fingernails, disorientation, drowsiness, and infectious diseases. Death is usually due to respiratory depression. An overdose of heroin is managed similar to an overdose with any narcotic. Naloxone (Narcan), a narcotic antagonist, is injected intramuscularly. Get a medical consultation if you suspect the patient is a current heroin addict (http://health.nytimes.com/health/guides/poison/heroin-overdose/over view.html).

XIII. Bisphosphonates

Q. What are bisphosphonates and indications for use?

A. In the mid-1990s bisphosphonates were first introduced and prescribed as alternates to hormone replacement therapies (HRTs) for osteoporosis and osteopenia to prevent spine and hip fractures and to treat osteolytic tumors and

Table 7.19   Bisphosphonates.

Generic name	Brand name	Generation 1st: non-nitrogen 2nd: nitrogen	Route of administration	Elimination half-life	Indication	Potency factor
Alendronate	Fosamax; Fosamax plus D	2nd	Oral	10 years	Osteoporosis	
Clodronate	Bonefos	1st	Oral	157 hours	Hypercalcemia (bone metastases); osteoporosis	
Etidronate disodium	Didronel	1st	Oral	1–6 hours	Paget's disease	1
Risedronate	Actonel	2nd	Oral	1.5 hours to 480 hours	Osteoporosis	10
Tiludronate	Skelid	1st	Oral	150 hours	Paget's disease	10
Ibandronate	Boniva	2nd	Oral/IV	37–157 hours	Osteoporosis	500
Pamidronate	Aredia	2nd	IV	21–35 hours	Hypercalcemia; with or without bone metastases	2,000
Zoledronate	Zometa	2nd	IV	0.24–1.87 hours; terminal 146 hours	Bone metastases	1,000
Pamidronate	Aredia	2nd	IV	21–35 hours	Bone metastases	100
Zoledronate	Zometa	2nd	IV	0.24–1.87 hours; terminal 146 hours	Bone metastases	10 000

possibly slow tumor development. Bisphosphonates are powerful inhibitors of bone resorption by decreasing the action of osteoclasts, which are cells that break down bone. Also, bisphosphonates inhibit the increased osteoclastic activity and skeletal calcium release into the bloodstream induced by various stimulatory factors released by tumors.

Q. What is a "newer" term used for bisphosphonates?

A. Antiresorptive agents are another term for bisphosphonates. The term "antiresorptive agents" was chosen by the American Dental Association Council on Scientific Affairs Expert Panel on Bisphosphonate-Associated Osteonecrosis of the Jaw because there are some drugs including denosumab (Prolia) that are not bisphosphonates that could cause osteonecrosis of the jaw (Hellstein *et al.*, 2011; Edwards *et al.*, 2008). See Table 7.19.

Q. How are bisphosphonates used in cancer therapy?

A. Generally, hypercalcemia with malignancy occurs in patients who have breast cancer, squamous cell tumors of the head and neck or lung, renal cell carcinoma and some blood malignancies such as multiple myeloma. Excessive release of calcium into the blood occurs as bone is resorbed resulting in pain. In patients with hypercalcemia of malignancy

(HCM) intravenous bisphosphonates decreased serum calcium and phosphorous and increased urinary calcium and phosphorous excretion.

Q. What is an oral adverse effect of bisphosphonates that is seen in dentistry?

A. There has been major dental concerns regarding the development of bisphosphonate- related osteonecrosis of the jaw (BRONJ) or antiresorptive agent-induced osteonecrosis (ARONJ). The mechanism of this adverse reaction is not clear. One proposed mechanism is that bone turnover is depressed; bisphosphonates inhibit bone removal or resorption of "old or diseased" bone by osteoclasts (remember bisphosphonates inhibit osteoclastic activity) thereby interfering with bone repair and bone turnover. The bisphosphonates irreversibly alter the metabolism of the osteoclasts which results in no or poor bone resorption even if the blood supply is adequate. This causes osteoblasts to build new bone around the diseased bone. However, one proposed mechanism is that if the necrotic bone cannot be resorbed by the osteoclasts (remember bisphosphonates inhibit osteoclastic activity) during healing, then the necrotic bone will inhibit healing and affect blood supply to the area.

Q. What are the risk factors for developing BRONJ?

A. Risk factors with the development of BRONJ include (Edwards *et al.*, 2011):

• Currently or history of taking bisphosphonates (especially IV formulations but also oral for more than two years)
• Individuals older than 65 years
• History of cancer (breast, lung, prostate, multiple myeloma or metastatic disease to the bone), osteoporosis, Paget's disease, chronic renal disease on dialysis.

The following are local dental risk factors for BRONJ in patients taking intravenous or oral (less likely than IV but still can occur) bisphosphonates:

• Periodontal surgery
• Extractions (highest incidence)
• Dental implant surgery
• Ill-fitting dentures that is irritating to the tissues
• Less likely with: endodontic therapy, orthodontics, scaling and root planing
• BRONJ can also occur spontaneously without any prior dental procedure.

Q. Are there any other medical/dental comorbidities related to the development of BRONJ?

A. Yes. Possible comobidities include diabetes mellitus, denture weaker, smoking and periodontitis. Corticosteroid use is no longer thought of as a risk factor (Edwards *et al.*, 2011; Barasch *et al.*, 2011).

Q. What are the clinical signs and symtptoms of BRONJ?

A. Osteonecrosis is necrosis or death of bone and can cause severe, extensive, and irreversible damage to the jaw bone (occurs more frequently in the mandible than maxilla). Oral lesions appear similar to those of radiation-induced osteonecrosis. Patients with BRONJ do not have a history of radiation to the jaws. There usually is a delayed or completely absent healing of the periodontium after dental extraction or surgery for more than 6 weeks or can occur spontaneously.
  The following are signs and symptoms of BRONJ:

• Irregular mucosal ulcer with exposed bone in the maxillofacial area
• Pain or swelling in the area
• Infection
• Pain
• Mobility of teeth
• Numbness or heavy sensation
• Bone sequestrum.

Q. Do patients taking oral bisphosphonates have the same incidence of developing BRONJ as patients taking intravenous (IV) bisphosphonates?

A. In 2007, The American Association of Oral and Maxillofacial Surgeons published a Position Paper on bisphosphonate-induced ONJ. They concluded that patients being treated with oral bisphosphonates are at a considerably lower risk for osteonecrosis than patient taking IV bisphosphonates. The concern is that once bone is exposed it will most likely become necrotic and infected. Once the bone is exposed it is difficult to treat. Patients who have been taking bisphosphonates for more than 6 months are at highest risk for developing BRONJ (Grewal & Fayans, 2008; Ruggiero *et al*., 2004).

Q. What is the most recent information regarding the incidence of developing BRONJ in patients taking oral bisphosphonates?

A. In 2011, Jeffcoat *et al*. reported that oral bisphosphonates do not increase the risk for osteonecrosis of the jaw but found a sixfold increased risk in patients taking intravenous bisphosphonates (Jeffcoat *et al*., 2011).

Q. When could BRONJ occur while a patient is taking a bisphosphonate?

A. A survey conducted in 2005 concluded that the mean time of onset of BRONJ is about 18 to 22 months after the initiation of bisphosphonate therapy, although most cases have occurred after prolonged therapy, up to 3 to 5 years after the start of oral bisphosphonates. According to the American Dental Association on Scientific Affairs antiresorptive drugs for low bone mass puts the patient at a lower risk of developing BRONJ but it still can occur (Edwards *et al*., 2011). Additionally, the Council concluded that the risk of developing BRONJ is less for patients not being treated for cancer (Edwards *et al*., 2011).

Q. Does the amount of accumulated bisphosphonate in the bone effect the poor healing response seen during dental treatment?

A. Yes. A recent model was developed that found that the total accumulated concentration of bisphosphonates in bone can predict toxic levels which could possibly result in poor healing of dental wounds (Jones *et al*., 2011; Landesberg *et al*., 2008).

Additionally, there may be a higher incidence in the development of BRONJ based on the size of the person's skeleton or the total quantity of bone mineral into which bisphosphonates concentrate (Jones *et al*., 2011). Basically, individuals with higher total bone mineral (larger skeletal frames versus smaller frames) content took longer to reach toxic concentrations of the bisphosphonate (Jones *et al*., 2011).

Q. Why is the mandibular especially prone to BRONJ?

A. The jaw bone is more prone to developing BRONJ because it has a higher turnover rate than long bones.

Q. Why is there a higher incidence of developing BRONJ in patients taking IV bisphosphonates rather than oral?

A. Because an IV dose of bisphosphonate is incorporated into the bone while in an oral dose very little is absorbed by the gastrointestinal tract into the bloodstream.

Q. How about implant surgery and the risk of BRONJ in patients taking oral or IV bisphosphonates?

A. Implant or any type of dental surgery including extractions is contraindicated in patients taking IV bisphosphonates for the past 6 months. Marx and colleagues suggested that there is an increased risk for implant failure or BRONJ around the implants once the oral bisphosphonate has been taken for more than 3 years. If a patient has been taking the drug for less than 3 years, then that patient, most likely, can be treated normally. However, with these patients, they should be informed of the small risk of BRONJ for every person taking bisphosphonates and that the risk increases after 3 years of drug use (http://cde.dentalaegis.com/courses/4443-bisphosphonates-101-an-update). Recently, it has been suggested that being on oral bisphosphonates for more than 2 years increases the risk of developing BRONJ (Edwards *et al*., 2011). So, not only is there about a 2.69 times higher risk for implants failure in middle-aged (>40 years) women taking oral bisphosphonates but there is also a risk, although low (<1%), for implant failure when oral bisphosphonates are started after successful implant placement (Yip *et al.*, 2012; Goss *et al.*, 2010).

Q. What is the half-life of oral bisphosphonates?

A. See Table 7.19 Once taken oral bisphosphonates accumulate slowly in the bone because an oral dose very little is absorbed by the gastrointestinal tract into the blood stream and slowly gets released from the bone when the drug is stopped. The half-life is the amount of time it takes the body to clear half of the medication. For example, the elimination half-life of Boniva is up to 157 hours, which is about 6.5 days. However, once the first 50% is gone by 6.5 days, it will take the body up to another 6.5 days to clear 50% of the remaining medication. Usually it takes about 5 half-lives to clear 99% of the medication. In the case of Boniva, it's about 32 days. Fosamax has the longest half-life so it takes many years (>10 years) for the drug to be totally eliminated from the body. Discontinuing an oral bisphosphonate may result in gradual improvement but may not reduce or eliminate the chance of developing BRONJ. The AAOMS states that discontinuation of oral bisphosphonates for 6–12 months may result in either spontaneous sequestration or resolution following debridement surgery (AAOMS, 2009).

Q. What are specific recommendation from the 2011 American Dental Association Council on Scientific Affairs for patients taking bisphosphonates for prevention and treatment of osteoporosis?

A. Currently, there is no established standard of care or protocol regarding dental treatment of patients on bisphosphonates. The American Dental Association Council on Scientific Affairs recommends the following regarding dental treatment in patients *without cancer* receiving antiresorptive therapy (Edwards *et al.*, 2011):

1) Inform patients about the risks of developing BRONJ with dental care while taking antiresorptive drugs. [Note that this Council refers to BRONJ as antiresorptive agent-induced osteonecrosis of the jaw (ARONJ)].
2) Dentists do not need to alter routine dental procedures.
3) Antiresorptive drug therapy for low bone mass puts the patient at low risk, but does not eliminate the chance of developing BRONJ.
4) A dental health program consisting of optimal oral hygiene care and regular dental appointments will help to minimize the risk of developing BRONJ (Nicolatou-Galitis *et al.*, 2011).
5) The dentist has to make the decision to treat or not treat the patient.
6) It is not advisable not to treat active dental disease including caries, abscesses or inflammatory periodontal diseases). Leaving untreated dental disease may exacerbate osteonecrosis and be a risk factor for BRONJ.
7) Best to prevent BRONJ by limiting extensive dental involvement.

Q. What are recommendations for patients without cancer concerning periodontal therapy?

A. It is recommended to treat periodontal diseases with nonsurgical therapy followed by a revaluation 4 to 8 weeks later (Edwards *et al.*, 2011; Segelnick & Weinberg, 2006). The Council says that periodontal surgery is not contraindicated but patients should be monitored regularly.

Q. What are the 2011 recommendations concerning implant placement?

A. Reports have documented that although there are cases of BRONJ at implant sites, the incidence is small. Additionally, there is a small incidence of implant failure in patient taking bisphosphonates (Edwards *et al.*, 2011; Fugazzotto *et al.*, 2007). Fugazotto *et al.* (2007) found that a history of oral bisphosphonate use for a mean time of 3.3 years was not a contributing factor to the development of BRONJ.

Q. What are the 2011 recommendations concerning extractions?

A. According to the American Dental Association Council on Scientific Affairs, extractions are a major risk factor for developing BRONJ, however, not contraindicated. It is recommended, if necessary, to perform endodontics followed by removal of the clinical crown. This would allow the root to exfoliate instead of doing an extraction (Edwards *et al.*, 2011).

Q. What are the current thoughts about restorative and prosthetic procedures in patients taking bisphosphonates?

A. According to the American Dental Association Council on Scientific Affairs (2011), all routine restorative procedures should be performed. Any irritating or rough area on dental prosthesis should be removed and smoothed (Edwards *et al.*, 2011). Additionally, malocclusion, occlusal trauma or masticatory forces do not increase the risk of developing BRONJ (Edwards *et al.*, 2011).

Q. What are the current thoughts about orthodontic procedures in patients taking bisphosphonates?

A. According to the American Dental Association Council on Scientific Affairs (2011), there are not enough studies concerning orthodontics increasing the risk of developing BRONJ. However, there are reports of inhibited tooth movement during orthodontic therapy but orthodontic therapy is not contraindicated (Edwards *et al.*, 2011; Rinchuse *et al.*, 2007).

Q. What is the only diagnostic test available to determine the risk of the patient of developing BRONJ?

A. There is only one test available that is a marker that measures bone metabolism or bone turnover and determines the risk for the development of BRONJ. This test was developed at University of Southern California and is called the CTx test and is done only at one lab in the US-Quest Diagnostics Lab in San Juan Capistrano, CA. The American Dental Association Council does not recognize or validate this test (Edwards *et al.*, 2011).

   The CTx test should be performed on any patient who has been taking an oral bisphosphonate for more than 3 years before any dental surgery, periodontal surgery or oral surgery. This test looks at the levels of the bone resorption marker serum β C-telopeptide which helps predict the risk of developing BRONJ. However, this test is not endorsed by any dental organization. The AAOMS recommends for patient taking IV bisphosphonates that all elective or emergency dental surgery that causes direct osseous trauma should not be performed. If an extraction is required it is recommended to cut down the crown of the tooth and perform root canal therapy instead (Marx *et al.*, 2007).

Q. How is the CTx test interpreted?

A. <100 pg/ml = high risk
100–150 pg/ml = moderate risk
>151 pg/ml = little or no risk.
When results are >450 pg/ml, this indicates that bone turnover is too rapid, which could potentially puts the patient at risk for BRONJ.

Q. How do we manage these patients?

A. Take a thorough medical history and written consent. Get a consultation from the patient's physician. The patient should be counseled on the practicality of developing ONJ. In 2006, the American Dental Association (ADA) Council on Scientific Affairs published its expert panel's recommendations on how to manage patients on oral bisphosphonates.

Q. What are recommendations for treating patients taking oral bisphosphonates and what is a 3 month drug holiday?

A. If on an oral bisphosphonate for <3 years = treat as usual.
   If on an oral bisphosphonate for >3 years = discontinue for 3 months before dental procedure and send for CTX testing. Once treatment is finished, extend the "drug holiday" for an additionally 3 months. This is referred to as a "3 month drug holiday" (Daniel *et al.*, 2011). However, the 2011 the ADA recommendations for managing the dental care of patients taking antiresorptive drugs for the prevention and treatment of osteoporosis states that "discontinuing bisphosphonate therapy may not eliminate the risk of developing BRONJ" (Edwards *et al.*, 2011).

Q. Is there a higher risk for implant failure in postmenopausal women?

A. A 2010 article reported that dental implant placement survival in postmenopausal women is the same regardless of whether they have a history of bisphosphonate use. Postmenopausal women taking bisphosphonate who have dental implant surgery are at low risk for BRONJ and a "drug holiday" would not be indicated in these patients (Koka *et al.*, 2010).

Table 7.20 Risk category stages of BRONJ with the appropriate management.

> *At risk category*: patients taken oral or IV bisphosphonates with no apparent signs or symptoms of BRONJ. No treatment is indicated besides oral hygiene instruction.
>
> *Stage 0*: no clinical evidence of necrotic bone, however there are non-specific clinical findings and symptoms. Management consists of pain medications and antibiotics.
>
> *Stage 1*: bone is exposed and or necrotic, but patient is asymptomatic and no infection is seen. Management consists of use of antibacterial oral rinse such as chlorhexidine, patient education and a follow-up 4 times a year.
>
> *Stage 2*: exposed and necrotic bone associated with an infection is seen. There is pain and erythema in the area of the exposed bone. Purulent exudates may or may not be evident. Management consists of oral antibiotics, oral antibacterial oral rinse, pain control, superficial debridement to relieve soft tissue irritation.
>
> *Stage 3*: Exposed and necrotic bone with pain, infection, and one or more the following: pathologic fracture, extraoral fistula, or osteolysis extending to the inferior boarder of the alveolar bone. Management consists of an antibacterial oral rinse, antibiotic therapy and pain control, and surgical debridement or resection for longer-term control of infection and pain.

Reprinted from American Association of Oral and Maxillofacial Surgeons (2009) with permission from John Wiley & Sons, Inc.

Q. If the patient develops BRONJ, what is its management?

A. It is very difficult to treat BRONJ and it is not reversible. If BRONJ is diagnosed it could last as few as 8 weeks to a life time. First, the bisphosphonate should be stopped.

The AAOMS has various risk category stages of BRONJ with the appropriate management (AAOMS, 2009) (Table 7.20).

Oral hygiene and conservative systemic antibiotic therapy is pivotal is healing an elimination of pain in these patients (Nicolatou-Galitis *et al.*, 2011). Systemic antibiotics (e.g., amoxicillin or levofloxacin (Levaquin) 500 mg every day and metronidazole 500 mg bid) to prevent secondary infection. Chlorhexidine gluconate 0.12% mouthrinse and irrigation with hydrogen peroxide and surgical debridement are also done. Hyperbaric oxygen is used to counteract the necrosis by promoting periosteal blood supply to the bone. Any movable segments of bony sequestrum should be removed without exposing uninvolved bone (AAOMS, 2009).

Q. Is BRONJ always evident immediately after a procedure?

A. No. Patients can stay asymptomatic for weeks to months and BRONJ is diagnosed only when it is seen that bone is exposed in the mouth during an examination. Diagnosis is difficult because BRONJ is not always seen on a radiograph.

Q. What are some guidelines to follow before a patient initiates oral bisphosphonate therapy?

A. Patients should have a complete dental examination and any major dental procedures including extractions and implants should be completed before bisphosphonate therapy is started. It is best to delay dental treatment until there is optimal dental health. While on bisphosphonate therapy patients should have routine maintenance dental visits. Meticulous oral hygiene should be reinforced with the patient (International Academy of Oral Medicine and Toxicology, 2007) (http://www.iaomt.org/articles/files/files302/Human%20Jawbone%20Osteonecrosis%208.08.pdf).

XIV. Tuberculosis

Q. Is a medical consult necessary for a patient presenting with a history of or currently with tuberculosis (TB)?

A. Yes. If the patient has active TB no dental treatment should be given to the patient. If the patient has been exposed and is taking isoniazid (INH) a medical consultation may be necessary because INH affects liver enzymes which may interfere with the metabolism of certain drugs including lidocaine as mentioned earlier.

Q. Is antibiotic prophylaxis required for patients exposed to but not having active TB?

A. No.

XV. Bariatric surgery

Q. If a patient has undergone bariatric (weight reduction) surgery does drug dosing need to be adjusted?

A. Yes. Altered drug absorption may occur after the Roux-en-Y gastric bypass surgical weight reduction procedure, which is a restrictive–malabsorptive procedure (the most commonly performed surgical procedure in obese people). This is can be a concern post-surgery because there is less surface area of the small intestine for drug absorption. For this reason many patients may develop nutritional deficiencies in especially in fat-soluble vitamins E and D and also iron and vitamin B_{12}. Drugs with long absorptive phases that remain in the intestine for extended periods are likely to exhibit decreased bioavailability in these patients (Padwal *et al.*, 2010; Miller & Smith, 2006). If you are concerned with altered drug absorption, it is recommended to use a drug that will have its active ingredient be released over and extended time (Seaman *et al.*, 2005). Also, since individual dose adjustments may be needed it is recommended to get a medical consultation from the patient's physician. These drugs include the following formulations: extended-release (ER), sustained-release (SR), delayed-release or long-acting (LA). Antibiotics that are supplied as delayed release include:

- Doryx Delayed-Release® (Doryx is a trade name for doxycycline)
  - Supplied: 75 mg, 100 mg cap; tab
  - Adults: 100 mg every 12 hours followed by a maintenance dose of 100 mg/day. The maintenance dose may be administered as a single dose or as 50 mg every 12 hours.
  - Children: The recommended dosage schedule for children weighing 4.5 kg (100 lb) or less is 2 mg/0.5 kg of body weight divided into two doses on the first day of treatment, followed by 1 mg/0.5 kg of body weight given as a single daily dose or divided into two doses on subsequent days. For more severe infections up to 2 mg/0.5 kg of body weight may be used. For children over 4.5 kg (100 lb), the usual adult dose should be used (http://www.rxlist.com/doryx-drug.htm).
  - Taken without regards to meals
  - Take with full glass of water
  - Do not take concurrently with antacids
  - If the capsule cannot be swallowed whole, it may be opened and sprinkle the contents over a spoonful of applesauce.
- ERYC® (erythromycin) Delayed-Release Capsules
  - Supplied: 250 mg cap
  - Adults: The usual dose is 250 mg every 6 hours taken one hour before meals. If twice-a-day dosage is desired, the recommended dose is 500 mg every 12 hours. Dosage may be increased up to 4 g/day, according to the severity of the infection.
  - Children: The usual dosage is 30 to 50 mg/kg/day in divided doses.

Additionally, it is best to use tablets that are enteric-coated to protect the small pouch size stomach. It must be kept in mind that tablets must break down or disintegrate and capsules must open up before it can be in a form that can be absorbed. Tablets can be crushed if desired or a chewable tablet prescribed. A solution/suspension is already in an easily absorbable liquid form.

When prescribing for dental indications the following antibiotics and analgesics can be prescribed in a liquid or suspension formulation (remember to confirm if there are any precautions or contraindications for any of the following drugs before prescribing):

1) Antibiotics available in liquid formulation for adult dosing are given in Table 7.21.
2) Anaglesics available in liquid form are given in Table 7.22.

Q. Are there any over-the-counter analgesic liquid formulations?

A. Yes. Extra Strength Tylenol acetaminophen Adult Liquid, Children's Tylenol acetaminophen Elixir, ibuprofen liquid suspension.

Table 7.21 Antibiotics available in liquid formulation for adult dosing.

Rx amoxicillin suspension (250 mg/5 ml)
Disp: 100 ml bottle
Sig: Take 4 teaspoonfuls po stat, followed by 2 teaspoonfuls q8h

NOTE: amoxicillin is also available as extended-release tablets and chewable tablets which can be given to this patient.

Rx amoxicillin/clavulanic acid (Augmentin) 250/62.5/5 ml
Disp: 100 ml bottle
Sig: Take 4 teaspoonfuls po stat, followed by 2 teaspoonfuls q8h

Rx penicillin VK 250 mg/5 ml
Disp: 100 ml bottle
Sig: Take 4 teaspoonfuls po stat, followed by 2 teaspoonfuls q6h

Rx clindamycin oral solution 75 mg/5 ml
Disp: 100 ml bottle
Sig: Take 2 to 4 teaspoonfuls po every 8 hours.

Rx azithromycin oral suspension
Disp: one single dose packet
Sig: Empty the entire contents of the packet into a glass of water (2 ounces) and mix. After swallow follow with 2 ounces of water to the glass and mix and drink. This suspension should be consumed immediately.

*One packet contains 1 g or 1000 mg of azithromycin.

Table 7.22 Analgesics available in liquid form.

Rx acetaminophen/codeine suspension (Schedule V) (Pregnancy C) (120 mg acetaminophen + 12 mg codeine/5 ml)
Disp: 8 fl. oz.
Sig: Take one tablespoonful (15 ml) every 4 hours as needed.

Rx acetaminophen/hydrocodone oral solution (Lortab Elixir) (hydrocodone bitartrate 7.5 mg and acetaminophen 500 mg/15 ml) (Schedule III)
Disp: 8 fl. oz. (note: do not write for 1 bottle because it is supplied as 1 pint)
Sig: Take one tablespoonful every 4 to 6 hours as needed for pain
(The total daily dosage for adults should not exceed 6 tablespoonfuls.)

Dental Therapeutics, 2010; Miller & Smith, 2006.

Q. Are there any problems with drug absorption in patients that had other types of bariatric surgery such as vertical-banded (stapled) gastroplasty and adjustable gastric banding?

A. The vertical-banded (stapled) gastroplasty and adjustable gastric banding are types of bariatric surgery that allows for weight loss by reducing stomach volume (restrictive procedures) and does by causing malabsorption as does Roux-en-Y gastric bypass. In restrictive procedures the smaller volume of the stomach can prevent adequate disintegration of the dosage formulation (tablet/capsule) needed for drug bioavailability. The same suggestions in the patient that had Roux-en-Y gastric bypass are also for the restrictive surgical procedure. (http://dig.pharm.uic.edu/faq/2011/Mar/faq3.aspx) (Weinberg & Segelnick, 2009).

XVI.   Pheochromocytoma

Q. What is pheochromocytoma?

A. Pheochromocytoma is a rare, benign tumor of the adrenal medulla that produces and secretes excess epinephrine and norepinephrine. Symptoms include increased blood pressure and heart rate.

Q. Is epinephrine contraindicated in patients presenting with pheochromocytoma?

A. Yes. Local anesthetics containing epinephrine is contraindicated in patients with pheochromocytoma.

References

American Academy of Periodontology (2004) Position Paper. Systemic Antibiotics in Periodontics. *Journal of Periodontology*, 75:1553–1565.

American Academy of Periodontology (1996) Periodontal management of patients with cardiovascular diseases. *Journal of Periodontology*, 67:627–635.

American Academy of Periodontology (2004) Task Force on Periodontal Treatment of Pregnant Women. *Journal of Periodontology*, January.

American Association of Oral and Maxillofacial Surgeons (2009) Position Paper on Bisphosphonate-Related Osteonecrosis of the Jaw – 2009 Update. Advisory Task Force on Bisphosphonate-Related Osteonecrosis of the Jaws. January.

American Dental Association (2002) Gingival retraction cord. *The Journal of the American Dental Association*, 133:653.

American Dental Association (2011) ADA Professional Product Review. Winter/January *The Journal of the American Dental Association*, 6:1–16.

American Dental Association Council on Scientific Affairs (2006) Dental management of patients receiving oral bisphosphonate therapy. *The Journal of the American Dental Association*, 137(8):1144–1150.

American Dental Association: American Academy of Orthopaedic Surgeons. Advisory Statement (2003) Antibiotic prophylaxis for dental patients with total joint replacements. *The Journal of the American Dental Association*, 134:895–898.

American Dental Hygiene Association 2011. Online. Available at www.adha.org/ce_course15/oral_antiplatelet_agents.htm (accessed 17 December 2011).

Ardekian, L., Gaspar, R., Peled, M., *et al.* (2000) Does low-dose aspirin therapy complicate oral surgical procedures? *The Journal of the American Dental Association*, 131:331–335.

Awtry, E.H. & Loscalzo, J. (2000) Aspirin. *Circulation*, 101:1206–1218.

Baddour, L.M., Epstein, A.E., Erickson, C.C., *et al.* (2011) A summary of the update on cardiovascular implantable electronic device infections and their management. *The Journal of the American Dental Association*, 142:159–165.

Barasch, A., Cunha-Cruz, J., Curro, F.A., *et al.* (2011) Risk factors for osteonecrosis of the jaws: a case-control study from the CONDOR dental PBRN. *Journal of Dental Research*, 90:439–444.

Bell, W.R. (1998) Acetaminophen and warfarin. Undesirable synergy. *Journal of the American Medical Association*, 279:702–703.

Bradley, J.G. & Davis, K.A. (2003) Orthostatic hypotension. *American Family Physician*, 68:2393–2399.

Brennan, M.T., Valerin, M.A., Noll, J.L., *et al.* (2008) Aspirin use and post-operative bleeding from dental extractions. *Journal of Dental Research*, 87:740–744.

Budenz, A.W. (2008) Local anesthetics and medically complex patients. *Journal of the California Dental Association*, 28:611–619.

Cardona-Tortajada, F., Sainz-Gómez, E., Figuerido-Garmendia, J. *et al.* (2009) Dental extractions in patients on antiplatelet therapy. A study conducted by the Oral Health Department of the Navarre Health Service (Spain). *Medicina Oral Patologia Oral y Cirugia Bucal*, 14:e588–592.

Cho, C.M., Hirsch, R. & Johnstone, S. (2005) General and oral health implications of cannabis use. *Australian Dental Journal*, 50:70–74.

Chobanian, A.V., Bakris, G.L., Black, H.R., *et al.* (2003) Seventh report of the Joint National Committee on Prevention, Detection, Evaluation, and Treatment of High Blood Pressure. *Hypertension*, 42:1206–1252.

Ciancio, S,G. (2004) Medications' impact on oral health. *Journal of the American Dental Association*, 135:1440–1448.

Daniel, R., Nowzari, H. & Garfunkel, A.A. (2011) Treatment in conjunction with bisphosphonate therapy. *Compendium*, 32:10–11.

Dajani, A.S., Taubert, K.A., Wilson, W. *et al.* (1997) Prevention of bacterial endocarditis. Recommendations by the American Heart Association. *Circulation*, 96:358–366.

Deacon, J.M., Pagliaro, A.J., Zelicof, S.B., *et al.* (1996) Prophylactic use of antibiotics for procedures after total joint replacement. *The Jounral of bone and joint surgery. American Volume*, 78:1755–1770.

Dental Therapeutics (2010) ADA Professional Product Review, Fall/October, 5(4):1–4.

Donaldson, M. & Goodchild, J.H. (2006) Oral health of the methamphetamine abuser. *American Journal of Health- System Pharmacy*, 63:2078–2082.

Edwards, B.J., Hellstein, J.W., Jacobsen, P.L., *et al.* (2008) American Dental Association Council on Scientific Affairs Expert Panel on Bisphosphonate-Associated Osteonecrosis of the Jaw. Updated recommendations for managing the care of patients receiving oral bisphosphonate therapy: an advisory statement from the American Dental Association Council on Scientific Affairs. *Journal of the American Dental Association*, 139:1674–1677.

Fugazzotto, P.A., Lightfoot, W.S., Jaffin, R., *et al.* (2007) Implant placement with or without simultaneous tooth extraction in patients taking oral bisphosphonates: postoperative healing, early follow-up, and the incidence of complications in two private practices. *Journal of Periodontology*, 78:1664–1669.

Ganda, K. (2008) Anticoagulants warfarin (Coumadin), standard heparin, and low molecular weight heparin (LMWH): assessment, analysis, and associated dental management guidelines. In: *Dentist's Guide to Medical Conditions and Complications*. Wiley-Blackwell, Ames, IA,pp. 169–174.

Gibson, N. & Ferguson, J.W. (2004) Steroid cover for dental patients on long-term steroid medication: proposed clinical guidelines based upon a critical review of the literature. *British Dental Journal*, 197:681–685.

Goodchild, J.H. & Donaldson, M. (2007) Methamphetamine abuse and dentistry: a review of the literature and presentation of a clinical case. *Quintessence International*, 38:583–590.

Goss, A., Bartold, M., Smabrook, P. & Hawker, P. (2010) The nature and frequency of bisphosphonate-associated ostenecrosis of the jaws in dental implant patients: a South Australian case series. *Journal of Oral and Maxillofacial Surgery*, 68:337–343.

Grewal, V.S. & Fayans, E.P. (2008) Bisphosphonate-associated osteonecrosis. A clinician's reference to patient management. *New York State Dental Journal*, 38–44.

Hassan, Y., Al Ramahi, R.J., Abd Aziz, N., *et al.* (2009) Drug use and dosing in chronic kidney disease. *Annals Academy Medicine Singapore*, 38:1095–1103.

Hellstein, J.W., Adler, R.A., Edwards, B., *et al.* (2011) Managing the care of patients receiving antiresorptive therapy for prevention of treatment of osteoporosis. Executive summary of recommendations from the American Dental Association Council on Scientific Affairs. *The Journal of the American Dental Association*, 142:1243–1251.

Horowitz, L.G. & Nersasian, R.R. (1978) A review of marijuana in relations to stress-response mechanisms in the dental patient. *The Journal of the American Dental Association*, 96(6):983–986.

Hughes, G.J., Patel, P. & Saxena, N. (2011) Effect of acetaminophen on International Nomralized Ratio: clinican awareness and patient education. *Pharmacotherapy*, 31(6):591–597.

Hylek, E.M., Heiman, H., Skates, S.J., *et al.* (1998) Acetaminophen and other risk factors for excessive warfarin anticoagulation. *Journal of the American Medical Association*, 279:657–662.

International Academy of Oral Medicine and Toxicology (2007) IAOMT Position Paper on Human Jawbone Osteonecrosis. March 6. Online. Available at http://www.iaomt.org/articles/files/files302/Human%20Jawbone%20Osteonecrosis%208.08.pdf) (accessed 26 December 2011).

Jeffocoat, M., Sedghizadeh, P.P. & Subramanian G. (2011) International Association of Dental Research (IADR) 89th General Session and Exhibition: Abstract 890. Presented March 17, 2011. San Diego, CA. *Journal of Dental Research* (Special Issue 90 Special Issue A).

Jeske, A.H. & Suchko, G.D. (2003) Lack of a scientific basis for routine discontinuation of oral anticoagulation therapy before dental treatment. *Journal of the American Dental Association*, 134:1492–1497.

Johnson, S.J. (2007) Opioid safety in patients with renal or hepatic dysfunction. Pain Treatment Topics (http://pain-topics.org/pdf/Opioids-Renal-Hepatic-Dysfunction.pdf) (accessed 26 December 2011).

Kassab, M.M., Radmer, T.W., Glore, J.W., *et al.* (2011) A retrospective review of clinical international normalized ratio results and their implications. *Journal of the American Dental Association*, 1252–1257.

Jones, A., Seghizadeh, P. & Khuat, C. (2011) New light shed on bisphosphonates and BRONJ. *Academy News. Academy of Osseointegration*, 22:8,10.

Kalmer J. (2009) Oral manifestations of drug reactions. Online. Available at http://emedicine.medscape.com/article/1080772-overview (accessed 26 December 2011).

Klasser, G.D. & Epstein, J.B. (2006) The methamphetamine epidemic and dentistry. *General Dentisty*, 54:431–439.

Koka, S., Babu, N.M.S. & Norell, A. (2010) Survival of dental implants in post-menopausal bisphosphonate users. *Journal of Prosthodontic Research*, 54:108–111.

Kuruvilla, M. & Gurk-Turner, C. (2001) A review of warfarin dosing and monitoring. *Proceedings (Baylor University Medical Center)*, 14:305–306.

Lamster, I.B., Lalla, E., Borgnakke, W.S., *et al.* (2008) The relationship between oral health and diabetes mellitus. *Journal of the American Dental Association*, 139(no. Suppl 5):19 s–24 s.

Landesberg, R., Cozin, M., Cremers, S., *et al.* (2008) Inhibition of oral mucosal cell wound healing by bisphosphonates. *Journal of Oral and Maxillofacial Surgery*, 61:1115–1117.

Lifshey, F.M. (2004) Evaluation of and treatment considerations for the dental patient with cardiac disease. *New York State Dental Journal*, 70:16–19.

Little, J.W., Miller, C., Robert, H. *et al.* (2002) Antithrombotic agents: implications in dentistry. *Oral Surgery Oral Medicine Oral Pathology Oral Radiology Endotontology*, 93:544–551.

Little, J.W., Jacobson, J.J. & Lockhart, P.B.. (2010) The dental treatment of patients with joint replacements. *Journal of the American Dental Association*, 141:667–671.

Lockart, P.B., Loven, B., Brennan, M.T., *et al.* (2007) The evidence base for the efficacy of antibiotic prophylaxis in dental practice. *Journal of the American Dental Association*, 138(4):458–474.

Madan, G.A., Madan, S.G., Madan, G., *et al* (2005) Minor oral surgery without stopping daily low-dose aspirin therapy: a study of 51 patients. *Journal of Oral and Maxillofacial Surgery*, 63:1262–1265.

Malamed, S.F. (1993) Physical evaluation and the prevention of medical emergencies: vital signs. *Anesthesia & Pain Control in Dentistry*, 2:107–113.

Marx, R.E., Cillo, J.E. Jr & Ulloa, J.J. (2007) Oral bisphosphonate-induced osteonecrosis: risk factors, prediction of risk using serum CTx testing, prevention, and treatment. *Journal of Oral and Maxillofacial Surgery*, 65:2397–410.

Mealey, B.L. & Oates, T.W. (2006) Diabetes mellitus and periodontal diseases. *Journal of Periodontology*, 77:1289–1303.

Michalowicz, B.S., DiAngelis, A.J., Novak, M.J., *et al.* (2008) Examining the safety of dental treatment in pregnant women. *Journal of the American Dental Association*, 139:686–695.

Miller, A.D. & Smith, K.M. (2006) Medication and nutrient administration after bariatric surgery. *American Journal of Health-System Pharmacy*, 63:1852–1857.

Miller, C.S. & McGarity, G.J. (2009) Tetracycline-induced renal failure after dental treatment. *Journal of the American Dental Association*, 140:56–60.

Muzzin, K.B. & O'Brien, C. (2010) Dealing with the devastation. How to provide oral heath care to patients with a history of meth-amphetamine abuse. *Dimensions of Dental Hygiene*, 8:42–45.

Napeñas, J.J., Hong, C.H.L., Brennan, M.T., *et al.* (2009) he frequency of bleeding complications after invasive dental treatment in patients receiving single and dual antiplatelet therapy. *Journal of the American Dental Association*, 140:690–695.

Nahas, G. & Latour, C. (1992) The human toxicity of marijuana. *Medical Journal of Australia*, 3:163–184.

New York State Department of Health (2006) Oral health care during pregnancy and early childhood. Practice Guidelines. August 2006.

Newton, T.F., De La Garza, R. 2nd, Kalechstein, A.D., *et al.* (2005) Cocaine and methamphetamine produce different patterns of subjective and cardiovascular effects. *Pharmacology, Biochemistry, and Behavior*, 82:90–97.

Nicolatou-Galitis, O., Papadopoulou, E., Sarri, T., *et al.* (2011) Osteoneocrosis of the jaw in oncology patients treated with bisphosphonates: prospective experience of a dental oncology referral center. *Oral Surgery Oral Medicine Oral Pathology Oral Radiology and Endodontology*, 112:195–202.

Padwal, R., Brocks, D. &Sharma, A.M. (2010) Systematic review of drug absorption following bariatric surgery and its theoretical implications. *Obesity Reviews*, 11:41–50.

Page, II R.L. (2005) Weighing the cardiovascular benefits of low-dose aspirin. *Pharmacy Times*, ACPE Program I.D. Number: 290–000–05-H01. Online. Available at www.pharmacytimes.com (accessed 26 December 2011).

Pallasch, T.J. (1998) Vasoconstrictors and the heart. *Journal of the California Dental Association*, 26:668–673, 676.

Pallasch, T.J. (1996) Pharmacokinetic principles of antimicrobial therapy. *Periodontology* 2000, 10:5–11.

Patel, R. & Paya, C.V.(1997) Infections in solid organ transplant recipients. *Clinical Microbiology Reviews*, 10:86–124.

Patrono, C., Collar, B., Dalen, J., *et al.* (1998) Platelet-active drugs: the relationships among dose, effectiveness, and side effects. *Chest*, 114:470S–488S.

Patrono, C., Coller, B., FitzGerald, G.A., *et al.* (2001) Platelet-active drugs: the relationhips among dose, effectiveness, and side effects. The Seventh ACCP Conference on Antithrombotic and Thrombolytic Therapy. *Chest*, 234S–264S.

Patrono, C., Coller, B., FitzGerald, G.A., *et al.* (2004) Platelet-active drugs: the relationships among dose, effectiveness, and side effects. The Seventh ACCP Conference on Antithrombotic and Thrombolytic Therapy. Chest, 234 S–264 S.

Pérusse, R., Goulet, J.P. & Turcotte, J.Y. (1992) Contraindications to vasoconstrictors in dentistry: Part II. *Oral Surgery Oral Medicine Oral Pathology*, 74:687–691.

Randall, C. (2007) Surgical management of the primary care dental patient on antiplatelet medication. 2007 UK Medicines Information. Online. Available at www.ukmi.nhs.uk/activities/specialistServices (accessed 26 December 2011).

Rees, S.R. & Gibson, J. (1997) Angioedema and swellings of the orofacial region. *Oral Diseases*, 3:39–42.

Rinchuse, D.J., Rinchuse, D.J., Sosovicka, M.F., *et al.* (2007) Orthodontic treatment of patients using bisphosphonates: a report of 2 cases. *American Journal of Orthodontics and Dentofacial Orthopedics*, 131:321–326.

Rubin, R., Salvati, E.A. & Lewis, R. (1976) Infected total hip replacement after dental procedures. *Oral Surgery Oral Medicine Oral Pathology*, 41:13–23.

Rubin, R.H., Young, L.S. & Rubin, R.H. (1994) Infection in the organ transplant recipient. In: *Clinical Approach to Infection in the Compromised Host*, 3rd edn (eds Rubin, R.H. & Young, L.S.), pp. 629–705. Plenum, New York.

Ruggiero, S.L., Mehrotra, B., Rosenberg, T.J., *et al.* (2004) Osteonecrosis of the jaws associated with the use of bisphosphonates: a review of 63 cases. *Journal of Oral and Maxillofacial Surgery*, 62:527–534.

Scully, C. & Bagan-Sebastian, J.V. (2004) Adverse drug reactions in the orofacial region. *Critical Reviews of Oral Biology & Medicine*, 15:221–240.

Scully, C. & Porter, S. (2003) Lumps and swelling of the mouth. In: *Orofacial Disease. Update for the Dental Clinical Team* (ed. Scully, C.). pp. 69–74. Churchill Livingstone, Philadelphia.

Seaman, J.S., Bowers, S.P., Dixon, P., *et al.* (2005) Dissolution of common psychiatric medications in a Roux-en-Y gastric bypass model. *Psychosomatics*, 46:250–253.

Segelnick, S.L. & Weinberg, M.A. (2006) Reevaluation of initial therapy: when is the appropriate time? *Journal of Periodontology*, 77:1598–1601.

Segelnick, S.L. & Weinberg, M.A. (2009) The periodontist's role in obtaining clearance prior to patients undergoing a kidney transplant. *Journal of Periodontology*, 80:874–877.

Ship. J.A. (2003) Diabetes and oral health: An overview. *Journal of the American Dental Association*, 134(Suppl 1):4s–10s.

Skaar, D.D., O'Connor, H., Hodges, J.S., *et al.* (2011) Dental procedures and subsequent prosthetic joint infections. *Journal of the American Dental Association*, 142:1343–1351.

Soave, R. (2001) Prophylaxis strategies for solid-organ transplantation. *Clinical Infectious Diseases*, 33 (Supplement 1):S26–S31.

Steinbacher, D.M. & Glick, M. (2001) The dental patient with asthma. *Journal of the American Dental Association*, 132:1229–1239.

Strassler, H.E. & Boksman, L. (2011). Tissue management, gingival retraction and hemostasis. *Oral Health Journal*. Online. Availabele from http://www.oralhealthgroup.com/news/tissue-management-gingival-retraction-and-hemostasis/1000519731/?type=Print%20 Archives (accessed 1 June 2012).

Weinberg, M.A. & Segelnick, S.L. (2009) Surgical procedures for weight loss. *US Pharmacist*, 34(12):HS-2–HS-10.

Weinberg, M.A. (2002) Fundamentals of drug action. In: *Oral Pharmacology*. (eds.Weinberg, M.A., Westphal, C. & Fine, J.B.), pp. 224, 337–368. Pearson Education Inc., New Jersey.

Wilson, W., Taubert, K.A., Gewitz, M., *et al.* (2007) Prevention of infective endocarditis: Guidelines from the American Heart Association Rheumatic Fever, Endocarditis, and Kawasaki Disease Committee, Council on Cardiovascular Disease in the Young, and the Council on Clinical Cardiology, Council on Cardiovascular Surgery and Anesthesia, and the Quality of Care and Outcomes Research Interdisciplinary Working Group. *Circulation*, 116:1736–1754.

Worrlax, J.D. & Flake, D. (2007) Alcoholic liver disease: Is acetaminophen safe? *Family Practice* 56:673–674.

Yagiela, J.A. (1999) Adverse drug interactions in dental practice: interactions associated with vasoconstrictors. *Journal of the American Dental Association*, 130:701–709.

Yagiela, J.A. & Haymore, T.L. (2007) Management of the hypertensive dental patient. *Journal of the California Dental Association*, 35:51–59.

Yajnik, S., Thapar, P., Lichtor, J.L., *et al.* (1994) Effects of marijuana history on the subjective, psychomotor, and reinforcing effects of nitrous oxide in humans. *Drug and Alcohol Dependence*, 36:227–36.

Yip, J.K., Borrell, L.N., Cho, S-C., Francisco, H. & Tarnow, D.P. (2012) Association between oral bisphosphonate use and dental implant failure among middle-aged women. *Journal of Clinical Periodontology*, 39:408–411.

Zucchelli, G., Pollini, F., Clauser, C., *et al.* (2000) The effect of chlorhexidine mouthrinses on early bacterial colonization of guided tissue regeneration. *Journal of Periodontology*, 71:263–271.

Chapter 8

Herbal and natural remedies

I. Herbal–drug interactions

Q. Do herbal products have any harmful effects?

A. One of the major skepticisms is whether these products are safe and effective. One of the most worrisome adverse effects of herbal products is anticoagulation. Most herbal medicines are unapproved drugs being sold as dietary supplements. In 1990, the Food and Drug Administration (FDA) classified herbal medicines as food supplements. The Dietary Supplement and Health Education Act (DSHEA) of 1994 classifies vitamins, minerals, amino acids, and herbs as dietary supplements, which allows the marketing of these "food supplements" without the approval of any government agency for testing for safety, efficacy, or standards of manufacturing. The FDA is only required to prove that these products are unsafe. Dietary supplements do not have to be tested prior to marketing, and the effectiveness of the product does not have to be demonstrated by the manufacturer. The product label must include a disclaimer that the product is not FDA evaluated or approved and it is not intended to diagnose, treat, or prevent any disease (Cupp, 1999). The DSHEA does not regulate the accuracy of the label; the product may or may not contain the product listed in the amounts claimed. Herbal products therefore cannot be marketed for the diagnosis, treatment, cure, or prevention of disease. However, these products can be labeled explaining their proposed effect on the human body (e.g., alleviation of fatigue) or their role in promoting general well-being (e.g., enhancement of mood). Dietary supplement labeling requires the wording "dietary supplement" as part of the product name, and it must include a "supplement facts" panel on the ingredients. Also, products derived from plants must designate the plant part and the Latin binomial.

Q. What are herbal medications made from?

A. Herbal medications are made from natural ingredients extracted from a plant and are produced either in the original form or refined, where the essential extract is removed from the plant, concentrated, and then added back into the original form to make it more concentrated. The active ingredients in an herbal product may be present in only one specific part of the plant or in all parts. For example, the active ingredient in ginger is composed of roots found below ground, whereas in St. John's wort it comes from leaves and stems that are above the ground. Every herb contains many active chemicals. Most of these chemicals have not been isolated and identified so that the strength of the product varies considerably, which makes standardization difficult. Additionally, the chemical composition of herbal supplements is unpredictable. Some standardizations are printed on the product label and may differ from one manufacturer to another.

Q. What are some adverse effects of herbal medications that are of concern especially for dental surgery?

A. Most reactions are due to filler substances added to the herbal product but not on the label. More commonly encountered adverse effects include sedation and bleeding, which manifests either via direct effects on capillaries, by interfering with platelet adhesion, or by increasing fibrinolytic activity. Caution should be used when nonsteroidal anti-inflammatory drugs (NSAIDs) are recommended to patients taking herbs that could increase bleeding, including

The Dentist's Drug and Prescription Guide, First Edition. Mea A. Weinberg and Stuart J. Froum.
© 2013 John Wiley & Sons, Inc. Published 2013 by John Wiley & Sons, Inc.

Table 8.1   Common herbal products taken by patients for dental problems.

Oral condition	Herbal supplement
Aphthous ulcer	Aloe vera, red raspberry
Caries	Licorice root
Oral inflammation in cancer patients	Chamomile, vitamin E
Oral fungal infections	Tea tree oil, garlic, cinnamon
Periodontal diseases	Coenzyme Q10, sanguinaria

Table 8.2   Common herbal–drug interactions in dentistry.

Herbal supplement	Interacting dental drug	How to manage
St. John's wort	Alprazolam (Xanax), diazepam, midazolam (Versed), ibuprofen, codeine, ketoconazole, clarithromvcin. ervthromvcin.	Don't take the two medications together. The active ingredient in St. John's wort has a half-life of 24 to 48 hours.
Khat	Penicillins (amoxicillin, ampicillin)	Avoid khat chewing or take the penicillin 2 hours after khat chewing.
Kava	Alprazolam	Avoid concurrent use because of additive effect.

Izzo & Ernst, 2001; Fugh-Berman, 2000; Cupp, 1999.

ginger, garlic, and ginkgo. Another adverse effect is an allergic reaction to the herb, which can manifest in the oral cavity (e.g., gingiva, tongue).

Q. What herbal products can be taken by patients for dental problems?

A. See Table 8.1.

Q. Are there any dental drug interactions with St. John's wort?

A. St. John's wort is indicated for depression. It has many drug interactions but none pertain to dentistry. Most of the drug interactions are primarily due to induction of CYP3A4 and also to induction of CPY1A2 and CYP2C9. These drugs include warfarin, cyclosporine, HIV protease inhibitors, theophylline, digoxin, and oral contraceptives, resulting in a decrease in concentration or effect of the medicines.

Q. What steps should be followed if you suspect that there could be a drug–herbal interaction?

A. Adjustment of the dosage of the herb, temporarily discontinue the herb, close monitoring of the patient, or change the drug therapy.

Q. What are some important drug–herbal product interactions in dentistry?

A. See Table 8.2.

II.   Implications in dentistry

Q. Why is it important to ask patients if they are taking any herbal medications?

A. Patients should be questioned about taking any herbal supplement. Prolonged bleeding may occur during dental procedures (e.g., surgery) in patients taking ginger, ginkgo, ginseng, St. John's wort, garlic, green tea, glucosamine/chondroitin, omega-3 fatty acids, and saw palmetto. Bleeding will most like be controlled in healthy patients. If the

Table 8.3 Dental-related adverse effects of herbal products.

Herbal product	Adverse effect
St. John's wort	Xerostomia
Echinacea	Tongue numbness
Garlic	Gingival bleeding
Feverfew	Gingival bleeding and mouth ulcerations
Ginger	Gingival bleeding
Ginkgo	Gingival bleeding
Ginseng	Gingival bleeding
Kava	Tongue numbness

patient is also taking aspirin or other blood thinner consult with the patient's physician. These medications should be stopped at least 7 days before periodontal/implant/extraction surgery.

Q. Can any herbal medications interfere with dental anesthesia?

A. Yes. There are many herbs that can as sedatives or stimulants that could modify anesthesia. Some herbs that can interact with dental anesthesia include valerian, kava, St. John's wort and ginseng (Tweddell & Boyle, 2009).

Q. Are there any dental-related adverse effects of herbal products?

A. Yes there are dental-related adverse effects (Cupp, 1999) – see Table 8.3.

Q. Which herbal products interact with warfarin and increase bleeding?

A. Many herbal supplements act similar to antiplatelet/anticoagulant drugs. Ginkgo (*Ginkgo biloba*), ginseng (*Panax ginseng*) licorice (*Glycyrrhiza*) garlic (*Allium sativum*), Dong quai (*Angelica sinensis*), Danshen (*Salvia miltiorrhiza*). These herbals should be discontinued before performing invasive dental procedures that could cause postoperative bleeding. It has been recommended to stop all herbals that can cause increased bleeding about 7–14 days prior to the dental procedure. No interactions were found for echinacea (*Echinacea angustifolia, E. purpurea, E. pallida*) and saw palmetto (*Serenoa repens*) (Izzo & Ernst, 2001).

Q. Are there any herbal drugs that could interfere with dental anesthesia?

A. Yes. Some herbals can be sedating or stimulating which can interfere with moderate sedation and general anesthesia with a potential for prolongation or interference with anaesthetic agents. Most likely there are no interactions with local dental anesthesia.

References

Cupp, M.J. (1999) Herbal remedies: adverse effects and drug interactions. *American Family Physicians*, 59:1239–1244.
Fugh-Berman, A. (2000) Herb–drug interactions. *Lancet*, 355:134–138.
Izzo, A.A. & Ernst, E. (2001) Interactions between herbal medicines and prescribed drugs: a systematic review. *Drugs*, 61:2163–2165.
Tweddell, P. & Boyle, C. (2009) Potential interactions with herbal medications and midazolam. *Dental Update*, 36(3):175–178.

Appendix 1

Smoking cessation therapy

Q. Can a dentist prescribe medications for smoking cessation?

A. Yes. Dentists are allowed and are encouraged to help patients with smoking cessation by counseling and prescribing smoking cessation medications.

Q. Should only one product be recommended or prescribed?

A. No. It is recommended to try different agents and combine them including behavioral therapy. Combination drug therapy is usually more effective than monotherapy, particularly for more heavily tobacco-dependent patients. These go-to combinations are nicotine replacement therapy (NRT) plus bupropion (Zyban), or high-dose NRT using a nicotine patch plus nicotine gum or lozenges (http://findarticles.com/p/articles/mi_hb4345/is_10_37/ai_n42054323/).

Q. Is Nicorette gum sugar-free?

A. Yes. Nicorette gum does not contain sugar.

Q. What is Chantix?

A. Chantix is varenicline, a nicotine receptor partial agonist and the first designer drug for tobacco dependence. One serious adverse effect is increased risk for suicide thoughts and actions. The dentist should know the following about Chantix: (1) patient has had depression or other mental health problems, because these symptoms may worsen while taking Chantix; (2) experienced nicotine withdrawal symptoms with prior quit attempts, with or without Chantix (quitting smoking, with or without Chantix, can result in nicotine withdrawal symptoms – such as depressed mood, agitation – or a worsening of existing mental health problems, such as depression; (3) patient has kidney problems or get kidney dialysis (a lower dose may be necessary and obtain a medical consult); (4) patient has a history of heart or blood vessel problems because these problems and any new or worse symptoms can occur while taking Chantix – obtain a medical consult; (5) if patient is pregnant or plans to become pregnant; and (6) if patient is breastfeeding (http://www.chantix.com/side-effects-safety-info.aspx?source=google&HBX_PK=s_+chantix+side+effects&HBX_OU=50&o=23 119569|166373525|0&skwid=43700003017636922).

Q. What are some medications that the dentist can recommend or prescribe for smoking cessation?

A. See Table A1.

Q. Can the patient smoke while using the patch or other products?

A. No. Smoking while using a nicotine patch or other nicotine products increases the incidence of nicotine overdose.

The Dentist's Drug and Prescription Guide, First Edition. Mea A. Weinberg and Stuart J. Froum.
© 2013 John Wiley & Sons, Inc. Published 2013 by John Wiley & Sons, Inc.

Table A1   Pharmacologic agents used for smoking cessation.

Product	Directions for use	Supplied	Adverse effects	Rx or OTC
Nicotine gum Generics Nicorette®	Do not smoke during treatment because of risk of nicotine overdose. Chew one piece of gum every 1–2 hours for weeks 1–6; every 2–4 hours for weeks 7–9; and every 4–8 hours for weeks 10–12. Do not eat or drink for 15 minutes before chewing gum, and do not eat or drink while chewing gum.	2 mg, 4 mg gum; starter kit has 108 pieces and refill kits have 48 pieces	Mouth soreness, sore jaw, dyspepsia (stomach pain or discomfort), bronchospasm, nausea, vomiting	OTC
Nicotine transdermal system Generics Nicotine Patch (generic) Nicoderm CQ® Nicotrol® Habitrol® Prostep®	Do not smoke during treatment because of risk of nicotine overdose. Nicoderm CQ: Use one patch daily; start at 21 mg/day for 6 weeks, then 14 mg/day for 2 weeks, then 7 mg/day for 2 weeks. Maximum therapy is 3 months. Habitrol: if you smoke >10 cigarettes a day: use 21 mg patch for 4 weeks, then the 14 mg patch for 2 weeks, and the a7 mg patch for 2 weeks. If you smoke ≤10 cigarettes a day start with 14 mg patch for 6 weeks, then 7 mg patch for 2 weeks. Treatment ends at 8 weeks.	Nicoderm CQ: (28-day supply): 21 mg, 14 mg, 7 mg patches Nicotrol: 15 mg (worn only while awake), 10 mg and 5 mg patches Habitrol: 21 mg, 14 mg, 7 mg Prostep: 22 mg or 11 mg patches	Local skin irritation, insomnia (difficulty in sleeping)	OTC
Nicotine lozenge Commit®	If patient smokes the first cigarette more than 30 minutes after awakening then use 2 mg lozenge; use 4 mg if smoke first cigarette within 30 minutes upon wakening. Maximum: not more than 20 lozenges a day. Allow lozenge to dissolve slowly over 20 to 30 minutes, swallow as little as possible	2 mg (72 pieces), 4 mg (72 pieces)	Xerostomia, indigestion and irritated throat	OTC

(continued)

Table A1   *(cont'd)*

Product	Directions for use	Supplied	Adverse effects	Rx or OTC
Nicorette®	If the first cigarette is smoked more than 30 minutes after waking up the 2 mg strength is used; if the first cigarette is smoked within 30 minutes after waking up then the 4 mg strength is used. Weeks 1 to 6: 1 lozenge every 1 to 2 hours. Weeks 7 to 9: 1 lozenge every 2 to 4 hours. Weeks 10 to 12: 1 lozenge every 4 to 8 hours.	2 mg lozenge 4 mg lozenge	Cardiovascular changes, increased heart rate, dizziness, nausea, vomiting, bronchospasm	OTC
Nicotine nasal spray Nicotrol NS	Start with two sprays in each nostril every hour, which may be increased to 80 sprays per day for heavy smokers; maximum dose: 40 doses/day. maximum therapy is 6 months. Taper after 4–6 weeks. Patient should tilt head back when using the spray	Prescription product Easy spray delivers 0.5 mg nicotine; available in 10-mL bottles	Irritation of nasal mucosa, cough, sneezing, bronchospasm in patients with pre-existing asthma Tolerance to adverse effects develops after the first week of using the inhaler. Contraindicated in patients with reactive airway disease (e.g. wheezing or allergic reactions) or chronic nasal disease such as nasal polyps or sinusitis.	Rx (prescription only)
Nicotine inhalation system Nicotrol Inhaler®	Less nicotine per puff is released with the inhaler than with a cigarette. Best effect is achieved by frequent continuous puffing for about 20 minutes (that is 6–16 cartridges per day; use 1 cartridge per hour). The recommended treatment is up to 3 months and, if needed, a gradual reduction over the next 6–12 weeks. Total treatment should not exceed 6 months. Avoid food and acidic drinks before and drinking use of inhaler	Prescription product Inhaler uses nicotine cartridges (10 mg/ cartridge) that provide about 20 minutes of active puffing, or approximately 80 deep draws	Irritation of mouth and throat, cough Contraindicated in patients with reactive airway disease	Rx (prescription only)

(continued)

Table A1   *(cont'd)*

Product	Directions for use	Supplied	Adverse effects	Rx or OTC
Oral medications (non-nicotine drugs Zyban®(bupropion HCl) (does not contain nicotine)	Patient should stop smoking within 2 weeks of start of therapy. Option 1: Initial dose is 150 mg/day for 3 days, THEN 150 mg twice a day (at least 8 hours apart). Option 2: 150 mg every morning (this option has fewer adverse effects and better tolerated). Maximum daily dose is 300 mg. Continue drug therapy for 7–12 weeks after the patient stops smoking and can be maintained up to 6 months. Can be used with nicotine patches.	Prescription 150 mg sustained-release tablets	Insomnia, xerostomia, anxiety Contraindicated in seizures, currently using Wellbutrin, eating disorder, alcohol dependence or head trauma. Additionally, blood pressure should be monitored	Rx (prescription only)
Chantix ® (varenicline) (does not contain nicotine)	FDA-approved in May 2006. Not used in patients younger than 18 years old. Caution in patients with renal impairment. Packs: first month: 1 card— 0.5 mg × 11 tabs and 3 cards – 1 mg × 14 tabs Bottles: 0.5 mg, 1.0 mg	Starting one week before the patient quits smoking. 0.5 mg/day for 3 days then 0.5 mg twice a day (am and pm) for the next 4 days. Then after the first 7 days, 1 mg twice a day No tapering needed. Approved for maintenance up to 6 months. Take after eating and with a full glass of water Do not double the dose if the dose if missed	Nausea, trouble sleeping, headache, **changes in behavior, hostility, agitation, depressed mood, suicidal thoughts or actions**	Prescription

Source: Fiore, M.C., Jaen, C.R., Baker, T.B., *et al.* (2008) Treating tobacco use and dependence: 2008 update. Clinical practice Guideline. US Department of Health and Human Services, Public Health Service, Rockville, MD, May 2008.

Q. How often is the Nicorette gum used?

A. The 2 mg gum (for smokers <25 cigarettes/day) and the 4 mg gum (for smokers ≥25 cigarettes/day). It is recommended to chew a piece every one to two hours during the first six weeks of quitting (a minimum of nine per day). An additional piece can be used if there is a craving. Not more than 24 pieces should be used in one day.

Q. How is the nicotine patch used?

A. If the patient smokes more than 10 cigarettes a day:

1. For the first 6 weeks, 21 mg per day.
2. For weeks 7 and 8, switch to a moderate-dosage patch, about 14 mg per day.
3. For weeks 9 and 10, move to a low-dosage patch that delivers 7 mg of nicotine per day (http://www.nicodermcq.com/quit-smoking-products/nicoderm-cq-steps.aspx).

If the patient smokes less than 10 cigarettes a day:

1. Begin with 14 mg for 6 weeks
2. Then switch to 7 mg for 2 weeks

Q. Are there any adverse effects of nicotine replacement therapy products?

A. Yes. (http://www.drugs.com/sfx/nicotine-side-effects.html)
   Patch: If increased heartbeat and dizziness occurs it is best to switch to a lower-dose patch. Other adverse effects include skin irritation (medical attention is needed if there is swelling or persistent redness lasting more than 4 days redness at the application site), abnormal dreams, headache, muscle aches, nausea and vomiting. If the patient has a history of heart disease, refer the patient to his/her physician.

- *Gum*: Abnormal dreams; diarrhea; difficulty sleeping; dry mouth; joint pain; muscle pain; nervousness, sweating, weakness, mouth, teeth, or jaw problems, allergic reaction, irregular or fast heartbeat, diarrhea, nausea, vomiting.
- *Lozenge*: warm or tingling sensation in the mouth, allergic reaction, persistent indigestion, irregular or fast heartbeat, pain, swelling or sores in the mouth.
- *Inhaler*: coughing; diarrhea; flu-like symptoms; headache; hiccups; indigestion; mouth or throat irritation; muscle aches; nausea; pain in the jaw and neck; runny nose, taste changes, allergic reaction, irregular or fast heartbeat.
- *Spray*: back pain, burning or irritation of the mouth, nose, or eyes, changes in taste and smell constipation, cough, earache, flushing of the face, gas, headache, hoarseness, indigestion, irritability, joint pain, sores in the mouth, ulcers or blisters in the nose, nose bleeding, nausea, runny nose, sneezing; sore throat; stuffy nose, watery eyes, irregular or fast heartbeat, memory loss.

Q. Are there any drug interactions with the smoking cessation products?

A. The following medications may need dosage adjustment when taking nicotine patch, gum, lozenge, or spray:

- Acetaminophen (Tylenol)
- Beta-blockers (atenolol, pindolol, metoprolol, timolol, nadolol, and propranolol)
- Caffeine (coffee, tea, colas)
- Furosemide (Lasix)
- Phenylephrine (Neo-Synephrine)
- Prazosin (Minipress)
- Theophylline
- Tricyclic antidepressants (amitriptyline, nortriptyline, imipramine).

Appendix 2

Oral manifestation of drugs

See Table A2.

Q. Are there any drugs that cause a "drug-induced vesiculobullous reaction"?

A. Yes. There are some drugs that induce the development of oral lesions that clinically and histologically resemble idiopathic vesiculobullous conditions such as lichen planus, lupus erythematosus (LE), pemphigoid, and erythema multiforme. A differential diagnosis of a vesiculobullous disorder is drug eruptions. So, if a patient is diagnosed with a bullous disorder make sure that a drug the patient is taking is not causing a drug-like reaction.

Q. What is the treatment for drug-induced vesiculobullous disorders?

A. Best to recommend contacting the patient's physician about the offending drug.

Q. Treatment is primarily symptomatic and depends on the individual case. Some patients require topical steroids and in severe cases systemic steroids or cyclosporine; contact the patient's physician.

Q. Do cardiovascular drugs have a high incidence of oral manifestations?

A. Yes. Cardiovascular drugs have a high incidence of oral manifestations, up to 14.1% (Habbab *et al.*, 2010). The incidence increases with the number of drugs taken and if the patient is diabetic.

Q. What is the definition of fixed drug eruptions?

A. Fixed drug eruptions or sometimes called contact stomatitis occurs when there is repeated ulceration at the same site in response to the same drug. It can be cause by many drugs including tetracycline or ingredients of products including toothpastes, oral rinses, chewing gum and dental materials (Scully & Bagan-Sebastian, 2004). Once the offending drug is determined the medications should be stopped.

Q. What prescription medications can be prescribed for severe decreased salivary flow because of radiation to the head and neck region or patients with Sjögren's syndrome?

A. Pilocarpine (Salagen) is only indicated for (1) the treatment of symptoms of dry mouth from salivary gland hypofunction caused by radiotherapy for cancer of the head and neck; and (2) the treatment of symptoms of dry mouth in patients with Sjögren's syndrome.

Q. What are common adverse effects of pilocarpine for the treatment of xerostomia?

A. Headache, visual disturbance, lacrimation, sweating, respiratory distress, gastrointestinal spasm, nausea, vomiting, diarrhea, atrioventricular block, tachycardia, bradycardia, hypotension, hypertension, shock, mental confusion, cardiac

The Dentist's Drug and Prescription Guide, First Edition. Mea A. Weinberg and Stuart J. Froum.
© 2013 John Wiley & Sons, Inc. Published 2013 by John Wiley & Sons, Inc.

Table A2   Oral manifestation of drugs.

Oral condition	Medication	Notes
Candidiasis (fungal/yeast infection) Shows up intraorally as a white plaque-like lesion that can be wiped off with gauze Fungal infections are found on the maxillary palatal gingival when patients do not remove their maxillary denture	Inhalation steroids (in asthma)	Patient should rinse mouth after use of asthma drugs
Tardive dyskinesia (abnormal mouth and tongue movements including lip-puckering and tongue protrusion)	Antipsychotics	There is no definitive treatment; patient management is important.
Esophageal burning/ulcers	Tetracycline/doxycycline	Take will full glass of water in an upright position.
Gingival enlargement	Phenytoin (Dilantin) Nifedipine (Procardia, Adalat) and other calcium channel blockers Cyclosporine	Keep meticulous oral hygiene; sometimes surgical removal of gingival is necessary but the enlargement will return
Gingival hemorrhages	Coumadin (Warfarin) Clopidogrel (Plavix)	Note petechiae on chart; consult with patient's physician
Hairy tongue	Mouthrinses Antibiotics (especially broad spectrum) Steroids	Brush tongue
Taste changes	Lithium Metronidazole (Flagyl)	Taste changes are transient for metronidazole (metallic taste) but chronic for lithium because the patient will be on lithium for a long time.
Exaggerated gag reflex	Digitalis/cardiac glycosides	Patient management with impression and radiographs.
Xerostomia	Many. See next	Many OTC products: Orajel Gel, spray, toothpaste, Biotène products, Osais moisturizing mouthrinse and saliva substitutes (e.g., Xero-Lube, Salivart) Prescription sialagogue may be beneficial; pilocarpine HCl (Salagen) and cevimeline (Evoxac).
Drug induced vesiculobullous conditions	Lichenoid (lichen-planus) reactions: beta-blockers, ACE inhibitors (captopril) and NSAIDs Pemphigoid-like reactions: amoxicillin, clondiine, furosemide, nadolol, penicillin VK Pemphigus-like reaction: Captopril, propranolol Erythema multiforme-like reactions: carbamazepine, clindamycin, codeine, diltiazem, nifedipine, tetracycline, verapamil	It must be determined that the oral lesions are actually due to a drug the patient is taking. Treatment depends on the individual case. The patient's physician may need to be contacted.

Adapted from: Ciancio, S.G. (2004) Medications' impact on oral health. *Journal of the American Dental Association*, 135:1440–1448.

arrhythmia, and tremors (http://www.drugs.com/pro/pilocarpine.html). Pilocarpine should be administered with caution to patients with known or suspected cholelithiasis or biliary tract disease.

Q. What is the dose of pilocarpine HCl?

A. Dose: Supplied: 5 mg tab; 5 mg tid or qid, may increase up to 10 mg tid. It can take up to 6 weeks to for the drug to have the maximum effect.

Q. What is the dose in patients with hepatic impairment?

A. In patients with moderate hepatic impairment, the starting dose should be 5 mg twice daily, followed by adjustment based on therapeutic response and tolerability. Patients with mild hepatic insufficiency (Child–Pugh score of 5 to 6) do not require dosage reductions. Consult with the patient's physician.

Q. Are there any drug interactions with pilocarpine?

A. Yes. Pilocarpine should be administered with caution to patients taking β-adrenergic antagonists because of the possibility of conduction disturbances. There are synergistic parasympathomimetic (anticholinergic) effects when administered concurrently with other anticholinergic drugs. Pilocarpine is a cholinergic agonist drug so it might antagonize the anticholinergic effects of drugs used concomitantly.

Q. What is cevimeline HCL (Evoxac)?

A. Cevimeline is indicated for symptoms of in patients with Sjögren's.

Q. What is the dose for cevimeline?

A. Dose: Supplied: 30 mg caps: 30 mg tid. It can take up to 6 weeks to for the drug to have the maximum effect.

Q. When is the best time during the day to take a sialogog such as pilocarpine or cevimeline?

A. It is advantageous to take a sialogog before meals to aid in chewing.

Q. What are common adverse effects of cevimeline?

A. Shortness of breath, wheezing, chest pain, uneven heart rate, stomach pain on the right side extending up to the shoulder, nausea, vomiting, bloating, and fever.

Q. Is cevimeline contraindicated in certain patients?

A. Yes. In patients with uncontrolled asthma, allergies to cevimeline, narrow-angle glaucoma, or inflammation of the iris.

Q. Are there any drug interactions with cevimeline?

A. Yes. Cevimeline should be administered with caution to patients taking β-adrenergic antagonists, because of the possibility of conduction disturbances. There is a synergistic effect with other cholinergic drugs. Cevimeline might interfere with desirable anticholinergic effects of drugs used concomitantly.

Q. Which drugs can cause xerostomia?

A. Classification of drugs causing xerostomia are listed in Table A3.

If medication cannot be changed or dose altered then increase water intake, or the patient can suck on sugarless candy or chew sugarless gum. Oral OTC products such as Oasis and Biotène (e.g., oral rinses, toothpaste, and gel) may be helpful.

Table A3   Common drugs that cause xerostomia.

Drug classification	Drugs
Antiacne	Isotretinoin (Accutane)
Antianxiety	Alprazolam (Xanax) Clorazepate (Tranxene) Diazepam (Valium) Hydroxyzine (Atarax, Vistaril) Lorazepam (Ativan) Oxazepam (Serax)
Anticonvulsants	Carbamazepine (Tegretol) Gabapentin (Neurontin) Lamotrigine (Lamictal)
Antidepressants	Amitriptyline (Elavil) Bupropion (Wellbutrin) Clomipramine (Anafranil) Desipramine (Norpramin) Doxepin (Sinequan) Fluoxetine (Prozac) Fluvoxamine (Luvox) Imipramine (Tofranil)
Antipsychotics	Clozapine (Clozaril), olanzapine (Zyprexa), lithium, haloperidol (Haldol)
Antihistamines	Diphendydramine (Benadryl), triprolidine/pseudoephedrine (Actifed), loratadine (Claritin), brompheniramine (Dimetane), brompheniramine/phenylpropanolamine (Dimetapp), promethazine (Phenergan)
Anticholinergic (Antispasmodic/ Anti-motion sickness)	Belladonna alkaloids (Bellergal), dicyclomine (Bentyl), hyoscyamine with atropine, Phenobarbital, scopolamine (Donnatal), scopolamine (Transderm-Scop)
Antidiarrheal	Loperamide (Imodium AD), diphenoxylate with atropine (Lomotil)
Bronchodilator	Ipratropium (Atrovent) Isoproterenol (Isuprel) Albuterol (Proventil, Ventolin)
Diuretics	Chlorothiazide (Diuril) Furosemide (Lasix) Hydrochlorothiazide (Hydrodiuril) Triamterene/hydrochlorothiazide (Dyazide)
Sedative/hypnotics	Temazepam (Restoril) Triazolam (Halcion)

Appendix 3

American Heart Association antibiotic prophylaxis guidelines

Table A4   Prophylactic antibiotic regimens for oral and dental procedures.

Situation	Drug	Regimen (to be taken 30 min to 60 min before dental procedure)
Oral Unable to take oral medications	Amoxicillin Ampicillin or cefazolin, or ceftriaxone*	adults: 2.0 g/children: 50 mg/kg adults: 2.0 g IM or IV/ children: 50 mg/kg IM or IV adults: 1 g IM or IV/ children: 50 mg/kg
Allergic to penicillins or ampicillin-oral	Cephalexin* or clindamycin or azithromycin or clarithromycin	adults: 2 g/children: 50 mg/kg adults: 600 mg/children: 20 mg/kg adults: 500 mg/children: 15 mg/kg
Allergic to penicillins or ampicillin and unable to take oral medications	cefazolin or ceftriaxone* or clindamycin	adults: 1 g IM or IV/children: 50 mg/kg IM or IV. adults: 600 mg IM or IV/children: 20 mg/kg IM or IV

*Cephalosporins should not be given to an individual with a history of anaphylaxis, angioedema, or urticaria with penicillins or ampicillin.
Reprinted from Wilson, W., Taubert, K.A., Gewitz, M., *et al*. (2007) Prevention of infective endocarditis: Guidelines from the American Heart Association Rheumatic Fever, Endocarditis, and Kawasaki Disease Committee, Council on Cardiovascular Disease in the Young, and the Council on Clinical Cardiology, Council on Cardiovascular Surgery and Anesthesia, and the Quality of Care and Outcomes Research Interdisciplinary Working Group. *Circulation*, 116:1736–1754 with permission from Lippincott, Williams & Wilkins.

The Dentist's Drug and Prescription Guide, First Edition. Mea A. Weinberg and Stuart J. Froum.
© 2013 John Wiley & Sons, Inc. Published 2013 by John Wiley & Sons, Inc.

Table A5   Suggested antibiotic prophylaxis regimens in patients at potential increased risk of hematogenous total joint infection.

Situation	Drug	Regimen
Standard general prophylaxis	Cephalexin or amoxicillin	2 g orally 1 h before dental procedure
Patients unable to take oral medications	Cefazolin or ampicillin	1 g IM or IV 1 h before procedure 2 g IM or IV 1 h before procedure
Allergic to penicillin	Clindamycin	600 mg orally 1 h before procedure
Allergic to penicillin and unable to take oral medications	Clindamycin	600 mg IV 1 h before procedure

Reprinted from Wilson, W., Taubert, K.A., Gewitz, M., *et al*. (2007) Prevention of infective endocarditis: Guidelines from the American Heart Association Rheumatic Fever, Endocarditis, and Kawasaki Disease Committee, Council on Cardiovascular Disease in the Young, and the Council on Clinical Cardiology, Council on Cardiovascular Surgery and Anesthesia, and the Quality of Care and Outcomes Research Interdisciplinary Working Group. *Circulation*, 116:1736–1754 with permission from Lippincott, Williams & Wilkins.

Appendix 4

List of tables

The Dentist's Drug and Prescription Guide, First Edition. Mea A. Weinberg and Stuart J. Froum.
© 2013 John Wiley & Sons, Inc. Published 2013 by John Wiley & Sons, Inc.

Appendix 5

Pharmacology pearls in dental practice

1) When writing a prescription do not abbreviate and write legibly in ink.
2) Avoid using premade ink stamps for the name of the drug and directions.
3) Avoid ambiguity when writing a prescription. If possible, avoid using decimal points. For example, if writing for 5 ml of a suspension, do no write 5.0 ml. Put a zero as a prefix: e.g., 0.5 mg rather than .5 mg.
4) When designating refills on the prescription either write for "NR" (no refills) or for the minimal amount.
5) When prescribing any medication to the dental patient reference the drug for any drug–drug or drug–food interactions.
6) Instruct the dental patient on how to take the medication prescribed. For example: take with food or without regards to meals, take with a full glass of water.
7) Always document in the treatment record anything told to the patient including how to take the medication and that there are no allergies or drug interactions.
8) One teaspoonful is equivalent to 5 mL or 5 cc.
9) Often a prescription is written in either teaspoons, milliliters (ml) or cubic centimeters (cc). However, the pharmacist will usually write milliliters.

The Dentist's Drug and Prescription Guide, First Edition. Mea A. Weinberg and Stuart J. Froum.
© 2013 John Wiley & Sons, Inc. Published 2013 by John Wiley & Sons, Inc.

Appendix 6

Dental drug formulary

Analgesics

Non-narcotics

Acetaminophen (Tylenol)
Aspirin
Celecoxib (Celebrex)
Diflunisal (Dolobid)
Ibuprofen (Motrin, Advil, Nuprin)
Ketorolac Nasal Spray (Sprix)
Ketorolac (Toradol)
Naproxen (Naprosyn)
Naproxen sodium (Aleve, Anaprox)

Narcotics

Acetaminophen/codeine (Tylenol No.3,4)
Hydrocodone/acetaminophen (Vicodin, Lorcet, Lortab)
Hydrocodone/ibuprofen (Vicoprofen)
Oxycodone/acetaminophen (Percocet)
Oxycodone/aspirin (Percodan)

Antibiotics

Penicillins

Penicillin VK
Amoxicillin (Trimox, Amoxil)
Amoxicillin/clavulanic acid (Augmentin)

Erythromycins

Clarithromycin (Zithromax)
Azithromycin (Biaxen)

The Dentist's Drug and Prescription Guide, First Edition. Mea A. Weinberg and Stuart J. Froum.
© 2013 John Wiley & Sons, Inc. Published 2013 by John Wiley & Sons, Inc.

Lincomycins

Clindamycin (Cleocin)

Tetracyclines

Tetracycline (Vibramycin)
Doxycycline (Doryx, doxycycline 20 mg, Atridox – not available generically)
Minocycline (Arestin)

Fluoroquinolones

Ciprofloxacin (Cipro)

Others

Metronidazole (Flagyl)

Topical antimicrobials

Chlorhexidine (Peridex, PeriGard, PerioChip)
Doxycycline hyclate (Atridox)
Minocycline HCl (Arestin)

Antifungal agents

Clotrimazole troche (Mycelex, Orvig – not available generically)
Fluconazole (Diflucan)
Nystatin Oral Suspension, pastilles (Mycostatin)

Antiviral agents

Acyclovir (Zovirax)
Docosanol (Abreva); OTC
Penciclovir (Denavir)
Valacyclovir (Valtrex)

References

Ciancio, S.G. (2004) Medications' impact on oral health. *Journal of the American Dental Association*, 135:1440–1448.
Habbab, K.M., Moles, D.R. & Porter, S.R. (2010) Potential oral manifestations of cardiovascular drugs. *Oral Diseases*, 16:769–773.
Scully, C. & Bagan-Sebastian, J.V. (2004) Adverse drug reactions in the orofacial region. *Critical Reviews in Oral Biology & Medicine*, 15:221–240.

Index

The Dentist's Drug and Prescription Guide, First Edition. Mea A. Weinberg and Stuart J. Froum.
© 2013 John Wiley & Sons, Inc. Published 2013 by John Wiley & Sons, Inc.